Dietary Supplements

Related titles

Foods, Nutrients and Food Ingredients with Authorised EU Health Claims
(ISBN 978-0-85709-842-9)

Human Milk Biochemistry and Infant Formula Manufacturing Technology
(ISBN 978-1-84569-724-2)

High Throughput Screening for Food Safety Assessment: Biosensor Technologies, Hyperspectral Imaging and Practical Applications
(ISBN 978-0-85709-801-6)

Woodhead Publishing Series in Food Science, Technology and Nutrition: Number 267

Dietary Supplements
Safety, Efficacy and Quality

Edited by

K. Berginc and S. Kreft

AMSTERDAM • BOSTON • CAMBRIDGE • HEIDELBERG
LONDON • NEW YORK • OXFORD • PARIS • SAN DIEGO
SAN FRANCISCO • SINGAPORE • SYDNEY • TOKYO

Woodhead Publishing is an imprint of Elsevier

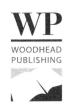

Woodhead Publishing is an imprint of Elsevier
80 High Street, Sawston, Cambridge, CB22 3HJ, UK
225 Wyman Street, Waltham, MA 02451, USA
Langford Lane, Kidlington, OX5 1GB, UK

Copyright © 2015 Elsevier Ltd. All rights reserved.

No part of this publication may be reproduced, stored in a retrieval system or transmitted in any form or by any means electronic, mechanical, photocopying, recording or otherwise without the prior written permission of the publisher.

Permissions may be sought directly from Elsevier's Science & Technology Rights Department in Oxford, UK: phone (+44) (0) 1865 843830; fax (+44) (0) 1865 853333; email: permissions@elsevier.com. Alternatively you can submit your request online by visiting the Elsevier website at http://elsevier.com/locate/permissions, and selecting Obtaining permission to use Elsevier material.

Notice
No responsibility is assumed by the publisher for any injury and/or damage to persons or property as a matter of products liability, negligence or otherwise, or from any use or operation of any methods, products, instructions or ideas contained in the material herein. Because of rapid advances in the medical sciences, in particular, independent verification of diagnoses and drug dosages should be made.

British Library Cataloguing-in-Publication Data
A catalogue record for this book is available from the British Library

Library of Congress Control Number: 2014944429

ISBN 978-1-78242-076-7 (print)
ISBN 978-1-78242-081-1 (online)

For information on all Woodhead Publishing publications visit our website at http://store.elsevier.com/

Typeset by Newgen Knowledge Works Pvt Ltd, India
Printed and bound in the United Kingdom

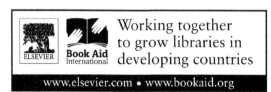

Contents

List of contributors	ix
Woodhead Publishing Series in Food Science, Technology and Nutrition	xi
Introduction	xxv

Part One General issues   1

1 Dietary supplement labelling and health claims   3
I. Pravst
- 1.1 Introduction: the regulatory situation in the European Union (EU)   3
- 1.2 Labelling requirements   4
- 1.3 Nutrition claims   6
- 1.4 Health claims   7
- 1.5 Borderline substances: between foods and medicine   18
- 1.6 Conclusions   20
- Acknowledgements   21
- References   21
- Appendix: abbreviations   24

2 Good manufacturing practice (GMP) in the production of dietary supplements   25
T. Sikora
- 2.1 Introduction   25
- 2.2 Key issues related to good manufacturing practice/good hygienic practice (GMP/GHP) implementation   26
- 2.3 Documentation of GMP   30
- 2.4 Benefits and drawbacks of GMP use in organisations   32
- 2.5 Summary   34
- References   35

3 Analysing the composition of fortified foods and supplements: the case of vitamins   37
S. Ötleş
- 3.1 Introduction   37
- 3.2 Extraction and purification methods   37
- 3.3 High performance liquid chromatography (HPLC)   38
- 3.4 Gas chromatography (GC)   39

3.5	Capillary electrophoresis (CE)	39
3.6	Spectroscopic methods	40
3.7	Microbiological methods	40
3.8	Immunoassays	41
3.9	Other methods	42
3.10	Future trends	43
	References	43

Part Two Drug–supplement interactions 45

4 Pharmacokinetic interactions between drugs and dietary supplements: herbal supplements 47
K. Berginc

4.1	Introduction	47
4.2	Herbals: introduction	49
4.3	*Hypericum perforatum* (St John's Wort (SJW))	51
4.4	*Allium sativum* (garlic)	51
4.5	*Ginkgo biloba* (ginkgo)	56
4.6	*Panax ginseng* (ginseng), *Piper methysticum* (kava kava) and *Serenoa repens* (saw palmetto)	57
4.7	*Echinacea purpurea* (purple coneflower), *Vaccinium macrocarpon* (cranberry) and *Silybum marianum* (milk thistle)	58
4.8	*Hydrastis canadensis* (goldenseal), *Valeriana officinalis* (valerian) and *Cimicifuga racemosa* (black cohosh)	59
4.9	*Glycine max* (soy), *Camellia sinensis* (green tea) and *Zingiber officinale* (ginger)	59
4.10	*Morinda citrifolia* (noni), *Aloe vera* (aloe), *Vitis vinifera* (grape seed) and *Curcuma longa* (turmeric)	60
4.11	*Stevia rebaudiana* (stevia), *Lepidium meyenii* (maca) and *Garcinia mangostana* (mangosteen)	61
4.12	Summary	62
	References	62

5 Pharmacokinetic interactions between drugs and dietary supplements: probiotic and lipid supplements 69
K. Berginc

5.1	Introduction	69
5.2	Probiotics and drug delivery in the colon	69
5.3	Probiotics: summary	73
5.4	Lipids and drug delivery	74
5.5	Lipidic excipients and drug release	74
5.6	Summary: pharmacokinetic drug–lipid interactions	76
	References	77

6	**Pharmacokinetic interactions between drugs and dietary supplements: carbohydrate, protein, vitamin and mineral supplements**	**85**
	K. Berginc	
	6.1 Introduction	85
	6.2 Carbohydrates as dietary supplements	85
	6.3 Carbohydrates as pharmaceutical excipients and prodrugs	90
	6.4 Carbohydrates: summary	91
	6.5 Proteins, peptides, and amino acids	91
	6.6 The impact of proteins on drug pharmacokinetics and their use as prodrugs	92
	6.7 Proteins: summary	93
	6.8 Vitamins	96
	6.9 Vitamins: summary	97
	6.10 Minerals and oligoelements	106
	6.11 Minerals: summary	117
	References	117
7	**Pharmacodynamic interactions between drugs and dietary supplements**	**127**
	S. Kreft	
	7.1 Introduction	127
	7.2 Vitamins	128
	7.3 Minerals	129
	7.4 Herbal supplements	130
	7.5 Antioxidants	133
	7.6 Conclusion	133
	References	133

Part Three Vitamins, minerals and probiotics as dietary supplements 137

8	**Vitamins/minerals as dietary supplements: a review of clinical studies**	**139**
	G.P. Webb	
	8.1 Introduction: efficacy in clinical trials does not guarantee practical impact	139
	8.2 Are some natural metabolites conditionally essential nutrients?	141
	8.3 Use of supplements to improve micronutrient adequacy	146
	8.4 Do folic acid supplements prevent neural tube defects (NTDs)?	149
	8.5 Do supplements of the ACE vitamins and selenium reduce cancer and heart disease mortality?	151
	8.6 Do vitamin C supplements prevent or ameliorate the common cold?	152
	8.7 Do vitamin D (and calcium) supplements improve bone health and have wider benefits?	153

	8.8	Can supplements of essential minerals reduce blood pressure?	157
	8.9	Should parents in areas without fluoridated water give their children fluoride supplements?	158
	8.10	Do micronutrients improve immune function in the elderly?	159
	8.11	Conclusions	160
		References	161

9 Reviewing clinical studies of probiotics as dietary supplements: probiotics for gastrointestinal disorders, *Helicobacter* eradication, lactose malabsorption and inflammatory bowel disease (IBD) — 171
M. Lunder

	9.1	Introduction	171
	9.2	Probiotics for gastrointestinal disorders	173
	9.3	Probiotics for *Helicobacter* eradication	179
	9.4	Probiotics for lactose malabsorption	180
	9.5	Probiotics for inflammatory bowel disease (IBD) and associated conditions	181
	9.6	Safety of probiotics	184
	9.7	Conclusions and future trends	185
		References	186

10 Reviewing clinical studies of probiotics as dietary supplements: probiotics for atopic and allergic disorders, urinary tract and respiratory infections — 199
M. Lunder

	10.1	Introduction	199
	10.2	Probiotics for atopic and allergic disorders	199
	10.3	Probiotics for urogenital infections	202
	10.4	Probiotics for respiratory tract infections	204
	10.5	Conclusions	205
		References	205

11 Reviewing clinical studies of probiotics as dietary supplements: probiotics for oral healthcare, rheumatoid arthritis, cancer prevention, metabolic diseases and postoperative infections — 211
M. Lunder

	11.1	Introduction	211
	11.2	Probiotics for oral healthcare	211
	11.3	Probiotics for rheumatoid arthritis	212
	11.4	Probiotics for cancer prevention	213
	11.5	Probiotics for metabolic diseases	214
	11.6	Probiotics for postoperative infections	216
	11.7	Conclusions	217
		References	218

Index — 225

List of contributors

K. Berginc Lek Pharmaceuticals d.d., Ljubljana, Slovenia

S. Kreft University of Ljubljana, Ljubljana, Slovenia

M. Lunder University of Ljubljana, Ljubljana, Slovenia

S. Ötleş Ege University, Izmir, Turkey

I. Pravst Nutrition Institute, Ljubljana, Slovenia

T. Sikora Cracow University of Economics, Kraków, Poland

G.P. Webb University of East London, London, UK

Woodhead Publishing Series in Food Science, Technology and Nutrition

1. **Chilled foods: A comprehensive guide**
   Edited by C. Dennis and M. Stringer
2. **Yoghurt: Science and technology**
   A. Y. Tamime and R. K. Robinson
3. **Food processing technology: Principles and practice**
   P. J. Fellows
4. **Bender's dictionary of nutrition and food technology Sixth edition**
   D. A. Bender
5. **Determination of veterinary residues in food**
   Edited by N. T. Crosby
6. **Food contaminants: Sources and surveillance**
   Edited by C. Creaser and R. Purchase
7. **Nitrates and nitrites in food and water**
   Edited by M. J. Hill
8. **Pesticide chemistry and bioscience: The food-environment challenge**
   Edited by G. T. Brooks and T. Roberts
9. **Pesticides: Developments, impacts and controls**
   Edited by G. A. Best and A. D. Ruthven
10. **Dietary fibre: Chemical and biological aspects**
    Edited by D. A. T. Southgate, K. W. Waldron, I. T. Johnson and G. R. Fenwick
11. **Vitamins and minerals in health and nutrition**
    M. Tolonen
12. **Technology of biscuits, crackers and cookies Second edition**
    D. Manley
13. **Instrumentation and sensors for the food industry**
    Edited by E. Kress-Rogers
14. **Food and cancer prevention: Chemical and biological aspects**
    Edited by K. W. Waldron, I. T. Johnson and G. R. Fenwick
15. **Food colloids: Proteins, lipids and polysaccharides**
    Edited by E. Dickinson and B. Bergenstahl
16. **Food emulsions and foams**
    Edited by E. Dickinson
17. **Maillard reactions in chemistry, food and health**
    Edited by T. P. Labuza, V. Monnier, J. Baynes and J. O'Brien
18. **The Maillard reaction in foods and medicine**
    Edited by J. O'Brien, H. E. Nursten, M. J. Crabbe and J. M. Ames

19 **Encapsulation and controlled release**
   Edited by D. R. Karsa and R. A. Stephenson
20 **Flavours and fragrances**
   Edited by A. D. Swift
21 **Feta and related cheeses**
   Edited by A. Y. Tamime and R. K. Robinson
22 **Biochemistry of milk products**
   Edited by A. T. Andrews and J. R. Varley
23 **Physical properties of foods and food processing systems**
   M. J. Lewis
24 **Food irradiation: A reference guide**
   V. M. Wilkinson and G. Gould
25 **Kent's technology of cereals: An introduction for students of food science and agriculture Fourth edition**
   N. L. Kent and A. D. Evers
26 **Biosensors for food analysis**
   Edited by A. O. Scott
27 **Separation processes in the food and biotechnology industries: Principles and applications**
   Edited by A. S. Grandison and M. J. Lewis
28 **Handbook of indices of food quality and authenticity**
   R. S. Singhal, P. K. Kulkarni and D. V. Rege
29 **Principles and practices for the safe processing of foods**
   D. A. Shapton and N. F. Shapton
30 **Biscuit, cookie and cracker manufacturing manuals Volume 1: Ingredients**
   D. Manley
31 **Biscuit, cookie and cracker manufacturing manuals Volume 2: Biscuit doughs**
   D. Manley
32 **Biscuit, cookie and cracker manufacturing manuals Volume 3: Biscuit dough piece forming**
   D. Manley
33 **Biscuit, cookie and cracker manufacturing manuals Volume 4: Baking and cooling of biscuits**
   D. Manley
34 **Biscuit, cookie and cracker manufacturing manuals Volume 5: Secondary processing in biscuit manufacturing**
   D. Manley
35 **Biscuit, cookie and cracker manufacturing manuals Volume 6: Biscuit packaging and storage**
   D. Manley
36 **Practical dehydration Second edition**
   M. Greensmith
37 **Lawrie's meat science Sixth edition**
   R. A. Lawrie

38 **Yoghurt: Science and technology Second edition**
  A. Y. Tamime and R. K. Robinson
39 **New ingredients in food processing: Biochemistry and agriculture**
  G. Linden and D. Lorient
40 **Benders' dictionary of nutrition and food technology Seventh edition**
  D. A. Bender and A. E. Bender
41 **Technology of biscuits, crackers and cookies Third edition**
  D. Manley
42 **Food processing technology: Principles and practice Second edition**
  P. J. Fellows
43 **Managing frozen foods**
  Edited by C. J. Kennedy
44 **Handbook of hydrocolloids**
  Edited by G. O. Phillips and P. A. Williams
45 **Food labelling**
  Edited by J. R. Blanchfield
46 **Cereal biotechnology**
  Edited by P. C. Morris and J. H. Bryce
47 **Food intolerance and the food industry**
  Edited by T. Dean
48 **The stability and shelf-life of food**
  Edited by D. Kilcast and P. Subramaniam
49 **Functional foods: Concept to product**
  Edited by G. R. Gibson and C. M. Williams
50 **Chilled foods: A comprehensive guide Second edition**
  Edited by M. Stringer and C. Dennis
51 **HACCP in the meat industry**
  Edited by M. Brown
52 **Biscuit, cracker and cookie recipes for the food industry**
  D. Manley
53 **Cereals processing technology**
  Edited by G. Owens
54 **Baking problems solved**
  S. P. Cauvain and L. S. Young
55 **Thermal technologies in food processing**
  Edited by P. Richardson
56 **Frying: Improving quality**
  Edited by J. B. Rossell
57 **Food chemical safety Volume 1: Contaminants**
  Edited by D. Watson
58 **Making the most of HACCP: Learning from others' experience**
  Edited by T. Mayes and S. Mortimore
59 **Food process modelling**
  Edited by L. M. M. Tijskens, M. L. A. T. M. Hertog and B. M. Nicolaï

60 **EU food law: A practical guide**
   Edited by K. Goodburn
61 **Extrusion cooking: Technologies and applications**
   Edited by R. Guy
62 **Auditing in the food industry: From safety and quality to environmental and other audits**
   Edited by M. Dillon and C. Griffith
63 **Handbook of herbs and spices Volume 1**
   Edited by K. V. Peter
64 **Food product development: Maximising success**
   M. Earle, R. Earle and A. Anderson
65 **Instrumentation and sensors for the food industry Second edition**
   Edited by E. Kress-Rogers and C. J. B. Brimelow
66 **Food chemical safety Volume 2: Additives**
   Edited by D. Watson
67 **Fruit and vegetable biotechnology**
   Edited by V. Valpuesta
68 **Foodborne pathogens: Hazards, risk analysis and control**
   Edited by C. de W. Blackburn and P. J. McClure
69 **Meat refrigeration**
   S. J. James and C. James
70 **Lockhart and Wiseman's crop husbandry Eighth edition**
   H. J. S. Finch, A. M. Samuel and G. P. F. Lane
71 **Safety and quality issues in fish processing**
   Edited by H. A. Bremner
72 **Minimal processing technologies in the food industries**
   Edited by T. Ohlsson and N. Bengtsson
73 **Fruit and vegetable processing: Improving quality**
   Edited by W. Jongen
74 **The nutrition handbook for food processors**
   Edited by C. J. K. Henry and C. Chapman
75 **Colour in food: Improving quality**
   Edited by D. MacDougall
76 **Meat processing: Improving quality**
   Edited by J. P. Kerry, J. F. Kerry and D. A. Ledward
77 **Microbiological risk assessment in food processing**
   Edited by M. Brown and M. Stringer
78 **Performance functional foods**
   Edited by D. Watson
79 **Functional dairy products Volume 1**
   Edited by T. Mattila-Sandholm and M. Saarela
80 **Taints and off-flavours in foods**
   Edited by B. Baigrie
81 **Yeasts in food**
   Edited by T. Boekhout and V. Robert

82 **Phytochemical functional foods**
   Edited by I. T. Johnson and G. Williamson
83 **Novel food packaging techniques**
   Edited by R. Ahvenainen
84 **Detecting pathogens in food**
   Edited by T. A. McMeekin
85 **Natural antimicrobials for the minimal processing of foods**
   Edited by S. Roller
86 **Texture in food Volume 1: Semi-solid foods**
   Edited by B. M. McKenna
87 **Dairy processing: Improving quality**
   Edited by G. Smit
88 **Hygiene in food processing: Principles and practice**
   Edited by H. L. M. Lelieveld, M. A. Mostert, B. White and J. Holah
89 **Rapid and on-line instrumentation for food quality assurance**
   Edited by I. Tothill
90 **Sausage manufacture: Principles and practice**
   E. Essien
91 **Environmentally-friendly food processing**
   Edited by B. Mattsson and U. Sonesson
92 **Bread making: Improving quality**
   Edited by S. P. Cauvain
93 **Food preservation techniques**
   Edited by P. Zeuthen and L. Bøgh-Sørensen
94 **Food authenticity and traceability**
   Edited by M. Lees
95 **Analytical methods for food additives**
   R. Wood, L. Foster, A. Damant and P. Key
96 **Handbook of herbs and spices Volume 2**
   Edited by K. V. Peter
97 **Texture in food Volume 2: Solid foods**
   Edited by D. Kilcast
98 **Proteins in food processing**
   Edited by R. Yada
99 **Detecting foreign bodies in food**
   Edited by M. Edwards
100 **Understanding and measuring the shelf-life of food**
   Edited by R. Steele
101 **Poultry meat processing and quality**
   Edited by G. Mead
102 **Functional foods, ageing and degenerative disease**
   Edited by C. Remacle and B. Reusens
103 **Mycotoxins in food: Detection and control**
   Edited by N. Magan and M. Olsen

104 **Improving the thermal processing of foods**
   Edited by P. Richardson
105 **Pesticide, veterinary and other residues in food**
   Edited by D. Watson
106 **Starch in food: Structure, functions and applications**
   Edited by A.-C. Eliasson
107 **Functional foods, cardiovascular disease and diabetes**
   Edited by A. Arnoldi
108 **Brewing: Science and practice**
   D. E. Briggs, P. A. Brookes, R. Stevens and C. A. Boulton
109 **Using cereal science and technology for the benefit of consumers: Proceedings of the 12th International ICC Cereal and Bread Congress, 24 – 26th May, 2004, Harrogate, UK**
   Edited by S. P. Cauvain, L. S. Young and S. Salmon
110 **Improving the safety of fresh meat**
   Edited by J. Sofos
111 **Understanding pathogen behaviour: Virulence, stress response and resistance**
   Edited by M. Griffiths
112 **The microwave processing of foods**
   Edited by H. Schubert and M. Regier
113 **Food safety control in the poultry industry**
   Edited by G. Mead
114 **Improving the safety of fresh fruit and vegetables**
   Edited by W. Jongen
115 **Food, diet and obesity**
   Edited by D. Mela
116 **Handbook of hygiene control in the food industry**
   Edited by H. L. M. Lelieveld, M. A. Mostert and J. Holah
117 **Detecting allergens in food**
   Edited by S. Koppelman and S. Hefle
118 **Improving the fat content of foods**
   Edited by C. Williams and J. Buttriss
119 **Improving traceability in food processing and distribution**
   Edited by I. Smith and A. Furness
120 **Flavour in food**
   Edited by A. Voilley and P. Etievant
121 **The Chorleywood bread process**
   S. P. Cauvain and L. S. Young
122 **Food spoilage microorganisms**
   Edited by C. de W. Blackburn
123 **Emerging foodborne pathogens**
   Edited by Y. Motarjemi and M. Adams
124 **Benders' dictionary of nutrition and food technology Eighth edition**
   D. A. Bender

125 **Optimising sweet taste in foods**
 Edited by W. J. Spillane
126 **Brewing: New technologies**
 Edited by C. Bamforth
127 **Handbook of herbs and spices Volume 3**
 Edited by K. V. Peter
128 **Lawrie's meat science Seventh edition**
 R. A. Lawrie in collaboration with D. A. Ledward
129 **Modifying lipids for use in food**
 Edited by F. Gunstone
130 **Meat products handbook: Practical science and technology**
 G. Feiner
131 **Food consumption and disease risk: Consumer–pathogen interactions**
 Edited by M. Potter
132 **Acrylamide and other hazardous compounds in heat-treated foods**
 Edited by K. Skog and J. Alexander
133 **Managing allergens in food**
 Edited by C. Mills, H. Wichers and K. Hoffman-Sommergruber
134 **Microbiological analysis of red meat, poultry and eggs**
 Edited by G. Mead
135 **Maximising the value of marine by-products**
 Edited by F. Shahidi
136 **Chemical migration and food contact materials**
 Edited by K. Barnes, R. Sinclair and D. Watson
137 **Understanding consumers of food products**
 Edited by L. Frewer and H. van Trijp
138 **Reducing salt in foods: Practical strategies**
 Edited by D. Kilcast and F. Angus
139 **Modelling microorganisms in food**
 Edited by S. Brul, S. Van Gerwen and M. Zwietering
140 **Tamime and Robinson's Yoghurt: Science and technology Third edition**
 A. Y. Tamime and R. K. Robinson
141 **Handbook of waste management and co-product recovery in food processing Volume 1**
 Edited by K. W. Waldron
142 **Improving the flavour of cheese**
 Edited by B. Weimer
143 **Novel food ingredients for weight control**
 Edited by C. J. K. Henry
144 **Consumer-led food product development**
 Edited by H. MacFie
145 **Functional dairy products Volume 2**
 Edited by M. Saarela
146 **Modifying flavour in food**
 Edited by A. J. Taylor and J. Hort

147 **Cheese problems solved**
   Edited by P. L. H. McSweeney
148 **Handbook of organic food safety and quality**
   Edited by J. Cooper, C. Leifert and U. Niggli
149 **Understanding and controlling the microstructure of complex foods**
   Edited by D. J. McClements
150 **Novel enzyme technology for food applications**
   Edited by R. Rastall
151 **Food preservation by pulsed electric fields: From research to application**
   Edited by H. L. M. Lelieveld and S. W. H. de Haan
152 **Technology of functional cereal products**
   Edited by B. R. Hamaker
153 **Case studies in food product development**
   Edited by M. Earle and R. Earle
154 **Delivery and controlled release of bioactives in foods and nutraceuticals**
   Edited by N. Garti
155 **Fruit and vegetable flavour: Recent advances and future prospects**
   Edited by B. Brückner and S. G. Wyllie
156 **Food fortification and supplementation: Technological, safety and regulatory aspects**
   Edited by P. Berry Ottaway
157 **Improving the health-promoting properties of fruit and vegetable products**
   Edited by F. A. Tomás-Barberán and M. I. Gil
158 **Improving seafood products for the consumer**
   Edited by T. Børresen
159 **In-pack processed foods: Improving quality**
   Edited by P. Richardson
160 **Handbook of water and energy management in food processing**
   Edited by J. Klemeš, R.. Smith and J.-K. Kim
161 **Environmentally compatible food packaging**
   Edited by E. Chiellini
162 **Improving farmed fish quality and safety**
   Edited by Ø. Lie
163 **Carbohydrate-active enzymes**
   Edited by K.-H. Park
164 **Chilled foods: A comprehensive guide Third edition**
   Edited by M. Brown
165 **Food for the ageing population**
   Edited by M. M. Raats, C. P. G. M. de Groot and W. A Van Staveren
166 **Improving the sensory and nutritional quality of fresh meat**
   Edited by J. P. Kerry and D. A. Ledward
167 **Shellfish safety and quality**
   Edited by S. E. Shumway and G. E. Rodrick
168 **Functional and speciality beverage technology**
   Edited by P. Paquin

169 **Functional foods: Principles and technology**
   M. Guo
170 **Endocrine-disrupting chemicals in food**
   Edited by I. Shaw
171 **Meals in science and practice: Interdisciplinary research and business applications**
   Edited by H. L. Meiselman
172 **Food constituents and oral health: Current status and future prospects**
   Edited by M. Wilson
173 **Handbook of hydrocolloids Second edition**
   Edited by G. O. Phillips and P. A. Williams
174 **Food processing technology: Principles and practice Third edition**
   P. J. Fellows
175 **Science and technology of enrobed and filled chocolate, confectionery and bakery products**
   Edited by G. Talbot
176 **Foodborne pathogens: Hazards, risk analysis and control Second edition**
   Edited by C. de W. Blackburn and P. J. McClure
177 **Designing functional foods: Measuring and controlling food structure breakdown and absorption**
   Edited by D. J. McClements and E. A. Decker
178 **New technologies in aquaculture: Improving production efficiency, quality and environmental management**
   Edited by G. Burnell and G. Allan
179 **More baking problems solved**
   S. P. Cauvain and L. S. Young
180 **Soft drink and fruit juice problems solved**
   P. Ashurst and R. Hargitt
181 **Biofilms in the food and beverage industries**
   Edited by P. M. Fratamico, B. A. Annous and N. W. Gunther
182 **Dairy-derived ingredients: Food and neutraceutical uses**
   Edited by M. Corredig
183 **Handbook of waste management and co-product recovery in food processing Volume 2**
   Edited by K. W. Waldron
184 **Innovations in food labelling**
   Edited by J. Albert
185 **Delivering performance in food supply chains**
   Edited by C. Mena and G. Stevens
186 **Chemical deterioration and physical instability of food and beverages**
   Edited by L. H. Skibsted, J. Risbo and M. L. Andersen
187 **Managing wine quality Volume 1: Viticulture and wine quality**
   Edited by A. G. Reynolds

188 Improving the safety and quality of milk Volume 1: Milk production and processing
Edited by M. Griffiths
189 Improving the safety and quality of milk Volume 2: Improving quality in milk products
Edited by M. Griffiths
190 Cereal grains: Assessing and managing quality
Edited by C. Wrigley and I. Batey
191 Sensory analysis for food and beverage quality control: A practical guide
Edited by D. Kilcast
192 Managing wine quality Volume 2: Oenology and wine quality
Edited by A. G. Reynolds
193 Winemaking problems solved
Edited by C. E. Butzke
194 Environmental assessment and management in the food industry
Edited by U. Sonesson, J. Berlin and F. Ziegler
195 Consumer-driven innovation in food and personal care products
Edited by S. R. Jaeger and H. MacFie
196 Tracing pathogens in the food chain
Edited by S. Brul, P. M. Fratamico and T. A. McMeekin
197 Case studies in novel food processing technologies: Innovations in processing, packaging, and predictive modelling
Edited by C. J. Doona, K. Kustin and F. E. Feeherry
198 Freeze-drying of pharmaceutical and food products
T.-C. Hua, B.-L. Liu and H. Zhang
199 Oxidation in foods and beverages and antioxidant applications Volume 1: Understanding mechanisms of oxidation and antioxidant activity
Edited by E. A. Decker, R. J. Elias and D. J. McClements
200 Oxidation in foods and beverages and antioxidant applications Volume 2: Management in different industry sectors
Edited by E. A. Decker, R. J. Elias and D. J. McClements
201 Protective cultures, antimicrobial metabolites and bacteriophages for food and beverage biopreservation
Edited by C. Lacroix
202 Separation, extraction and concentration processes in the food, beverage and nutraceutical industries
Edited by S. S. H. Rizvi
203 Determining mycotoxins and mycotoxigenic fungi in food and feed
Edited by S. De Saeger
204 Developing children's food products
Edited by D. Kilcast and F. Angus
205 Functional foods: Concept to product Second edition
Edited by M. Saarela

206 **Postharvest biology and technology of tropical and subtropical fruits Volume 1: Fundamental issues**
Edited by E. M. Yahia
207 **Postharvest biology and technology of tropical and subtropical fruits Volume 2: Açai to citrus**
Edited by E. M. Yahia
208 **Postharvest biology and technology of tropical and subtropical fruits Volume 3: Cocona to mango**
Edited by E. M. Yahia
209 **Postharvest biology and technology of tropical and subtropical fruits Volume 4: Mangosteen to white sapote**
Edited by E. M. Yahia
210 **Food and beverage stability and shelf life**
Edited by D. Kilcast and P. Subramaniam
211 **Processed Meats: Improving safety, nutrition and quality**
Edited by J. P. Kerry and J. F. Kerry
212 **Food chain integrity: A holistic approach to food traceability, safety, quality and authenticity**
Edited by J. Hoorfar, K. Jordan, F. Butler and R. Prugger
213 **Improving the safety and quality of eggs and egg products Volume 1**
Edited by Y. Nys, M. Bain and F. Van Immerseel
214 **Improving the safety and quality of eggs and egg products Volume 2**
Edited by F. Van Immerseel, Y. Nys and M. Bain
215 **Animal feed contamination: Effects on livestock and food safety**
Edited by J. Fink-Gremmels
216 **Hygienic design of food factories**
Edited by J. Holah and H. L. M. Lelieveld
217 **Manley's technology of biscuits, crackers and cookies Fourth edition**
Edited by D. Manley
218 **Nanotechnology in the food, beverage and nutraceutical industries**
Edited by Q. Huang
219 **Rice quality: A guide to rice properties and analysis**
K. R. Bhattacharya
220 **Advances in meat, poultry and seafood packaging**
Edited by J. P. Kerry
221 **Reducing saturated fats in foods**
Edited by G. Talbot
222 **Handbook of food proteins**
Edited by G. O. Phillips and P. A. Williams
223 **Lifetime nutritional influences on cognition, behaviour and psychiatric illness**
Edited by D. Benton
224 **Food machinery for the production of cereal foods, snack foods and confectionery**
L.-M. Cheng

225 **Alcoholic beverages: Sensory evaluation and consumer research**
   Edited by J. Piggott
226 **Extrusion problems solved: Food, pet food and feed**
   M. N. Riaz and G. J. Rokey
227 **Handbook of herbs and spices Second edition Volume 1**
   Edited by K. V. Peter
228 **Handbook of herbs and spices Second edition Volume 2**
   Edited by K. V. Peter
229 **Breadmaking: Improving quality Second edition**
   Edited by S. P. Cauvain
230 **Emerging food packaging technologies: Principles and practice**
   Edited by K. L. Yam and D. S. Lee
231 **Infectious disease in aquaculture: Prevention and control**
   Edited by B. Austin
232 **Diet, immunity and inflammation**
   Edited by P. C. Calder and P. Yaqoob
233 **Natural food additives, ingredients and flavourings**
   Edited by D. Baines and R. Seal
234 **Microbial decontamination in the food industry: Novel methods and applications**
   Edited by A. Demirci and M.O. Ngadi
235 **Chemical contaminants and residues in foods**
   Edited by D. Schrenk
236 **Robotics and automation in the food industry: Current and future technologies**
   Edited by D. G. Caldwell
237 **Fibre-rich and wholegrain foods: Improving quality**
   Edited by J. A. Delcour and K. Poutanen
238 **Computer vision technology in the food and beverage industries**
   Edited by D.-W. Sun
239 **Encapsulation technologies and delivery systems for food ingredients and nutraceuticals**
   Edited by N. Garti and D. J. McClements
240 **Case studies in food safety and authenticity**
   Edited by J. Hoorfar
241 **Heat treatment for insect control: Developments and applications**
   D. Hammond
242 **Advances in aquaculture hatchery technology**
   Edited by G. Allan and G. Burnell
243 **Open innovation in the food and beverage industry**
   Edited by M. Garcia Martinez
244 **Trends in packaging of food, beverages and other fast-moving consumer goods (FMCG)**
   Edited by N. Farmer

245 New analytical approaches for verifying the origin of food
  Edited by P. Brereton
246 Microbial production of food ingredients, enzymes and nutraceuticals
  Edited by B. McNeil, D. Archer, I. Giavasis and L. Harvey
247 Persistent organic pollutants and toxic metals in foods
  Edited by M. Rose and A. Fernandes
248 Cereal grains for the food and beverage industries
  E. Arendt and E. Zannini
249 Viruses in food and water: Risks, surveillance and control
  Edited by N. Cook
250 Improving the safety and quality of nuts
  Edited by L. J. Harris
251 Metabolomics in food and nutrition
  Edited by B. C. Weimer and C. Slupsky
252 Food enrichment with omega-3 fatty acids
  Edited by C. Jacobsen, N. S. Nielsen, A. F. Horn and A.-D. M. Sørensen
253 Instrumental assessment of food sensory quality: A practical guide
  Edited by D. Kilcast
254 Food microstructures: Microscopy, measurement and modelling
  Edited by V. J. Morris and K. Groves
255 Handbook of food powders: Processes and properties
  Edited by B. R. Bhandari, N. Bansal, M. Zhang and P. Schuck
256 Functional ingredients from algae for foods and nutraceuticals
  Edited by H. Domínguez
257 Satiation, satiety and the control of food intake: Theory and practice
  Edited by J. E. Blundell and F. Bellisle
258 Hygiene in food processing: Principles and practice Second edition
  Edited by H. L. M. Lelieveld, J. Holah and D. Napper
259 Advances in microbial food safety Volume 1
  Edited by J. Sofos
260 Global safety of fresh produce: A handbook of best practice, innovative commercial solutions and case studies
  Edited by J. Hoorfar
261 Human milk biochemistry and infant formula manufacturing technology
  Edited by M. Guo
262 High throughput screening for food safety assessment: Biosensor technologies, hyperspectral imaging and practical applications
  Edited by A. K. Bhunia, M. S. Kim and C. R. Taitt
263 Foods, nutrients and food ingredients with authorised EU health claims: Volume 1
  Edited by M. J. Sadler
264 Handbook of food allergen detection and control
  Edited by S. Flanagan

265 **Advances in fermented foods and beverages: Improving quality, technologies and health benefits**
Edited by W. Holzapfel
266 **Metabolomics as a tool in nutrition research**
Edited by J.-L. Sébédio and L. Brennan
267 **Dietary supplements: Safety, efficacy and quality**
Edited by K. Berginc and S. Kreft
268 **Grapevine breeding programs for the wine industry: Traditional and molecular technologies**
Edited by A. G. Reynolds
269 **Handbook of natural antimicrobials for food safety and quality**
Edited by M. Taylor
270 **Managing and preventing obesity: Behavioural factors and dietary interventions**
Edited by T. P. Gill
271 **Electron beam pasteurization and complementary food processing technologies**
Edited by S. D. Pillai and S. Shayanfar
272 **Advances in food and beverage labelling: Information and regulations**
Edited by P. Berryman
273 **Flavour development, analysis and perception in food and beverages**
Edited by J. K. Parker, S. Elmore and L. Methven
274 **Rapid sensory profiling techniques and related methods: Applications in new product development and consumer research**
Edited by J. Delarue, B. Lawlor and M. Rogeaux
275 **Advances in microbial food safety: Volume 2**
Edited by J. Sofos
276 **Handbook of antioxidants in food preservation**
Edited by F. Shahidi
277 **Lockhart and Wiseman's crop husbandry including grassland: Ninth edition**
H. J. S. Finch, A. M. Samuel and G. P. F. Lane
278 **Global legislation for food contact materials: Processing, storage and packaging**
Edited by J. S. Baughan
279 **Colour additives for food and beverages: Development, safety and applications**
Edited by M. Scotter
280 **A complete course in canning and related processes 14th Edition Volume 1**
Revised by S. Featherstone
281 **A complete course in canning and related processes 14th Edition Volume 2**
Revised by S. Featherstone
282 **A complete course in canning and related processes 14th Edition Volume 3**
Revised by S. Featherstone

Introduction

Food supplements (or dietary supplements) are an important but also controversial group of products. Professionals and the public are not always adequately informed about their role and status. On the one hand, they are regulatorily regarded as a food but, on the other hand, they are produced in pharmaceutical form (tablets, capsules) and widely perceived as medicines.

The use of food supplements and functional foods has risen substantially in the past 5–10 years among a wide range of consumers, including:

- those with particular health problems (e.g. the elderly and patients with chronic conditions)
- healthy subjects with particular food requirements (e.g. athletes and pregnant women)
- the wider public, concerned about an unhealthy diet and lifestyle.

They can be used to meet a wide range of needs, including as self-medication to compensate for dissatisfaction with health services and the high costs associated with purchasing some drugs for treatment. They are available from a wide range of outlets, including pharmacies, health food stores, and through online channels.

The USA, Europe and Japan collectively still hold the major share of the global market, with growth rates of 9% a year, but this is expected to change owing to the growth of Asian and Chinese markets. The maturing Baby Boomers aged from 42 to 60 years (making up 78 million of the American population) have been suggested as the main reason for high increases in sales, especially in USA. Empowered with the choice of taking control over their health management, more and more consumers are declaring themselves as supplement users. The supplement industry is expected to continue to grow at current rates, but only for the products compliant with the relevant regulations (i.e. good manufacturing practices (GMP), pharmacovigilance systems), owing to an increasingly educated consumer base. Most importantly, supplement users have recognized the importance of scientific evidence supporting health claims for products, purchasing those backed by a wide range of credible clinical studies over those lacking evidence to support a particular health claim. Products such as soy, saw palmetto, green tea, garlic, ginseng, ginkgo, grass, flax seed and oil, aloe, turmeric, stevia, cranberry products, lutein, lycopene, vitamins E and A, calcium and magnesium minerals, coenzyme Q, and glucosamine will most likely be among the top sellers in the future, based on current market research. Food supplements with high antioxidant content have the highest commercial interest world-wide.

Food supplements typically contain concentrated phytochemicals, vitamins, minerals, and pro- and pre-biotics formulated into tablets or other forms which enable administration of the prescribed dose. Owing to their natural origin, the consumers of these products usually do not question their quality, safety and efficacy. Unfortunately, such a widely held view is often misleading. Food supplements are intended to supplement the diet with nutrients and to support the physiological functions of the body, not to cure or prevent diseases. However, in real life they are frequently used also for self-medication.

Self-medication with food supplements can put users at high risk of unwanted side effects triggered by pharmacokinetic and/or pharmacodynamic interactions. Some countries have recognized the need for adequate regulations and guidelines, implementing GMPs for food supplement production, including establishing pharmacovigilance systems for these products. Unfortunately, law enforcement evolves at different speed in different countries. The United States and Europe are in the forefront, followed by Asian countries, which are just beginning to establish their regulatory framework, and by countries in Latin America, some of which have the most outdated legislation.

This book provides a summary of the most important clinical studies involving dietary supplement–drug pharmacokinetic and pharmacodynamic interactions, evidence supporting supplement efficacy and the lessons learnt. Chapters also deal with more specific issues, such as the analytics associated with testing supplement composition. The book aims to raise awareness among food supplement consumers about the advantages and drawbacks in self-medicating with these products. It also provides a reference for those working in the fields of nutrition and health care, as well as those involved in the supplement industry (food technologists, nutritionists, dietitians, food scientists, pharmacologists and regulatory bodies).

Part One

General issues

Dietary supplement labelling and health claims

I. Pravst
Nutrition Institute, Ljubljana, Slovenia

1.1 Introduction: the regulatory situation in the European Union (EU)

In the EU, food supplements are regulated as food and covered by general food and specific food supplements legislation. To ensure the protection of consumers and facilitate their choices, products must be safe and appropriately labelled. The quality and safety of food supplements is the full responsibility of the producer, but can be controlled by national authorities.

While in different EU member states food supplements are regulated by local regulations, these regulations should be in harmony with EU Directive 2002/46/EC of the European Parliament and of the Council on the approximation of the laws of the member states relating to food supplements (EC, 2002). Food supplements are considered as foodstuffs whose purpose is to supplement the normal diet and which are concentrated sources of nutrients or other substances with a nutritional or physiological effect, alone or in combination, marketed in dose form, such as capsules, pastilles, tablets, pills and other similar forms, sachets of powder, ampoules of liquids, drop-dispensing bottles, and other similar forms of liquids and powders designed to be taken in measured small unit quantities.

However, the labelling of food supplements also needs to be in line with general food labelling. EU member states harmonised their local regulations in the year 2000 according to Directive 2000/13/EC on the approximation of the laws of the member states relating to the labelling, presentation and advertising of foodstuffs (EC, 2000). In 2011, a harmonised EU Regulation (EU) No 1169/2011 on the provision of food information to consumers was adopted (EC, 2011b) and from the end of 2014 it will be in use instead of Directive 2000/13/EC.

Since food supplements are usually composed of vitamins, minerals or other food substances, a number of other regulations are also applicable. These include:

- Regulation (EC) No 1925/2006 on the addition of vitamins and minerals and of certain other substances to foods (EC, 2006b),
- Regulation (EC) No 258/97 concerning novel foods and novel food ingredients (EC, 1997).

It should be noted that only authorised forms of vitamins and minerals can be used in food supplements in the EU, and they are listed in Annex II of EU Directive 2002/46/EC (EC, 2002). However, the addition of other substances is regulated in Regulation

(EC) No 1925/2006 (EC, 2006b), which established the Community Register on the addition of vitamins and minerals and of certain other substances to foods (EC, 2013b). There are strict rules about the inclusion of new substances in this list of authorised substances, and all new applications are subject to evaluation of their safety by the European Food Safety Authority (EFSA). A number of substances are allowed outside the EU, but are not authorised for use within the EU, thereby limiting imports of such food supplements.

The use of nutrition and health claims on foods (including food supplements) was harmonised in the EU in 2006 by Regulation (EC) No 1924/2006 on nutrition and health claims made on foods (NHCR) (EC, 2006a). Only authorised nutrition and health claims are allowed. All health claims require specific authorisation by the EC through the comitology procedure, following scientific assessment and verification of each claim by EFSA.

1.2 Labelling requirements

Because regulatory food supplements are considered as foods, their labelling should be in line with general food labelling requirements and specific requirements for food supplements.

1.2.1 General labelling requirements

In line with general food labelling provisions and definitions, the labelling of food supplements is compulsory as concerns both information on the identity, composition, properties or other characteristics, and information on the protection of consumers' health and the safe use of the food supplement. The list of compulsory information on labelling includes: (a) the name of the food supplement; (b) the list of ingredients; (c) any ingredient or processing aid causing allergies or intolerances that is used in the manufacture or preparation of a product and is still present in the finished product, even if in an altered form; (d) the quantity of certain ingredients or categories of ingredients; (e) the net quantity of the product; (f) the date of minimum durability or the "use by" date; (g) any special storage conditions and/or conditions of use; (h) the name or business name and address of the food business operator; and (i) instructions for use.

It should be noted that the list of ingredients must include all of the food's ingredients, in descending order of weight, as recorded at the time of their use in the manufacture of the food. Ingredients must be designated by their specific name. All additives must be labelled with their function (i.e. sweetener, colour, carrier, etc.) according to the list of functional classes of food additives (EC, 2008, 2011b). All ingredients present in the form of engineered nanomaterials must be clearly indicated on the list of ingredients. The names of such ingredients must be followed by the word "nano" in brackets. All substances which can cause allergies or intolerances must also be labelled.

Food supplements must be labelled "food supplement." The labelling, presentation and advertising must not attribute to food supplements the property of preventing, treating or curing a human disease, or refer to such properties. The labelling of products must also include: (a) the names of the categories of nutrients or substances that characterise the product; (b) the portion of the product recommended for daily consumption; (c) a warning not to exceed the stated recommended daily dose; (d) a statement to the effect that food supplements should not be used as a substitute for a varied diet; and (e) a statement to the effect that the products should be stored out of reach of young children.

Food supplements are purchased by consumers for supplementing dietary intakes. To ensure that this aim is achieved, if vitamins and minerals are labelled, these compounds must be present in the product in significant amounts. The labelling, presentation and advertising of food supplements must not include any wording stating or implying that a balanced and varied diet cannot provide appropriate quantities of nutrients in general.

1.2.2 Composition

In addition to the above mentioned list of all the ingredients, food supplements must also be labelled with the content of all the nutrients and substances with a nutritional or physiological effect. These must be in numerical form and defined per portion of the product as recommended for daily consumption. Information on the content of vitamins and minerals must also be expressed as a percentage of the reference values (Table 1.1), either in text or graphical form. The labelled composition must be in average values, based on the manufacturer's analysis of the product. However, poor

Table 1.1 **Vitamins and minerals which must be declared and their nutrient reference values (NRVs)**

Vitamin	NRV	Mineral	NRV
Vitamin C	80 mg	Potassium	2000 mg
Niacin	16 mg	Calcium	800 mg
Vitamin E	12 mg	Chloride	800 mg
Pantothenic acid	6 mg	Phosphorus	700 mg
Riboflavin	1.4 mg	Magnesium	375 mg
Vitamin B6	1.4 mg	Iron	14 mg
Thiamin	1.1 mg	Zinc	10 mg
Vitamin A	800	Fluoride	3.5 mg
Folic acid	200 µg	Manganese	2 mg
Vitamin K	75 µg	Copper	1 mg
Biotin	50 µg	Iodine	150 µg
Vitamin D	5 µg	Selenium	55 µg
Vitamin B12	2.5 µg	Molybdenum	50 µg
		Chromium	40 µg

quality of a significant proportion of supplements in relation to the content of the labelled ingredients has been reported (Lockwood, 2011; Pravst and Zmitek, 2011).

1.3 Nutrition claims

The regulation defines a *nutrition claim* as any claim stating, suggesting or implying that a food has particular beneficial nutritional properties owing to the calorific value or composition with respect to the presence (or absence) of specific nutrients or other substances. Nutrition claims are permitted only if they are listed in the Annex of Regulation (EC) No 1924/2006 and provided they are in accordance with the set conditions of use (EC, 2006a). Some examples of authorised nutrition claims and the conditions applying to them are listed in Table 1.2. Any claim considered to have the same meaning for consumers as a nutrition claim included on the list is subject to the same conditions of use indicated therein.

A claim that a food contains a nutrient or another substance for which certain conditions are not specified in regulation, or any claim likely to have the same meaning for the consumer, may be made only where the nutrient or other substance is contained in the final product in a significant quantity that will produce the nutritional or physiological effect claimed as established by generally accepted scientific evidence. To ensure that claims are truthful, it is necessary for the substance that is the subject of the claim to be present in the final product in quantities that are sufficient to produce the nutritional or physiological effect claimed.

Table 1.2 **Examples of nutrition claims**

Nutrition claim	Conditions of use
Source of vitamins and/or minerals	A claim that a food is a source of vitamins and/or minerals, and any claim likely to have the same meaning for the consumer, may be made only where the product contains at least a significant amount of such a nutrient.[a]
High in vitamins and/or minerals	A claim that a food is high in vitamins and/or minerals, and any claim likely to have the same meaning for the consumer, may be made only where the product contains at least twice the value of a "source of vitamins/minerals."
Contains other substances	A claim that a food contains a nutrient or another substance, for which specific conditions are not specified in regulation, or any claim likely to have the same meaning for the consumer, may be made only where the nutrient or other substance is contained in the final product in a significant quantity that will produce the nutritional or physiological effect claimed as established by generally accepted scientific evidence.

[a] A significant amount of vitamins and minerals in a food supplement is considered to be 15% of the nutrient reference values as recommended for daily consumption on the labelling as mentioned in Table 1.1.

Source: EC, 2006a.

1.4 Health claims

Regulation (EC) No 1924/2006 defines a *health claim* as any claim which states, suggests or implies that a relationship exists between a food category, a food or one of its constituents, and health. All health claims must be authorised and included in the list of authorised claims. The quantity of the food and pattern of consumption required to obtain the claimed beneficial effect must be included in the labelling and reasonably expected to be consumed in the context of a varied and balanced diet. The claim must be specific, based on generally accepted scientific data and well understood by the average consumer. Reference to general, non-specific benefits of the nutrient or food for overall good health or health-related well-being may be made only if it is accompanied by a specific health claim (EC, 2006a). All authorised health claims are listed in a public *Community Register of nutrition and health claims made on foods*, which includes the wordings of claims and the conditions applying to them, together with any restrictions. Basically, the regulation distinguishes three categories of health claims (Table 1.3). General function claims describe the role of a food in body functions, including the sense of hunger or satiety and not referring to children; disease risk reduction claims state that the consumption of a food or food constituent significantly reduces a risk factor in the development of a human disease. The regulation also mentions claims referring to children's development and health, for which no further definition is given.

Table 1.3 **Types of health claims according to EC regulations**

General function health claims		Claims referring to children's development and health	Reduction of disease risk claims
Based on generally accepted scientific evidence	Based on new evidence		
Claims not referring to children. Claims describing the role of a nutrient or other substance in the growth, development and functions of the body, psychological and behavioural functions, slimming or weight control, etc.	General function health claims based on newly developed scientific evidence	No further definition provided	Claims that state, suggest or imply that the consumption of a food category, a food or one of its constituents significantly reduces a risk factor in the development of a human disease

Source: EC, 2006a.

1.4.1 Labelling requirements when health claims are used

When health claims are made for food supplements, four pieces of compulsory information must be provided on the labelling: (a) a statement indicating the importance of a varied and balanced diet and a healthy lifestyle; (b) the quantity and pattern of consumption required to obtain the claimed beneficial effect; (c) where appropriate, a statement addressed to persons who should avoid using the food; and (d) an appropriate warning for products that are likely to present a health risk if consumed in excess. Manufacturers should be aware of their responsibilities under the general food law, and comply with the fundamental requirement to market food which is safe and not harmful to health and to utilise such statements on their own recognisance (EC, 2013a).

The NHCR allows the use of easy, attractive statements which make reference to the general, non-specific benefits of a product for overall good health or health-related well-being, without an authorisation procedure. While the use of such statements could be helpful to consumers in conveying more consumer-friendly messages, they could easily be misunderstood, possibly leading people to imagine different health benefits from those that actually pertain (EC, 2013a). For this reason, such statements should be accompanied by permitted health claims. A specific health claim must be made *next to* or *following* such a general statement. The specific claims should bear some relevance to the general reference. To avoid misleading consumers, the manufacturer has a responsibility to demonstrate the link between the reference to the general, non-specific benefits of the food and the specific, accompanying and permitted health claim (EC, 2013a).

1.4.2 Review of authorised health claims

The EFSA's opinions related to the evaluation of health claims were reviewed in 2011 (Pravst, 2012a), but not all scientifically substantiated claims have been authorised by the EC. Authorisation may legitimately be withheld if health claims do not comply with other general and specific requirements of the NHCR, even in the case of a favourable scientific assessment (EC, 2012a). Indeed, in the process of authorising health claims, some claims were not included in the list of authorised health claims for public health reasons. For example, in evaluating a health claim on the effect of sodium in maintaining normal muscle function, a cause-and-effect relationship has been established. However, the use of such a claim would convey a conflicting and confusing message to consumers because it would encourage the consumption of a nutrient for which, on the basis of generally accepted scientific advice, authorities are informing consumers that their intake should be reduced. Therefore, such a claim would be ambiguous or misleading (EC, 2012a). In some other cases, public health risks were avoided by establishing proper conditions of use (EC, 2012a; Cappuccio and Pravst, 2011), while in others there are still some unresolved issues (Ritz *et al.*, 2012; Pravst, 2011, 2013).

There are currently about 250 claims in the EU Register of approved health claims, most of which are general function health claims and are based on generally accepted scientific evidence (EC, 2013c). Claims can be used on food supplements if the product meets all requirements of the NHCR and any specific requirements set for each specific claim in the authorisation process. In most cases, common conditions of use of health claims for vitamins and minerals are that a product contains a significant amount of a nutrient (see Tables 1.1 and 1.2). In Table 1.4, authorised claims are reviewed with a focus on the wording of a claim. It is noted that some regulatory limits might apply in some EU countries for the use of some ingredients for which claims are made (see Section 1.5).

Some claims were not included in a review if they were clearly not meant for use on food supplements. This is also the case of olive oil phenolic compounds (conventionally called olive oil polyphenols), which are currently the only non-essential food constituent for which antioxidant properties were confirmed in the health claim evaluation process (Martin-Pelaez *et al.*, 2013). On the basis of an established cause-and-effect relationship, the claim that "olive oil polyphenols contribute to the protection of blood lipids from oxidative stress" is allowed on olive oil which contains at least 5 mg of hydroxytyrosol and its derivatives (e.g. oleuropein complex and tyrosol) per 20 g of olive oil. To make the claim, information must be given to the consumer that the beneficial effect is obtained with a daily intake of 20 g of olive oil. Such a condition obviously cannot be met with food supplements.

1.4.3 Health claims approval process and scientific substantiation

All health claims on the EU market prior to 2006 were included in the evaluation process. The regulation requires the authorisation of all health claims by the EC through the comitology procedure, following the scientific assessment and verification of a claim by the EFSA (Pravst, 2010). Lists of general function claims then on the market were provided by EU member states and included in a consolidated list of about 4600 general function claims, which entered the EFSA's evaluation process. The evaluation of most claims was concluded in 2011 with 341 scientific opinions having been published, and scientific advice provided for 2758 general function health claims, about 20% of which were favourable (Pravst, 2012a). While some claims were withdrawn, about 1500 claims on so-called *botanicals* have been placed on hold by the EC pending further consideration of how to proceed with these (see Section 1.5.3).

On the other hand, all general function health claims based on new evidence, claims referring to children's development and health, and reduction of disease risk claims are submitted directly by companies. In cases where a health claim substantiation is based on (unpublished) proprietary data, and where a claim cannot be substantiated without such proprietary data, the applicant can request 5 years of protection of such data (Pravst, 2012a).

Scientific substantiation of claims is performed by taking into account the totality of the available pertinent scientific data and weighing up the evidence, in particular whether: (a) the effect is relevant to human health; (b) there is an established cause-and-effect relationship between the consumption of the food and the claimed effect in humans; (c) the effect has been shown on a study group which is representative

Table 1.4 Review of authorised health claims

Ingredient	Wording	Conditions[a]
Immune system, oxidative stress and regeneration of vitamin E		
Copper, Folate, Iron, Selenium, Vitamin A, Vitamin B12, Vitamin B6, Vitamin C, Vitamin D, Zinc	Contribute to the normal function of the immune system	
Vitamin C	Contributes to maintaining the normal function of the immune system during and after intense physical exercise	200 mg
Copper, Manganese, Riboflavin, Selenium, Vitamin C, Vitamin E, Zinc	Contribute to the protection of cells from oxidative stress	
Vitamin C	Contributes to the regeneration of the reduced form of vitamin E	
Brain, psychological and neurological functions		
Biotin, Copper, Iodine Magnesium, Niacin, Potassium, Riboflavin, Thiamine, Vitamin B12, Vitamin B6, Vitamin C	Contribute to normal functioning of the nervous system	
Biotin, Folate, Magnesium, Niacin, Thiamine, Vitamin B12, Vitamin B6, Vitamin C	Contribute to normal psychological function	
Iodine, Iron, Zinc	Contribute to normal cognitive function	
Pantothenic acid	Contributes to normal mental performance	
Docosahexaenoic acid (DHA)	Contributes to maintenance of normal brain function	250 mg
Calcium	Contributes to normal neurotransmission	
Folate, Iron, Magnesium, Niacin, Pantothenic acid, Riboflavin, Vitamin B12, Vitamin B6, Vitamin C	Contribute to the reduction of tiredness and fatigue	
Bone, teeth and calcium levels		
Calcium	Is needed for the maintenance of normal bones and teeth	
Magnesium, Phosphorus, Vitamin D	Contribute to the maintenance of normal bones and teeth	
Manganese, Protein, Vitamin K, Zinc	Contribute to the maintenance of normal bones	

Table 1.4 Continued

Ingredient	Wording	Conditions[a]
Vitamin C	Contributes to normal collagen formation for the normal function of bones and teeth	
Fluoride	Contributes to the maintenance of tooth mineralisation	
Vitamin D	Contributes to normal absorption/utilisation of calcium and phosphorus	
Vitamin D	Contributes to normal blood calcium levels	
Collagen, connective tissue and mucous membranes		
Vitamin C	Contributes to normal collagen formation for the normal function of blood vessels, bones, teeth, cartilage, gums and skin	
Copper	Contributes to maintenance of normal connective tissues	
Manganese	Contributes to the normal formation of connective tissue	
Biotin, Niacin, Riboflavin, Vitamin A	Contribute to the maintenance of normal mucous membranes	
Skin, hair and nails		
Biotin, Selenium, Zinc	Contribute to the maintenance of normal hair	
Selenium, Zinc	Contribute to the maintenance of normal nails	
Biotin, Iodine, Niacin, Riboflavin, Vitamin A, Zinc	Contribute to the maintenance of normal skin	
Vitamin C	Contributes to normal collagen formation for the normal function of skin	
Copper	Contributes to normal hair and skin pigmentation	
Muscle mass and function		
Calcium, Magnesium, Potassium, Vitamin D	Contribute to (the maintenance of) normal muscle function	
Protein	Contributes to a growth in muscle mass	
Protein	Contributes to the maintenance of muscle mass	
Cell specialisation and division, cell membranes and DNA synthesis		
Vitamin A, Calcium	Have a role in the process of cell specialisation	
Calcium, Folate, Iron, Magnesium, Vitamin B12, Vitamin D, Zinc	Have a role in the process of cell division	

Continued

Table 1.4 Continued

Ingredient	Wording	Conditions[a]
Phosphorus	Contributes to normal function of cell membranes	
Zinc	Contributes to normal DNA synthesis	
Digestion		
Chloride	Contributes to normal digestion by production of hydrochloric acid in the stomach	
Calcium	Contributes to the normal function of digestive enzymes	
Vision and metabolism of vitamin A		
DHA, Riboflavin, Vitamin A, Zinc	Contribute to the maintenance of normal vision	DHA: 250 mg
Zinc	Contributes to normal metabolism of vitamin A	
Blood, oxygen transport and iron absorption and metabolism		
Calcium, Vitamin K	Contribute to normal blood clotting	
Riboflavin	Contributes to the maintenance of normal red blood cells	
Folate	Contribute to normal blood formation	
Iron, Vitamin B12, Vitamin B6	Contribute to normal red blood cell formation	
Iron	Contributes to normal formation of haemoglobin	
Iron	Contributes to normal oxygen transport in the body	
Riboflavin	Contributes to the normal metabolism of iron	
Vitamin A	Contributes to normal iron metabolism	
Copper	Contributes to normal iron transport in the body	
Vitamin C	Increases iron absorption	
Water-Soluble Tomato Concentrate[b] (WSTC I and II)	Helps maintain normal platelet aggregation, which contributes to healthy blood flow	WSTC I: 3g[b] WSTC II: 150 mg[b]
Blood pressure		
Potassium	Contributes to the maintenance of normal blood pressure	
DHA/eicosapentaenoic acid (EPA)		3 g
Blood cholesterol or triglyceride levels		
Beta glucans[c], Chitosan, Glucomannan, Guar gum hydroxypropyl methylcellulose (HPMC), Pectins	contribute to the maintenance of normal blood cholesterol levels	3–10 g (fibre dependent)

Table 1.4 Continued

Ingredient	Wording	Conditions[a]
Plant sterols/stanols, Monascus purpureus (red yeast rice) Beta glucans[c] Plant sterols, Plant sterols/stanol esters	Have been shown to lower/reduce blood cholesterol. High cholesterol is a risk factor in the development of coronary heart disease.	0.8 g Monacolin K: 10 mg 3 g[c] 1.5–2.4 g
DHA/EPA	Contributes to the maintenance of normal blood glucose levels	2 g
Blood glucose levels		
Chromium	Contributes to the maintenance of normal blood glucose levels	
Heart DHA contributes to the maintenance of normal blood triglyceride levels		
DHA and EPA, Thiamine	Contribute to the normal function of the heart	EPA + DHA: 250 mg
Liver		
Choline	Contributes to the maintenance of normal liver function	82.5 mg
Thyroid gland		
Iodine, Selenium	Contribute to the normal thyroid function	
Hormonal activity/synthesis		
Iodine	Contributes to the normal production of thyroid hormones	
Vitamin B6	Contributes to the regulation of hormonal activity	
Pantothenic acid	Contributes to normal synthesis and metabolism of steroid hormones, vitamin D and some neurotransmitters	
Zinc	Contributes to the maintenance of normal testosterone levels in the blood	
Fertility, reproduction and pregnancy		
Zinc	Contributes to normal fertility and reproduction	
Selenium	Contributes to normal spermatogenesis	
Folate	Contributes to maternal tissue growth during pregnancy	
Performance		
Creatine	Increases physical performance in successive bursts of short-term, high intensity exercise	Creatine: 3 g[d]

Continued

Table 1.4 Continued

Ingredient	Wording	Conditions[a]
Macronutrients and energy-yielding metabolism		
Biotin, Calcium, Copper, Iodine, Iron, Magnesium, Manganese, Niacin, Pantothenic acid, Phosphorus, Riboflavin, Thiamine, Vitamin B12, Vitamin B6, Vitamin C	Contribute to normal energy-yielding metabolism	
Biotin, Chromium, Zinc	Contribute to normal macronutrient metabolism	
Choline	Contributes to normal lipid metabolism	
Vitamin B6	Contributes to normal protein and glycogen metabolism	
Magnesium, Zinc	Contribute to normal protein synthesis	
Zinc	Contributes to normal metabolism of fatty acids	
Amino acids and homocysteine metabolism/synthesis		
Molybdenum	Contributes to normal sulphur amino acid metabolism	
Folate	Contributes to normal amino acid synthesis	
Vitamin B6	Contributes to normal cysteine synthesis	
Betaine, Choline, Folate, Vitamin B12, Vitamin B6	Contribute to normal homocysteine metabolism	Betaine: 500 mg[c]
Electrolyte balance and acid-base metabolism		
Zinc	Contributes to normal acid-base metabolism	
Magnesium	Contributes to electrolyte balance	
Claims referring to children's development and health		
Iodine	Contributes to the normal growth of children	
Calcium, Phosphorus, Protein, Vitamin D	Is needed for normal growth and development of bone in children	
Iron	Contributes to normal cognitive development of children	
Essential fatty acids	Are needed for normal growth and development of children	
DHA	Maternal intake contributes to the normal brain development of the foetus and breastfed infants	200 mg[i]
DHA	Maternal intake contributes to the normal development of the eye of the foetus and breastfed infants	200 mg[i]

Table 1.4 Continued

Ingredient	Wording	Conditions[a]
Other claims		
Activated charcoal	Contributes to reducing excessive flatulence after eating	1 g[f]
Melatonin	Contributes to the alleviation of subjective feelings of jet lag	0,5 mg[g]
Melatonin	Contributes to the reduction of time taken to fall asleep	1 mg[h]
Lactase enzyme	Improves lactose digestion in individuals who have difficulty digesting lactose	4500 FCC units

[a] Common conditions regarding the use of health claims are that the product contains a significant amount of a nutrient (eligible for the nutrition claim "source of"), except where different conditions are noted.
[b] General function health claims based on newly developed scientific evidence with a request for restricted use of scientific evidence for a period of 5 years from the date of authorisation (2009). The beneficial effect can be obtained with a daily consumption of 3 g WSTC I or 150 mg WSTC II in food supplements when taken with a glass of water or other liquid.
[c] Beta-glucans from barley or oats.
[d] Only for foods targeting adults performing high intensity exercise
[e] A daily intake in excess of 4 g may significantly increase blood cholesterol levels.
[f] The beneficial effect is obtained when 1 g of activated charcoal is consumed at least 30 min before and 1 g shortly after a meal.
[g] The beneficial effect is obtained when 0.5 mg of melatonin is taken close to bedtime on the first day of travel and on the following few days after arrival at the destination.
[h] The beneficial effect is obtained with an intake of 1 mg of melatonin close to bedtime.
[i] The beneficial effect is obtained with a daily intake of 200 mg of DHA in addition to the recommended daily intake of omega-3 fatty acids for adults.

of the target population; and (d) the quantity of the food and pattern of consumption required to obtain the claimed effect can reasonably be achieved as part of a balanced diet. Useful guidance has been provided by the EFSA for applicants to prepare an application for authorisation of a health claim and about the evaluation of health claims (EFSA, 2011a, d). Guidance related to specific health-related issues has also been released to help applicants substantiate health claims: (a) gut and immune function (EFSA, 2011c); (b) antioxidants, oxidative damage and cardiovascular health (EFSA, 2011b); (c) appetite ratings, weight management, and blood glucose concentrations (EFSA, 2012a); (d) bone, joints, skin and oral health (EFSA, 2012b); (e) physical performance (EFSA, 2012d); and (f) functions of the nervous system, including psychological functions (EFSA, 2012c).

The key questions addressed by the EFSA in the scientific evaluation of health claims are whether: (a) the food/constituent is sufficiently defined and characterised; (b) the claimed effect is sufficiently defined, and if it is a beneficial physiological effect; and (c) pertinent human studies have been presented to substantiate the claim. If this is the case, the EFSA weighs up the evidence of all pertinent studies presented (EFSA, 2011a).

1.4.3.1 The wording of a health claim

A health claim must reflect the scientific evidence and must be well understood by the average consumer. In the scientific evaluation process, the EFSA can propose changing the wording to reflect the scientific evidence, but such wording is sometimes hard for the general population to understand. An example of such a procedure is a health claim for a specific water-soluble tomato concentrate and the maintenance of a healthy blood flow (EFSA, 2009; Pravst, 2010). The applicant proposed a claim that the product *helps to maintain a healthy blood flow and benefits circulation*. The EFSA considered that this wording did not reflect the scientific evidence because only measures of platelet aggregation have been used, whereas blood flow and circulation also depend on many other factors. They suggested a different wording to reflect the scientific evidence (*helps maintain normal platelet aggregation*), although the Commission later reworded it to be understood by consumers (*helps maintain normal platelet aggregation, which contributes to healthy blood flow*) (Pravst, 2010). When discussing the wording of health claims, it should also be noted that, as regards reduction of disease risk claims, the wording should refer to the specific risk factor for the disease and not to the disease alone. Further information in relation to consumer understanding of health claims can be found in the review by Nocella and Kennedy (2012).

1.4.3.2 Characterisation

To enable the scientific evaluation of a health claim application and control of the products on the market by authorities, the food constituents should be sufficiently characterised. In the scientific evaluation process this characterisation is needed to identify the food or food constituent, to define the appropriate conditions of use, and to connect it with the scientific studies provided. A lack of characterisation has been one of the most common reasons for the EFSA's non-favourable opinions regarding general function claims.

Beside the physical and chemical properties and the composition, the analytical methods must also be provided (EFSA, 2011a). In cases where variations in composition could occur, variability from batch to batch should be addressed together with stability with respect to storage conditions during shelf life (EFSA, 2011a). Where applicable, it is useful to show that a constituent is bioavailable and to provide a rationale of how the constituent reaches the target site. There are no specific requirements on the type of evidence to provide such a rationale; therefore this should be done on case-by-case basis with respect to the nature of the constituent. If a claim is made for a specific combination of constituents, such a combination must be characterised in detail, particularly in relation to the active constituents.

For microorganisms, genetic typing should be performed at the strain level with internationally accepted molecular methods and the naming of strains according to the International Code of Nomenclature. Depositing samples in an internationally recognised culture collection for control purposes has been suggested (EFSA, 2011a). The stability of the microorganisms and the influence of the food matrix on their activity should be studied.

For plant products, the scientific name of the plant should be specified, together with the part of the plant used and details of the preparation used, including details of the extraction, drying, etc. It is beneficial when the applicant can show that the composition of the plant-derived product can be controlled by analyses of specific chemical ingredients, for which biological activity is shown.

1.4.3.3 Specific conditions of use and the target population

To ensure that the health claim is not misleading to the consumer, specific conditions of use are set during the authorisation process. Conditions are proposed by the applicant and evaluated in the evaluation process by the EFSA. The conditions should ensure that the nutrient or other substance of which the claim is made is contained in the final product in a quantity that will produce the claimed effect. If needed, the pattern of consumption must be specified together with possible warnings, restrictions on use and directions for use.

The target population must be specified and, in relation to this, it is critical that the specific study group in which the evidence was obtained is also representative of the target population for which the claim is intended (Pravst, 2010). In cases where studies are not performed on a representative sample of the target population, evidence must be provided that an extrapolation can be performed. It is important to mention that patients are usually not considered an appropriate study group. However, judgement on this is made on a case-by-case basis. Subjects with untreated hypertension were found to be an appropriate study population for substantiation of a claim (for the general population) on maintaining normal blood pressure. Similarly, studies using irritable bowel syndrome (IBS) patients are considered pertinent for substantiating claims on bowel function and gastro-intestinal discomfort for the general population (Pravst, 2012a).

1.4.3.4 Scientific substantiation of the claimed effect

The relevance of the claimed effect on human health and human data are critical for substantiating a claim. Studies need to be carried out with the subject product/constituents with similar conditions of use in a study group representative of the population group and using an appropriate outcome measure of the claimed effect (EFSA, 2011a; Meoni *et al.*, 2013). Using appropriate outcome measures can be a challenge because a limited number of validated biomarkers are available (Cazaubiel and Bard, 2008). Biomarkers are characteristics that are objectively measured and evaluated as indicators of normal biological processes, pathogenic processes or pharmacologic responses to therapeutic intervention. Well-performed human intervention trials are particularly important for successful substantiation. Double-blind, randomised, placebo-controlled trials are considered the *gold standard* for all types of claims, except for claims about generally accepted functions of nutrients (Pravst, 2010). During scientific evaluation, such trials are critically assessed to ensure that there are no weaknesses. In some cases, non-blind studies are also acceptable, particularly in the case of non-processed foods where blinding is not possible. However, blinding is necessary when testing the efficiency of food supplements. Human observational studies and data from studies in animals or model systems are considered only as supporting evidence.

1.5 Borderline substances: between foods and medicine

With the possibility of health claims on foods, the borderline between foods and medicine is becoming ever thinner. The concept of foods is moving beyond providing basic nutritional needs, and this is also often the case with food supplements. It is clear that when products are intended to cure diseases, these are classified as medicine. However, it is less clear in what conditions substances used in such medicine can be used in foods.

1.5.1 Vitamins, minerals and other natural compounds with a nutritional or physiological effect

A healthy diet consisting of foods with functional properties can help promote well-being and even reduce the risk of developing certain diseases (Howlett, 2008). Such properties are usually related to the chemical composition of foods and food supplements are often a source of concentrated constituents which are found in traditional foods. In the EU, the maximum levels of such compounds are not harmonised, not even for vitamins and minerals. While in most EU countries tolerable upper intake levels (UL) (Table 1.5) are considered a maximum limit for the use of vitamins and minerals with foods (total intake with food and food supplements), some countries have defined limits in national regulations. Therefore some EU-approved health claims cannot be

Table 1.5 **Tolerable UL for vitamins and minerals (adults)**

Vitamin or mineral	UL
Vitamin A	3000 µg
Vitamin D	50 µg
Vitamin E	300 mg
Vitamin B6	25 mg
Niacin	900 mg
Folic acid	1000 µg
Calcium	1500 mg
Copper	5 mg
Iodine	600 µg
Zinc	25 mg
Selenium	300 µg
Molybdenum	600 µg

Source: EFSA, 2006.

used in all EU countries. The claim concerning the role of vitamin C in maintaining normal function of the immune system during and after intense physical exercise may be used only for products which provide a daily intake of 200 mg vitamin C. In some EU countries, such a level of vitamin C is allowed only in drugs.

The use of other substances with a nutritional or physiological effect is even less harmonised (Eisenbrand, 2008). While in some countries this area is also regulated by national regulations, the Commission and the majority of EU member states believe that the current legislation is sufficient to provide consumer protection (FSA, 2010). Nevertheless, the lack of legislation has contributed to the fact that products containing such ingredients are poorly controlled in the markets of many EU countries.

1.5.2 Drug compounds

Some health claims were approved for compounds which can be found in medicine. It should be explained that the use of substances in food supplements is governed by specific EU and national legislation, and that the inclusion of a compound in the list of permitted health claims does not constitute authorisation of the marketing of the substance on which the claim is made, a decision on whether the substance can be used in foodstuffs, or a classification of a certain product as a foodstuff (EC, 2012a; Eussen *et al.*, 2011). This is also the case for red yeast rice (*Monascus purpureus*) which contains Monacolin K (authorised claim: *contributes to the maintenance of normal blood cholesterol levels*, see Table 1.4). Monacolin K is synonymous with lovastatin, an inhibitor of cholesterol synthesis which is contained, as an active substance, in a number of prescription medicinal products. The health claim could only be used for products providing a daily intake of 10 mg of Monacolin K from red yeast rice; however, in a decision of the European Court of Justice, such a level of Monacolin K is possible only in medicinal products (ECJ, 2009).

There are also country-to-country differences regarding the use of health claims for substances which can be found in medicine – similarly as with the case of vitamins. For example, two health claims have been authorised for melatonin (*alleviation of subjective feelings of jet lag* and *contribution to the reduction of time taken to fall asleep*, see Table 1.4). In some countries, melatonin can be found in food supplements, while in others it is allowed only in medicine.

1.5.3 Botanicals

Botanicals are plant and herbal substances with a long tradition of being used in both food and medicine. As a medicinal product, botanicals can be registered using a simplified traditional use registration and sold as traditional herbal medicinal products (THMP) (EC, 2004; Calapai, 2013). For such products, there is no requirement for clinical trials on the effectiveness of the product, although products must have sufficient safety data and their production must comply with good manufacturing practices (GMP). About 750 such products were on the EU market at the beginning of 2012 (EC, 2012b).

On the contrary, when botanicals are used as food supplements there is no special requirement regarding manufacturing practices other than for foods alone, although the final product should be safe for use and labelled in line with the legislation pertaining to food, including the regulation on health claims. The use of botanicals in foods (food supplements) is not yet harmonised in the EU, and member states are using different approaches as to which botanicals can be used in foods, and in what conditions. However, the use of health claims on foods is harmonised and claims must be substantiated by scientific evidence of the highest possible standard. Contrary to THMP, traditional use is not accepted as sufficient evidence for the use of claims on food supplements. In scientific assessments, a number of health claims applications for botanicals have therefore received negative opinions (Pravst, 2012b).

The difference in dealing with the *evidence of traditional use* between food and medicinal legislation has caused a wide debate within the EU. The EC noted that the same botanicals are sometimes used in both foods and medicines, and consumers may sometimes struggle to perceive the difference between certain claims or indications of their physiological effect. The Commission therefore decided to launch a reflection on whether this difference should be maintained or not (EC, 2012b). In 2010 the EFSA was asked to discontinue its assessment of health claims for botanicals, with the result that these, together with a number of already assessed botanicals, have been put on hold (EC, 2011a). Two possible solutions for these claims have been suggested by the Commission. One is to continue the scientific evaluations by applying the same criteria and standards as for other food ingredients. In practice, this would mean negative opinions for the vast majority of claims made for botanicals. The other solution is to adopt a regulation and establish different rules that recognise their traditional use. In this case, the use of botanicals in the EU market would also have to be harmonised.

No further decision has been accepted and, while claims for botanicals are still *on hold*, they may continue to be used at the full responsibility of the producers (EC, 2012a). Such claims also need to be in line with the general requirements of the NHCR and should not be misleading to consumers.

1.6 Conclusions

In the EU food supplements are regulated as food and covered by general food legislation and Directive 2002/46/EC on food supplements. To ensure the protection of consumers and facilitate their choices, products must be safe and appropriately labelled. The quality and safety of food supplements is the full responsibility of the producer but can be controlled by national authorities. The labelling of food supplements is regulated by both specific and broader food regulations. Health claims regulation was accepted in the EU in 2006, and all health claims require scientific assessment by the EFSA and authorisation by the EC. Only authorised health claims are allowed, with the exception of some claims which are in the evaluation process. To avoid misleading consumers, specific labelling requirements apply when health claims are used. For the authorisation of a new health claim, an applicant needs to prepare a scientific dossier in which the health claim is scientifically substantiated. In cases where a health claim substantiation is based on (unpublished) proprietary data, and if a claim cannot be substantiated without such proprietary data, the applicant can request 5 years of protection of such data. Studies need to be carried out with the subject product with similar conditions of use in a study group representative of the target population group and using an appropriate outcome measure of the claimed effect. Well-performed human intervention trials are particularly important for successful substantiation while human observational studies and data from studies in animals or model systems are considered only as supporting evidence.

Acknowledgements

We thank Murray Bales for help with language editing of the text. The work was supported by grants ARRS-MKO (V7-1107) and Nutrition Institute Research Fund (NIRF 2013).

References

Calapai, G. (2013) Research and development for botanical products in medicinals and food supplements market. *Evidence-Based Complementary and Alternative Medicine*, 2013, 649720.
Cappuccio, F. P. and Pravst, I. (2011) Health claims on foods: Promoting healthy food choices or high salt intake? *British Journal of Nutrition*, 106, 1770–1771.
Cazaubiel, M. and Bard, J. M. (2008) Use of biomarkers for the optimization of clinical trials in nutrition. *Agro Food Industry Hi-Tech*, 19, 22–24.
EC (1997) Regulation (EC) No 258/97 concerning novel foods and novel food ingredients. Available from: http://eur-lex.europa.eu/LexUriServ/LexUriServ.do?uri=CONSLEG:1997R0258:20090807:EN:PDF (Accessed: 31 March 2014).
EC (2000) Directive 2000/13/EC on the approximation of the laws of the Member States relating to the labelling, presentation and advertising of foodstuffs. Available from: http://eur-lex.europa.eu/LexUriServ/LexUriServ.do?uri=CONSLEG:2000L0013:20110120:EN:PDF (Accessed: 31 March 2014).
EC (2002) Directive 2002/46/EC of the European parliament and of the Council on the approximation of the laws of the Member States relating to food supplements. Available from: http://eur-lex.europa.eu/LexUriServ/LexUriServ.do?uri=CONSLEG:2002L0046:20111205:EN:PDF (Accessed: 31 March 2014).
EC (2004) Directive 2004/24/EC amending, as regards traditional herbal medicinal products, Directive 2001/83/EC on the Community code relating to medicinal products for human use. Available from: http://eur-lex.europa.eu/LexUriServ/LexUriServ.do?uri=OJ:L:2004:136:0085:0090:EN:PDF (Accessed: 31 March 2014).

EC (2006a) Regulation (EC) No 1924/2006 on nutrition and health claims made on foods. Available from: http://eur-lex.europa.eu/LexUriServ/LexUriServ.do?uri=CONSLEG:2006R1924:20121129:EN:PDF (Accessed: 31 March 2014).

EC (2006b) Regulation (EC) No 1925/2006 on the addition of vitamins and minerals and of certain other substances to foods. Available from: http://eur-lex.europa.eu/LexUriServ/LexUriServ.do?uri=CONSLEG:2006R1925:20111205:EN:PDF (Accessed: 31 March 2014).

EC (2008) Regulation (EC) No 1333/2008 on food additives. Available from: http://eur-lex.europa.eu/LexUriServ/LexUriServ.do?uri=CONSLEG:2008R1333:20130206:EN:PDF (Accessed: 31 March 2014).

EC (2011a) Questions and Answers on the list of permitted Health Claims – MEMO/11/868. Available from: http://europa.eu/rapid/pressReleasesAction.do?reference=MEMO/11/868 (Accessed: 31 March 2014).

EC (2011b) Regulation (EU) No 1169/2011 of the European Parliament and of the Council of 25 October 2011 on the provision of food information to consumers. Available from: http://eur-lex.europa.eu/LexUriServ/LexUriServ.do?uri=CONSLEG:2011R1169:20111212:EN:PDF (Accessed: 31 March 2014).

EC (2012a) Commission Regulation (EU) No 432/2012 establishing a list of permitted health claims made on foods, other than those referring to the reduction of disease risk and to children's development and health. Available from: http://eur-lex.europa.eu/LexUriServ/LexUriServ.do?uri=OJ:L:2012:136:0001:0040:EN:PDF (Accessed: 31 March 2014).

EC (2012b) Discussion paper on health claims on botanicals used in foods (DG SANCO). Available from: http://izbamleka.pl/wp-content/uploads/2012/09/instrukcja.pdf (Accessed: 31 March 2014).

EC (2013a) Commission implementing decision 2013/63/EU adopting guidelines for the implementation of specific conditions for health claims laid down in Article 10 of Regulation (EC) No 1924/2006. Available from: http://eur-lex.europa.eu/LexUriServ/LexUriServ.do?uri=OJ:L:2013:022:0025:0028:EN:PDF (Accessed: 31 March 2014).

EC (2013b) Community Register on the addition of vitamins and minerals and of certain other substances to foods. Available from: http://ec.europa.eu/food/food/labellingnutrition/vitamins/comm_reg_En.pdf (Accessed: 31 March 2014).

EC (2013c) EU Register of nutrition and health claims made on foods. Available from: http://ec.europa.eu/nuhclaims/ (Accessed: 31 March 2014).

ECJ (2009) Case C-140/07: Hecht-Pharma GmbH v Staatliches Gewerbeaufsichtsamt Lüneburg. Directive 2001/83/EC – Articles 1(2) and 2(2) – Concept of "medicinal product by function" – Product in respect of which it has not been established that it is a medicinal product by function – Account taken of the content in active substances. European Court reports, P I-00041. Available from: http://eur-lex.europa.eu/LexUriServ/LexUriServ.do?uri=CELEX:62007CJ0140:EN:NOT (Accessed: 31 March 2014).

EFSA (2006) Tolerable Upper Intake Levels for Vitamins and Minerals. Available from: http://www.efsa.europa.eu/en/ndatopics/docs/ndatolerableuil.pdf (Accessed: 31 March 2014).

EFSA (2009) Water-soluble tomato concentrate (WSTC I and II) and platelet aggregation. *The EFSA Journal*, 1101, 1–15.

EFSA (2011a) General guidance for stakeholders on the evaluation of Article 13.1, 13.5 and 14 health claims. *EFSA Journal*, 9, 2135.

EFSA (2011b) Guidance on the scientific requirements for health claims related to antioxidants, oxidative damage and cardiovascular health. *EFSA Journal*, 9, 2474.

EFSA (2011c) Guidance on the scientific requirements for health claims related to gut and immune function. *EFSA Journal*, 9, 1984.

EFSA (2011d) Scientific and technical guidance for the preparation and presentation of an application for authorisation of a health claim (revision 1). *EFSA Journal*, 9, 2170.

EFSA (2012a) Guidance on the scientific requirements for health claims related to appetite ratings, weight management, and blood glucose concentrations. *EFSA Journal*, 10, 2604.

EFSA (2012b) Guidance on the scientific requirements for health claims related to bone, joints, skin, and oral health. *EFSA Journal*, 10, 2702.

EFSA (2012c) Guidance on the scientific requirements for health claims related to functions of the nervous system, including psychological functions. *EFSA Journal*, 10, 2816.

EFSA (2012d) Guidance on the scientific requirements for health claims related to physical performance. *EFSA Journal*, 10, 2817.

Eisenbrand, G. (2008) Evaluation of food supplements containing other ingredients than vitamins and minerals. *Deutsche Lebensmittel-Rundschau*, 104, 161–166.

Eussen, S. R. B. M., Verhagen, H., Klungel, O. H., Garssen, J., van Loveren, H., van Kranen, H. J. and Rompelberg, C. J. M. (2011) Functional foods and dietary supplements: Products at the interface between pharma and nutrition. *European Journal of Pharmacology*, 668, Supplement 1, S2–S9.

FSA. The use of substances other than vitamins and minerals (URL: http://www.food.gov.uk/safereating/chemsafe/supplements/other/, Accessed 31 March 2014). 2010. London, Food Standards Agency.

Howlett, J. (2008) *Functional Foods: From Science to Health and Claims,* ILSI Europe, Brussels.

Lockwood, G. B. (2011) The quality of commercially available nutraceutical supplements and food sources. *Journal of Pharmacy and Pharmacology*, 63, 3–10.

Martin-Pelaez, S., Covas, M. I., Fito, M., Kusar, A. and Pravst, I. (2013) Health effects of olive oil polyphenols: Recent advances and possibilities for the use of health claims. *Molecular Nutrition & Food Research*, 57, 760–771.

Meoni, P., Restani, P. and Mancama, D. T. (2013) Review of existing experimental approaches for the clinical evaluation of the benefits of plant food supplements on cardiovascular function. *Food and Function*, 4, 856–870.

Nocella, G. and Kennedy, O. (2012) Food health claims: What consumers understand. *Food Policy*, 37, 571–580.

Pravst, I. (2010) The evaluation of health claims in Europe: What have we learned? *Agro Food Industry Hi-Tech*, 21, 4–6.

Pravst, I. (2011) Risking public health by approving some health claims? – The case of phosphorus. *Food Policy*, 36, 725–727.

Pravst, I. (2012a) *Functional Foods in Europe: A Focus on Health Claims. Scientific, Health and Social Aspects of the Food Industry* (ed. by B. Valdez) InTech, Rijeka.

Pravst, I. (2012b) Health claims: An opportunity for science. *Agro Food Industry Hi-Tech*, 23, 2–3.

Pravst, I. (2013) Health: EU fructose claim ignores risks. *Nature*, 504, 376.

Pravst, I. and Zmitek, K. (2011) The coenzyme Q10 content of food supplements. *Journal fur Verbraucherschutz und Lebensmittelsicherheit-Journal of Consumer Protection and Food Safety*, 6, 457–463.

Ritz, E., Hahn, K., Ketteler, M., Kuhlmann, M. K. and Mann, J. (2012) Phosphate additives in food – a health risk. *Dtsch Arztebl Int*, 109, 49–55.

Appendix: abbreviations

DHA	Docosahexaenoic acid
DNA	Deoxyribonucleic acid
EC	European Commission
EFSA	European Food Safety Authority
EPA	Eicosapentaenoic acid
EU	European Union
FCC	Food Chemicals Codex
GMP	Good Manufacturing Practices
HPMC	Hydroxypropyl methylcellulose
IBS	Irritable Bowel Syndrome
NHCR	Regulation (EC) 1924/2006 on nutrition and health claims on foods
NRV	Nutrient reference value
THMP	Traditional herbal medicinal products
UL	Tolerable upper intake level

Good manufacturing practice (GMP) in the production of dietary supplements

2

T. Sikora
Cracow University of Economics, Kraków, Poland

2.1 Introduction

Good practice (GP) codes were first developed in the 1960s with the aim of providing clear procedures for safe and hygienic manufacturing. In general terms, GMP may be defined as a set of rules developed through experience. GMP involves performing all production activities in accordance with defined requirements within the field of construction, modifying technology, equipment, operational practice and manufacturing methods, as necessary to manufacture food of appropriate quality.

The basic criterion for a quality assurance (QA) system is that products are manufactured and controlled according to defined standards guaranteeing uniformity and reproducibility of the product. Such a system has to be embedded in the organisational structure of an enterprise, with a defined hierarchy of goals and precisely established scope of responsibility, especially in managerial posts. Quality-orientated activities in the manufacturing process must be planned, coordinated and controlled according to strictly defined procedures and instructions, preventing errors. It can be summarised by the motto: "*do it the first time you try*" (GMP Guidebook, 2002).

GMP is a system covering the whole process from the procurement and storage of raw materials, through production, packaging, labelling and storage of the final product, to quality control and distribution, including internal audits. A properly planned system guarantees that each operation is performed in accordance with written procedures and properly reviewed. To sum up, it may be stated that the general GMP rule is to ensure uniformity. Each activity must be performed exactly as indicated in the procedure, and recorded in an appropriate document and confirmed (GMP Guidebook, 2002 – guidebooks used for the implementation of GMP are generally targeted at the food industry, but the hints given in this publication may be used in all kinds of production, e.g. pro-/pre-biotics, teas and herbal supplements as well as different kinds of foodstuffs). GPs contain guidelines aimed at guaranteeing minimum acceptable standards and conditions for product manufacture and storage; they do not have any official status, but their implementation is often recommended. GMP for specific food groups contains additional aspects typical for such product groups (Luning *et al.*, 2002).

The rules of good manufacturing practice (GMP) are applied in various fields of business activity. GMP is a set of verified, effective rules of conduct and manufacturing conditions, designed to ensure specified results, e.g. an appropriate level of product quality or safety. GMP, as applicable to particular business types, is usually described in their relevant codes or guidebooks. Most often GMP requirements are applied voluntarily; however, in some areas they have been set down in legislation and thus have become mandatory. To meet the requirements at the design stage, appropriate functional solutions are introduced to enable employees to maintain the required hygiene standards.

When it was realised that quality is created not in the quality control department but at the manufacturing stage, the rules were formulated and GMP started to be regarded as the way to ensure the quality of dietary supplements. In Section 2.2 key issues of GMP implementation will be explained. Subsequently, the GMP manual will be presented in Section 2.3. The chapter will conclude by outlining their benefits and disadvantages, with the example of the Polish manufacturers of dietary supplements in Section 2.4.

2.2 Key issues related to good manufacturing practice/ good hygienic practice (GMP/GHP) implementation

Among key issues related to GMP/GHP implementation are: legal requirements, stages of GMP implementation, the role of the management board during quality assurance, defining the tasks and scope of GMP, hygiene requirements that should be met, and documentation of GMP.

2.2.1 Legal requirements

Due to numerous connections between GMP and good hygienic practice (GHP) in food processing, it is reasonable that these practices are incorporated within one set of rules. Consequently, GHP is implemented simultaneously within GMP within enterprises (Figure 2.1).

The GMP/GHP rules have been described in the first part of CAC/PRC 1-1969 Rev. 4 2003, Recommended International Codes of Practice – General Principles of Food Hygiene, Codex Alimentarius. They are also included in the annex to Regulation 852/2004.

According to Art. 8 of EC Regulation 852/2004 in EU countries, the food sectors should develop and share GP guidelines:

- after obtaining the opinion of the parties whose interests may be significantly affected, such as appropriate agencies and consumer groups,
- after considering appropriate codes of practice from Codex Alimentarius.

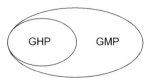

Figure 2.1 Connections between GHP and GMP.

Detailed descriptions of the actions that should be taken by enterprises as regards rooms, personnel, transport, food products and packaging are included in the annexes to Regulation 852/2004. In accordance with EC Regulation 852/2004, food sector enterprises should maintain and keep documentation related to their actions in an appropriate manner and for an appropriate period of time, proportionately to the nature and volume of their activity. Annex II to Regulation 852/2004 defines general hygiene requirements for all food sector enterprises.

2.2.2 Stages of GMP implementation

QA may be realised by answering three questions (von Bockelmann, 1995):

1. Where are we?
2. Where do we want to go?
3. How do we want to get there?

2.2.2.1 Stage 1: Where are we?

Having made the decision to implement the GMP standard in an organisation, there must be an assessment of the present situation. Firstly, there must be a zero audit which will provide an estimate of the elements of the system already functioning and those which have yet to be implemented or updated. (In an organisation that does not yet have such a system, there are always some elements of the system that should be used). Implementation of GP in an organisation should be evolutionary and not revolutionary, to be more readily accepted by the employees.

2.2.2.2 Stage 2: Where do we want to go?

The ultimate goal should be specified. It is also necessary to define the time-frame and necessary means to complete the scheduled activities, as well as the benefits that can be achieved by implementing GPs.

2.2.2.3 Stage 3: How do we get there?

Depending on the scope of planned works, it is necessary to consider the following activities:

- educating and training the staff,
- improvement of procedures,
- improvement of processes, and
- improving the initial condition (of raw materials).

The process of improving the functioning standard (of GP) in an organisation is a continuous and indefinite process.

2.2.3 Role of management board in quality assurance (QA)

The responsibility for quality rests with the company management, but all employees at all organisational levels have to contribute to achieving the desired quality.

Among the tasks of the management board, assuming the members have appropriate knowledge, we can list:

- planning quality-orientated activities within the enterprise,
- preparing organisational structures in which each member will have a defined post and responsibilities related to it, as well as procedures, processes and resources,
- creating operational rules for the quality system,
- actions aimed at QA,
- raising employees' qualifications and awareness of quality through regular training,
- continuous system improvement.

Such actions may bring numerous benefits, most of all raising the company's reputation in the market and increasing customer trust, which in turn increases sales volumes. One of the undisputed advantages of the involvement of senior executives in quality management is to develop employee trust in the site management system, increasing productivity through their greater commitment to the company as well as their inventiveness improving cycles, costs and parameters of process flows.

2.2.4 Quality assurance in the food production/industry

QA is a quality management tool, comprising organisational structures, processes and documentation. In the food industry, the QA system is supposed to guarantee the following (The Rules..., 1997):

- appropriate quality of food (safe, reproducible and complying with the specifications),
- the development and manufacture of food products consistent with GMP and other GPs,
- precisely defined production and control activities, consistent with GMP requirements,
- a defined scope of responsibility on particular levels of management,
- supply and application of appropriate initial and packaging materials,
- all required controls of semi-finished products (interim process controls, calibrations, validations),
- production consistent with valid procedures,
- good distribution practice (GDP),
- appropriate storage (good storage practice (GSP)) and transport (good transport practice (GTP)) of food products throughout their shelf life,
- internal audits aimed at refining and verifying the effectiveness of the QA system.

Summing up, QA is a way of thinking, both for the company as a whole and for individual employees. GMP must be applied throughout the production process. Production comprises all stages, from the purchase of raw materials to the completion of the production stage, distribution and delivery to the consumer.

The basic criterion of the QA system is that the products are manufactured and controlled in accordance with predefined standards ensuring the uniformity and reproducibility of a product. Such a system must be embedded in the organisational structure of the enterprise, with a defined hierarchy of goals and precisely planned areas of responsibility, especially at the managerial level.

2.2.5 Ten rules of GMP

The most important requirements of GMP for employees may be summed up in ten basic GMP rules, as follows (Turlejska *et al.*, 1998):

1. Before you start any work, make sure you have the required procedures and instructions.
2. Always follow the instructions exactly, do not use "shortcuts." If you are uncertain, ask your superiors or check the relevant documentation.
3. Before you start work, make sure that you have the appropriate raw material or semi-finished product.
4. Make sure that the technical condition of devices and equipment are appropriate and that they are clean.
5. Work in such a manner as to minimise the risk of contaminating the product, the premises, the equipment and devices.
6. Be careful and avoid errors.
7. Report to the management any irregularities or deviations from assumed production process parameters.
8. Take care of personal hygiene and keep your own post clean and tidy.
9. Record all parameters of the process flow precisely.
10. Take responsibility for your actions.

2.2.6 Tasks and scope of GMP

A very important aspect of the GMP system implementation is the rule of double-checking. It is applicable principally to the critical activities (process stages, process conditions, required examinations) ensuring that the performance of an activity is checked by another, independent person and then recorded in a defined document.

The main tasks of GMP are as follows:

- ensuring the quality of the product,
- preventing mistakes,
- preventing and minimising the risk of cross-contamination (contamination of a raw material or product with another raw material or product),
- ensuring the reproducibility of a series, defining the amount of e.g. active substance, raw material or packaging material (used to package the product) utilised in a process made up of one or more operations so that it can be regarded as uniform.

To fulfil these tasks, manufacturing processes must be performed in properly prepared rooms and premises, equipped with the required devices and machines. The manufacturer must also have well-trained staff. It is vital that hygiene is considered, in the context of both employees' personal and workplace hygiene and general production hygiene. Every enterprise should have a pre-planned hygiene monitoring system, and the results of measurements and analyses should be recorded in written reports proving the realisation of a sanitary programme.

The basic GMP requirements refer to the following scope (Kołożyn-Krajewska and Sikora, 2010):

- appropriate location of the site and whether production rooms are appropriate for a particular type of production,

- whether the equipment and devices are appropriate and properly maintained,
- appropriate on-site ventilation,
- appropriate inventory of equipment, chemical substances and food products,
- efficient lighting,
- sewage and water service,
- good technical maintenance of the whole facility,
- whether the control and measuring instruments are reliable,
- whether materials used for production have appropriate quality and are properly secured against contamination,
- whether all technological processes, washing and disinfection instructions and procedures are always current,
- whether materials and products (raw or otherwise) are properly stored and transported,
- whether the staff have appropriate qualifications,
- whether no deviations are made from the instructions,
- whether each mistake in production is checked and relevant root causes are analysed,
- whether the site is properly secured against pests,
- whether the documentation is transparent.

2.2.7 Hygienic requirements concerning food production

GHP comprises all actions that must be performed and conditions that must be met at all stages of food production.

Production hygiene depends on many factors, among others (Kołożyn-Krajewska and Sikora, 2010):

- functional site design,
- trace of production flow: straight – one way route,
- reduction of unnecessary movement of staff between work centres, especially between clean and dirty zones,
- reduction of the possibility of cross-contamination,
- separating functional zones: clean and dirty,
- appropriate conditions for unit operations,
- keeping the site clean and tidy,
- using raw materials manufactured in appropriate hygienic conditions,
- appropriate work organisation,
- considering hygiene aspects in machine and device design,
- applying verified procedures for cleaning and disinfecting rooms and devices,
- ensuring personal hygiene of the staff,
- appropriate staff training.

2.3 Documentation of GMP

Each organisation should define the scope and application of GMP rules, considering those that follow from legal regulations and those that are not mandatory but may have an influence on ensuring product safety. The appropriate procedures and instructions to be followed should be set out. Documenting the GMP/GHP system involves the development of complete documentation – the GMP/GHP Code (Manual). The prepared documentation must take into account all activities performed in the plant to ensure good hygiene. The related documents describe what is done, as well as specifying in detail how a given operation should be performed, together with any reports, protocols, minutes and records that document the performance of such activities. Another issue is developing templates to record the performance of given activities. It is very important to emphasise the correct completion of the forms, to create accurate records. From experience in GMP operation and functioning, the greatest number of irregularities are found in this area (Kołożyn-Krajewska and Sikora, 2010).

One of the key areas in ensuring QA systems function properly in an enterprise is well-kept documentation. Each stage of the business activity, and each phase, has its own documentation. An effective QA system relies on all steps in the production process being fully documented.

The basic GMP documentation includes the following (GMP Guidebook, 2002):

- specifications (e.g. for the raw materials used in production, packaging materials and the final products),
- operational instructions related to the materials used in production,
- packaging instructions related to the packaging materials,
- reports on performed operations, examinations, tests, etc. Here we can list: batch tickets (batch production records), which comprise the production process together with packaging; reports on the follow-up checks on raw materials, packaging materials and final products; claim and return registers and reports following internal inspections,
- standard operational procedures for all activities that affect the quality of the manufactured pharmaceutical product which have not been included in previous documents.

There should be a specialist on site who will supervise the coherence and consistency of the documentation.

The essence of a properly functioning GMP system is the staff. Consequently, it is very important that senior management take care of their personnel through planned and systematic training. The better educated the team is, the better its performance, and the money invested in the training will pay dividends. Regular audits ensure compliance with implemented GMP rules. They are a planned way of obtaining information by the management and vice versa – involve a constant conscientiousness to obey implemented rules of GMP.

It is necessary to document that everything has been done in accordance with the specifications qualifications and validations and that the assumed goals have been achieved. Validation processes require the involvement of experienced employees with specialist training. Since each proof has to be supported with relevant measurements, a group of measurement technicians (lab assistants) have to be part of each validation team – these are calibration specialists who have access to a well-equipped metrological, analytical and microbiological laboratory. In summary, GMP includes in its scope the resources, processes and methods related to manufacturing. It is directed towards ensuring a proper flow of the technological process, resulting in a product of guaranteed quality.

The GMP Code (Manual) is the document forming the basis for all actions related to hygiene, and should contain a set of instructions regarding the hygiene maintenance of the premises, machines, staff, training plans and medical check-ups, as well as the templates (forms) confirming the execution of these instructions. This Manual

Table 2.1 Example of table of contents of a GMP Code valid for a plant

1. Table of contents	13. Leisure room
2. Used abbreviations and definitions	14. Employees and guests
3. Scope of application	15. Protection against pest
4. Legal basis	16. Cleaning, washing and disinfection
5. Documentation management	17. Waste management
6. Location and surroundings	18. Withdrawing a hazardous product
7. Buildings and premises	19. Identification and traceability
8. Raw materials, additions and materials	20. Measuring equipment
9. Machines, devices and equipment	21. Water and sewage
10. Technological process	22. Trainings
11. Storage	23. Documentation and records
12. Distribution and transport	

Source: Dzwolak, 2005.

should also contain, as related documents, a set of certificates, analytical methods and informative materials concerning the means of cleaning, disinfecting, and de-infesting other materials used in the plant to maintain hygiene (Table 2.1).

2.4 Benefits and drawbacks of GMP use in organisations

GMP in organisations brings both benefits and drawbacks. In this chapter these two characteristics are described.

2.4.1 Benefits

Proper implementation of GMP in companies provides many benefits, both as regards the manufacturing process and, in turn, refinement of the manufactured product. It also creates opportunities for organisational development by increasing its competitiveness. GMP makes it cheaper and safer, preventing quality irregularities rather than analysing their root causes afterwards.

GMP focuses on correcting errors. It requires an internal audit, which highlights what is defective in an enterprise and provides guidelines for future action. The GMP is therefore consistent with the main idea of the quality management system. It provides the employees with clearly defined responsibilities in a particular organisation and, as a result, people act according to certain procedures and instructions. It minimises the risk of errors and ensures greater safety during production, especially when using raw materials that are life threatening in higher concentrations. Other important benefits of implementing GMP are as follows (GMP Guidebook, 2002):

- protection of the recipients' interests by increasing product safety,
- protection of the entrepreneur's interests by possessing a documented production process or a documented service delivery process,

- reducing the risk of transmitting diseases,
- greater personnel involvement – identification with the company,
- qualified personnel – training,
- proper resource management,
- preventing lawsuits due to product liability,
- increasing trust among contractors, customers, suppliers and controlling entities,
- improving organisational culture.

2.4.2 Drawbacks

When considering the many benefits of GMP implementation, one should also mention its drawbacks. One of them is the lack of comparable models of manufacturing plant, equipment, technology or documentation. Many authors of GMP guidebooks and guidelines describe extensively what to do, what to have, and what to install during the system implementation, but they do not define in detail how to achieve them. How a given enterprise implements GMP is largely an individual issue, and depends on the vision and competence of the management and, of course, on available funds.

All GMP elements are interrelated, and an error in any one of them affects the whole system. Any action in any one element of the system causes a reaction elsewhere. For example, using raw materials bought from unqualified suppliers in a technological process becomes particularly visible in manufacture, where it is then necessary to change the process parameters to achieve the stipulated product specification. Even if the product quality is satisfactory, it is an accidental, not a planned result. Generally speaking, the GMP system is like a chain made up of many links, and one broken link destroys the whole chain. All the links are equally important.

Implementing the GMP system involves constant refinement, which in turn becomes a never-ending quest for perfection. What is good today will become obsolete tomorrow and, as such, will have to be changed. Changes are forced by competition. One can never say that a given enterprise has fully achieved GMP – one can only state that it conforms to a particular GMP criterion. Consequently, we speak of constant GMP implementation in an organisation.

2.4.3 Benefits and drawbacks of GMP implementation in practice

Implementation of GMP within EU countries is a legal requirement, ensuring an implementation level of almost 100% among companies producing dietary supplements. The implementation and functioning of GMP has practical benefits, as we will see in the example of the ABC Company. Observing a hygiene regime, controlling the manufacturing stage, only using qualified suppliers, and conducting analytical examinations of particular raw materials by qualified chemists using high-quality equipment are just some of the points that prove the indisputable quality of the company's products. Product stability is also tested during the products' shelf life. Improved organisation in the plant warehouses, stable storage conditions, with particular attention to products that have to be kept in special premises with defined temperature and humidity – all these contribute to a reduction in the number of returns and claims, and the implementation of GTP ensures the correct conditions of product loading and transport.

An effective GMP creates opportunities for company development, making the enterprise more competitive. Properly operating GMP, good laboratory practice (GLP) and GTP systems enable the company to secure more and more profitable contracts. The employees have clearly defined goals within a given organisational unit; they act in accordance with predefined procedures and instructions. Such conduct minimises the risk of errors in production and improves safety in the workplace Thanks to this fact, greater personnel involvement is achieved. The staff identify with the company and its benefits. Through regular training, the enterprise continuously raises the qualifications of its staff.

However, the implementation of GMP rules also entails certain problems. One of them is conducting the validation process. As regards the validation of analytical methods, there are no great concerns. However, it is different in relation to the production process or cleaning validation. Although the company has qualified personnel, the performance of some validation activities slows down or interrupts production, resulting in significant financial expense. In future, a separate validation department will have to be set up in the company to take care of the process validation as well as premises and equipment qualification. Another issue is observing all procedures related to the documentation. Not all employees fill in the documentation due to their own workload, and strict observance of rules regarding documentation in the GMP system generates a lot of work. Another obstacle is the physical arrangement of the premises within the plant. Due to limited space, the company may have problems adjusting the rooms to comply with the GMP guidelines related to the organisation of the premises. However, ABC is a developing company and it plans to expand.

The employees' attitude to the work may also be a problem in implementing the GMP system. On the one hand, there will be staff who are enthusiastic about the system, while on the other hand there will be people who are constantly treating the system as a "whim." Training is designed to avoid such situations, but still there will be still some employees who treat each change as something bad, and regard the QA Department as "the people who have nothing better to do, but come up with new ways of complicating people's life and work."

2.5 Summary

The present chapter has outlined the problem of GMP implementation in the food industry. The key issues of GMP implementation have been presented, including legal requirements, stages of implementation, and the role of the management board, as well as the scope of GMP. The next section presented the documentation and GMP manual, which was followed by a discussion on the benefits and drawbacks concerning the use of GMP in organisations.

GMP implementation is now mandatory in all food production companies, which involves expenditure on their part. The costs of implementing GMP in the production of dietary supplements are difficult to estimate, because they depend on the infrastructure, employee training and facility equipment, as well as on the size of the plant. The costs of implementation and maintenance of GMP may be divided into the following groups:

- preliminary audit costs,
- training costs,
- implementation costs,
- validation costs,
- plant adjustment costs,
- maintenance costs.

Quality Control does not guarantee the elimination of errors because it is impossible to examine all samples. Consequently, total manufacturing control from selecting qualified raw material suppliers, through a proper technological process and sampling in the subsequent stages, up to correct packaging and storage of the finished product, is becoming obligatory, ensuring that the product is of indisputable quality. Even a trace of contamination or wrongly packaged product may lead to tragedy. A properly implemented GMP system creates opportunities for company development, which in turn increases its prestige.

The consumer, the final beneficiary of a dietary supplement, is often unable to evaluate the quality of the product himself. However, errors that may occur during the production of such supplements lead to the creation of a defective product, which may become a threat to the consumer's health or life.

The main drawback of GMP may be its changeability due to the constant quest for perfection, implementing new technological, scientific and organisational solutions. One cannot produce safe food without implementing GMP rules in the manufacturing plant. Applying GMP rules in everyday manufacturing practice allows companies to:

- reduce the risk of food contamination,
- improve the quality of the final products,
- reduce the number of claims and production losses,
- organise corporate documentation,
- reduce the need to supervise the staff.

The implementation of GMP may be described by the following motto: *"GMP is an endless journey, but made with better and better means of transport"*.

References

Bockelmann von, B. (1995), "Total Quality Management" *Von Bockelmann Hygiene* (not published).
Dzwolak, W. (2005), "GMP/GHP in production of safe food" Olsztyn, BD Long (*in Polish*).

"GMP Guidebook" (2002), Warszawa, POLFARMED.
Kołożyn-Krajewska, D. and Sikora T. (2010), Food safety management. Theory and practice, Warszawa, C.H. Beck (*in Polish*).
Luning, P. A., Marcelis, W. J. and Jongen, W. M. F. (2002), *"Food Quality Management: A Techno-Managerial Approach"* Wageningen, Wageningen Academic Publishers.
Recommended International Code of Practice: General Principles of Food Hygiene, CAC/RCP 1-1969. Rev.3 (1997), amended 1999.
The Rules Governing Medical Products in the European Union (1997), *Good Manufacturing Practice*, Vol. 4.
Turlejska, H., Szponar, L. and Pelzner, U. (1998), "GMP in food production and processing enterprises" Warszawa, IŻŻ (*in Polish*).

Analysing the composition of fortified foods and supplements: the case of vitamins

S. Ötleş
Ege University, Izmir, Turkey

Note: This chapter is based on material from Chapter 8 "Vitamin analysis in fortified foods and supplements" by S. Ötleş, originally published in *Food fortification and supplementation*, ed. Peter Berry Ottaway, Woodhead Publishing Limited, 2008, ISBN: 978-1-84569-144-8.

3.1 Introduction

Standard and official analytical methods for detecting vitamins involve pre-treatment of the sample through complex chemical, physical or biological reactions to eliminate interferences commonly found, followed by individual methods for each different vitamin. These methods include spectrophotometric, polarographic, fluorometric, enzymatic and microbiological procedures. Besides colorimetric methods, there are numerous non-spectrophotometric methods, and their number and kind are increasing rapidly. These include titrimetry, voltammetry, fluorometry, potentiometry, radio-immunoassay (RIA), enzyme-linked immunosorbent assay (ELISA), kinetic-based chemiluminescence (CL), flow injection analyses and chromatography (Otles, 2005).

3.2 Extraction and purification methods

Extraction and purification of vitamins in foods, whether inherently present or added during food manufacture, is a challenging task owing to the sensitivity of these compounds to light, oxygen, heat and pH. As a result, some authors have recommended chemical methods alone. Other authors have opted to perform these procedures by means of an acid phosphatase or a takadiastase, sometimes combined with a b-glucosidase treatment. In some cases, the enzymatic treatments were preceded by mineral acid hydrolysis.

The first step in the analysis is extraction from the food sample, which is done with either strong acid or alkali or a solvent, combined with heat, in order to produce a fluid for testing. The next step is enzyme treatment, to release any of the water-soluble vitamins bound to the proteins and other components in the food matrix.

The conventional method for the isolation of fat-soluble vitamins from a simple food matrix includes solvent extraction, using such compounds as hexane, ethanol, methanol, tetrahydrofuran and petroleum ether. Complex food matrices are usually saponified prior to extraction, in order to disrupt the matrix and degrade triacylglycerols to glycerol. Soaps may be produced from the resulting free fatty acids.

Solid phase extraction (SPE) techniques have also been developed to replace many traditional liquid–liquid extraction methods for vitamins in aqueous samples. SPE is applied as an isolation method of the two sub-components of vitamins (water-soluble and fat-soluble), should both exist in the same sample. Modern supercritical fluid extraction (SFE) offers shorter extraction times, potentially higher selectivity and increased sample throughput (due to available automated instruments) compared to conventional solvent extraction techniques (Agostini *et al.*, 1997; Augustine *et al.*, 1985; Beney *et al.*, 1996).

3.3 High performance liquid chromatography (HPLC)

HPLC is a form of column chromatography used frequently in biochemistry and analytical chemistry. It is sometimes referred to as high pressure liquid chromatography. HPLC is a popular method of analysis because it is easy to use and not limited by the volatility or stability of the sample compound. More sophisticated methods, such as high pressure liquid chromatography which separates the fat- and/or water-soluble vitamins in a pre-treated food sample, followed by spectrophotometric or fluorometric methods, can also be used.

HPLC combined with a UV-Vis detector is the most common method for identification and quantification of fat- and water-soluble vitamins in foods. In the past, reversed-phase columns that were capable of tolerating high organic mobile phases, needed for the analysis of fat-soluble vitamins, could not tolerate the high aqueous conditions needed for retention of water-soluble vitamins. Conversely, reversed-phase columns that could tolerate high aqueous mobile phases lacked the hydrophobicity needed to adequately retain and separate fat-soluble vitamins. A highly versatile column capable of tolerating a wide range of mobile phase conditions is therefore required (Binkley *et al.*, 2008; Carter *et al.*, 2004; Hollis, 2004; Horst *et al.*, 1981; Jones, 1978; Terry *et al.*, 2005).

For vitamin analysis there is wide range of HPLC techniques, including reversed phase (RP-HPLC), normal phase (NP-HPLC), ion-exchange (IEC), paired ion (PIC) with different columns (C_{18}, NH_2) and detections (UV, fluorescence, coulochemical). Most of the published methods involve the use of complex buffered mobile phases. Several bonded and stationary phases and column packing materials have been developed, and a number of detection methods can be applied: UV–Vis absorbance with a single or variable wavelength or photodiode array, fluorometric and electrochemical. The HPLC method used to determine vitamins and their isomers has high sensitivity, good selectivity and the capability to simultaneously identify multiple components (Augustine *et al.*, 1981, 1984; Bognar, 1981).

3.4 Gas chromatography (GC)

GC procedures were developed for water- and fat-soluble vitamins before the development of HPLC. GC can be used to determine the homologues of certain vitamins together with their isomers. Trimethylsilyl (TMS), and other derivatives of vitamins, are suitable for flame ionisation detection (FID) on capillary columns. Application of GC to the determination of vitamin C has occurred on a limited scale, and a few papers have been published on its application to foods and supplements.

Utilisation of GC creates a high risk of thermal degradation of vitamins, even when derivatisation is done prior to GC separation. An example of this is GC-based vitamin K applications, which, due to high retention times and possible on-column degradation, are not very well suited for GC analysis. GC, however, results in some interesting features when used in conjunction with specific and sensitive detectors, such as gas chromatography-mass spectrometry (GC-MS), gas chromatography-electron capture detector (GC-ECD) and gas chromatography-selected ion monitoring (GC-SIM) (Bates, 2000; Kalcher and Vengust, 2007; Nakata and Tsuchida, 1980).

3.5 Capillary electrophoresis (CE)

CE is a fairly recent analytical technique that allows for the rapid and efficient separation of sample components based on differences in their electrophoretic characteristics as they migrate or move through narrow-bore capillary tubes. In spite of considerable developments, CE still suffers from problems of poor peak shape, lack of sensitivity and poor robustness. It has not yet been accepted in the food industry, owing to the absence of well-validated analytical procedures applicable to a broad range of food products.

In recent reports, a number of CE techniques, such as capillary zone electrophoresis (CZE), micellar electrokinetic chromatography (MEKC), microemulsion electrokinetic chromatography (MEEKC) and in-capillary enzyme reaction methods, have emerged as potential alternative techniques for determining and monitoring vitamins in samples. These reports relate to CE-based methods for vitamin forms in foods, biological samples and pharmaceuticals. To our knowledge, no extensive CZE methods are available for the simultaneous separation and quantification of vitamin esters in samples. Separation of L-ascorbic acid (L-AA) and D-isoascorbic acid (D-IAA) in a model system by CZE has, however, been described.

High performance capillary electrophoresis (HPCE) is a relatively new separation technique which has several advantages compared to RP-HPLC. These advantages include the possibility for higher efficiency, higher resolution and method simplification. Various techniques have also been developed for charged as well as uncharged analytes in free zone capillary electrophoresis (FZCE) and micellar electrokinetic capillary chromatography (MECC).

Vitamins have been characterised in different kinds of pharmaceutical formulations, such as tablets, injections, syrup and gelatine capsules, using MEKC or CZE methods. Over the last decade CZE with laser induced fluorescence (CE-LIF) detection has gained much in popularity. While high resolutions can be obtained in the separation of both ionogenic and neutral compounds, LIF detection is recognised to be an extremely sensitive detection method. More recently, the experimental conditions in CE with LIF detection have been optimised and successfully applied to the analysis of milk and wine samples. The widespread use of multi-vitamin preparations has stimulated research on accurate, efficient and easy methods for quality control. Use of CE for the purpose of simultaneous determination of fat- and water-soluble vitamins has been undertaken with CZE or MEKC. Methods based on CE have the capability of rapid, high-resolution separation of analytes from extremely low sample volumes, and are suitable for simultaneous determination (Altria *et al.*, 1998; Boonkerd *et al.*, 1994; Cataldi *et al.*, 2003).

3.6 Spectroscopic methods

At present, the most common methods used for the characterisation of diverse products are fluorometry, spectrophotometry and other spectroscopic methods (Fourier transform infrared-photoacoustic (FTIR-PAS) and FT-Raman spectroscopy).

Fluorometry is particularly useful in pharmaceutical analysis, and the lack of fluorescence of many compounds has led to the development of reagents which aid the formation of fluorescent derivatives. The most widely used method for thiamin determination is the so-called thiochrome method, which involves its oxidation in alkaline solution and extraction of the thiochrome formed from the aqueous phase into an organic phase, which is then measured fluorometrically. Riboflavin is usually assayed fluorometrically by measurement of its characteristic yellowish green fluorescence. Niacin is determined by first hydrolysing the samples with sulphuric acid to liberate nicotinic acid from combined forms. The pyridine ring of the nicotinic acid is opened with cyanogen bromide, and the fission product is coupled with sulphanilic acid to yield a yellow dye at 470 nm. For routine analysis of fat-soluble vitamins in different samples, the first procedure liberates the vitamins from the sample by saponification, but it is not needed when extracting vitamins from biological fluids. It is followed by extraction and evaporation and, for accurate quantitation, by fluorometry or spectrophotometry (Amin, 2001; Antonelli *et al.*, 2002; Barrales *et al.*, 1998).

3.7 Microbiological methods

Microbiological assay is applicable only to B vitamins. The rate of growth of a species of microorganism that requires a vitamin is measured in growth media that contain various known quantities of a foodstuff preparation with unknown amounts of the vitamin. Microbiological methods use test microorganisms, such as bacteria, protozoa or yeast, where growth is proportional to the presence of a specific vitamin. Turbidity measurement and such other parameters as gravimetry, acid production or gas production monitor the growth.

A related technique is the radiometric-microbiological assay based on the measurement of a 14C-labelled metabolite, normally $14CO_2$ formed by the test microorganism from a 14C-labelled substrate. Microbiological assays have the advantage of specificity and sensitivity, but they are highly time-consuming compared to the physicochemical methods and, in the former case, the analytical protocol must be strictly followed due to the variability in microbiological techniques. There are no microbiological methods for fat-soluble vitamins.

The first assays developed for the vitamin B group were animal assays, followed by microbiological methods. Vitamin B_6 (*Saccharomyces carlsbergensis* as the test organism), folic acid (*Lactobacillus casei*), vitamin B_{12} (*Lactobacillus leichmannii*), pantothenic acid (*Lactobacillus plantarum*) and biotin (*Allescheria boydii*) are usually assayed microbiologically. Novel microbiological assays for vitamins in test kit format have been marketed by different companies. These kits can be used in place of traditional microbiological determinations and have a much shorter application time.

The microtitre plates for these microbiological determinations are coated with specific microorganisms, which grow according to the presence/absence of vitamins in the sample. After placing the sample, standard and assay medium into the wells, the plates are incubated and subsequently evaluated using a microtitre plate reader. These test kits provide a fast and easy method for determining the content of vitamins in food products, feed and pharmaceutical products (Augustine *et al.*, 1985; Fennema, 1985; Machlin, 1984).

3.8 Immunoassays

Immunoassays are quick and accurate tests that can be used on-site to detect specific molecules. Immunoassays rely on the inherent ability of an antibody to bind to the specific structure of a molecule. Antibodies are proteins generated in response to the invasion of a foreign molecule (antigen). Antibodies are found in blood and tissue fluids and will bind to the antigen wherever it is encountered. Because immunoassays are developed to the specific 3D structure of an antigen, or analyte, they are highly specific and will bind only to that structure.

In addition to the binding of an antibody to its antigen, the other key feature of all immunoassays is a means to produce a measurable signal in response to the binding. Most, though not all, involve chemically linking antibodies to antigens with some kind of detectable label. A large number of labels exist in modern immunoassays, and they allow for detection through different means. They may either emit radiation, produce a colour change in a solution, fluoresce under light, or be induced to emit light. Common labels for immunoassays include:

- Immunoassays which employ enzymes are referred to as ELISAs, or sometimes enzyme immunoassays (EIA). Enzymes used in enzyme-linked immunosorbent assays (ELISAs) include horseradish peroxide (HRP), alkaline phosphate (AP) or glucose oxidase. These enzymes allow for detection often because they produce detectable colour change in the presence of certain reagents. In some cases these enzymes are exposed to reagents which cause them to produce light or chemiluminesce.
- Fluorogenic reporters such as phycoerythrin are used in a number of common immunoassays. Protein microarrays are a type of immunoassay that often employ fluorogenic reporters.
- DNA reporters are a newer approach to immunoassays and involve combining real-time quantitative polymerase chain reaction (RT qPCR) and traditional immunoassay techniques. Called real-time immunoquantitative polymerase chain reaction (PCR) (iqPCR), the label used in these assays is DNA.

Immunoassays can be used to detect such vitamins as vitamin D. Circulating 25-hydroxyvitamin D (25-OH-D) is widely recognised as the best indicator of vitamin D status. In blood circulation, the two major vitamin D metabolites are 25-hydroxyvitamin D_3 (25-OH-D_3) and 25-hydroxyvitamin D_2 (25-OH-D_2). In immunoassay techniques, a measure of total metabolite concentration and equivalent detection of both 25-OH-D_2 and 25-OH-D_3 can be challenging, as antigen binding shows a higher affinity for 25-OH-D_3 than 25-OH-D_2. Reports have shown inter-laboratory and inter-method variations in results for vitamin D determinations (Otles, 2005; Terry et al., 2005).

There is on-going debate as to which is the better method of 25-OH-D measurement for routine clinical laboratory and research use. It is clear that both immunoassays and LC-MS/MS have advantages and limitations. The strengths of the measurement of 25-OH-D by immunoassays are convenience, speed, turnaround and cost (Wagner et al., 2009; Wootton, 2005). Both immunoassays and LC-MS/MS are useful for measuring 25-OH-vitamin D, provided these methods are correctly standardised and, in particular, sample pre-treatment is carefully done (Koivula et al., 2013).

3.9 Other methods

The use of mass spectrometry (MS) is gaining ground, and can be combined with several other separation techniques, such as GLC, HPLC and CE. The coupled technique liquid chromatography/mass spectrometry (LC–MS) enables the separation of these non-volatile thermally labile substances for introduction into the mass spectrometer for reliable identification. Although the assay of vitamins is important in food analysis, due to their important biological activity in humans, few papers dealing with the LC–MS analysis of fat-soluble and water-soluble vitamins have been published recently. Nevertheless, the few studies on the LC–MS analysis of these natural compounds have revealed that this coupled technique has considerable potential in vitamin characterisation and determination.

Other methods include titrimetry, voltammetry, potentiometry, RIA, kinetic-based CL, flow injection analyses, competitive protein binding assays (CPBA) and radioreceptor assay (RRA) (Aboul-Kasim 2000; Arya and Jain, 2000; Careri et al., 2002).

3.10 Future trends

The literature contains numerous references to the determination of fat- and water-soluble vitamins in fortified foods and supplements using a wide variety of techniques. Many of these methods, however, suffer from lack of selectivity, are complicated and tedious procedures, and require the use of either expensive instrumentation or dangerous reagents. There is therefore a need for more economic and safe methodologies for the characterisation of vitamins in food products and supplements.

References

Aboul-Kasim, E. (2000), Anodic adsorptive voltammetric determination of the vitamin B_1 (thiamine), *J. Pharmaceut. Biomed. Anal.*, 22, 1047.
Agostini, T. and Godoy, H. (1997), Simultaneous determination of nicotinamide, nicotinic acid, riboflavin, thiamin, and pyridoxine in enriched Brazilian Foods by HPLC, *J. High Resol. Chromatogr.*, 20, 245.
Altria, K., Kelly, M. and Clark, B. (1998), Current applications in the analysis of pharmaceuticals by capillary electrophoresis, *Trends Anal. Chem.*, 17(4), 204.
Amin, A. (2001), Colorimetric determination of tocopheryl acetate (vitamin E) in pure form and in multi-vitamin capsules, *Eur. J. Pharmaceut. Biopharmaceut.*, 51, 267.
Antonelli, M., D'Ascenzo, G., Lagana, A. and Pusceddu, P. (2002), Food analyses: a new calorimetric method for ascorbic acid (vitamin C) determination, *Talanta*, 58(5), 961–967.
Arya, S. and Jain, P. (2000), Non-spectrophotometric methods for the determination of Vitamin C, *Anal. Chim. Acta*, 417, 1.
Augustin, J., Klein, B., Becker, D. and Venugopal, P. (1985), *Methods of Vitamin Assay*, John Wiley & Sons, New York, 1.
Augustine, J., Beck, C. and Marousek, G. (1981), Quantitative determination of ascorbic acid in potatoes and potato products by HPLC, *J. Food Sci.*, 46(1), 312.
Augustin, Y. (1984), Simultaneous determination of thiamine and riboflavin in foods by LC, *J. Assoc. Off. Anal. Chem.*, 67(5), 1012.
Barrales, O., Fernandez, D. and Diaz, M. (1998), A selective optosensor for UV spectrophotometric determination of thiamine in the presence of other vitamins B, *Anal. Chim. Acta*, 376, 227.
Bates, C.J. (2000), Vitamins: fat and water soluble: analysis, In R.A.Meyers, ed. *Encyclopedia of Analytical Chemistry*, John Wiley, & Sons Ltd, Chichester, 7390–7425.
Beney, P., Breuer, G., Jacobs, G., Larabee-Zierath, D., Mollenhauer, P., Norton, K. and Wichman, M. (1996), Review, evaluation and application of solid phase extraction methods, *Hotline*, 35(6), 1.
Binkley, N., Krueger, D., Gemar, D. and Drezner, M.K. (2008), Correlation among 25-hydroxyvitamin D assays, *J. Clin. Endocrinol. Metab.*, 93, 1804–1808.
Binkley, N., Krueger, D., Cowgill, C.S., Plum, L., Hansen, K.E., Deluca, H.F. and Dresner, M.K. (2004), Assay variation confounds the diagnosis of hypovitaminosis D: a call for standardization, *J. Clin. Endocrinol. Metab.*, 89, 3152–3157.
Bognar, A. (1981), Bestimmung von riboflavin und thiamin in lebensmitteln mit hilfe der HPLC, *Deutsche Lebensmittel-Rundschau*, 77(12), 431.

Boonkerd, S., Detaevernier, M. and Michotte, Y. (1994), Use of capillary electrophoresis for the determination of vitamins of the B group in pharmaceutical preparations, *J. Chromatogr. A*, 670, 209.

Careri, M., Bianchi, F. and Corradini, C. (2002), Recent advances in the application of mass spectrometry in food-related analysis, *J. Chromatogr. A*, 970, 3.

Carter, G.D., Carter, R., Jones, J. and Berry, J. (2004), How accurate are assays for 25-hydroxyvitamin D? Data from the international vitamin D external quality-assessment scheme, *Clin. Chem.*, 50, 2195–2197.

Cataldi, T., Nardiello, D., Carrara, V., Ciriello, R. and Benedetto, G. (2003), Assessment of riboflavin and flavin content in common food samples by capillary electrophoresis with laser-induced fluorescence detection, *Food Chem.*, 82(2), 309.

Fennema, O.R. (1985), *Food Chemistry*, 2nd Edition, Marcel Dekker, Inc., New York, 477.

Hollis, B.W. (2004), The determination of circulating 25-hydroxyvitamin D: no easy task, *J. Clin. Endocrinol. Metab.*, 89, 3149–3151.

Horst, R.L., Rheinhardt, T.A., Beitz, D.C. and Likedike, E.T. (1981), A sensitive competitive protein binding assay for vitamin D in plasma, *Steroids*, 37, 581–591.

Jones, G. (1978), Assays of vitamin D2 and D3, and 25-hydroxyvitamin D2 and D3 in human plasma by high-performance liquid chromatography, *Clin. Chem.*, 24, 287–298.

Kalcher, G.T. and Vengust, A. (2007), Stability of vitamins in premixes, *Anim. Feed Sci. Technol.*, 132(1–2), 148.

Koivula, M.K., Matinlassi, N., Laitinen, P. and Risteli, J. (2013), Four automated 25-OH total vitamin D immunoassays and commercial liquid chromatography tandem-mass spectrometry in Finnish population, *Clin Lab.*, 59(3–4), 397–405.

Machlin, L.J. (1984), *Handbook of Vitamins*, Marcel Dekker, Inc., New York, 1.

Nakata, H. and Tsuchida, E. (1980), Determination of vitamin K1 in photodegradation products by GLC, *Methods Enzymol.*, 67, 148.

Otles, S. (2005), *Methods of Analysis of Food Components and Additives*, Taylor & Francis, Boca Raton, 1.

Terry, A.H., Sandrock, T. and Meikle, A.W. (2005), Measurements of 25-hydroxyvitamin D by the Nichols ADVANTAGE, DiaSorin LIASION, DiaSorin RIA and liquid chromatography-tandem mass spectography, *Clin. Chem.*, 51, 1565–1566.

Wagner, D., Hanwell, H.E. and Vieth, R. (2009), An evaluation of automated methods for measurement of serum 25-hydroxyvitamin D, *Clin. Biochem.*, 42(15), 1549–1556.

Wootton, A.M. (2005), Improving the measurement of 25-hydroxyvitamin D, *Clin. Biochem. Rev.*, 26(1), 33–36.

Part Two

Drug–supplement interactions

Pharmacokinetic interactions between drugs and dietary supplements: herbal supplements

K. Berginc
Lek Pharmaceuticals d.d., Ljubljana, Slovenia

4.1 Introduction

Pharmacokinetics (PK) denotes the action of biological systems on drug absorption, distribution, metabolism and excretion (i.e. ADME – Figure 4.1), which directly relates to the amount of drug present in the blood stream or other body fluids (Henderson *et al.*, 2002). Interference from a concomitantly ingested xenobiotic (i.e. drug, food, dietary supplement (DS)) with a drug's ADME may bear clinical significance, when drug plasma concentrations reach either toxic or sub-therapeutic levels (Kuhn, 2002). The extent of PK interactions depends on intervening factors that may be either drug- (dose, dose regimen, route of administration, therapeutic range, time of intake), patient- (race, age, weight, gender, state of health, pathology, genetic polymorphism, lifestyle), or xenobiotic-dependent (the amount and duration of exposure) (Skalli *et al.*, 2007; Tomlinson *et al.*, 2008; Gurley *et al.*, 2008a). Patients subjected to complex treatment algorithms and polypharmacotherapy, elderly, pregnant and lactating women, cancer and HIV patients, people awaiting surgery, chronic patients, patients prescribed drugs with narrow therapeutic indices, and therapy non-responders are the most vulnerable population to abrupt alterations in drug PKs (Mallet *et al.*, 2007; Skalli *et al.*, 2007; Hermann and von Richter, 2012; (CDER), 2012; Bressler, 2005).

PK interactions are evaluated with *in vitro/in vivo* animal studies or in human trials. While *in vitro* research screens which DS may affect drug PKs, identifies PK targets susceptible to modulation by xenobiotics, and creates a platform for subsequent clinical studies, only the latter may provide a definitive means for determining whether statistically significant changes in drug plasma levels translate into clinically relevant outcomes (Butterweck *et al.*, 2004; Gurley *et al.*, 2008a). It is not uncommon for human trials to refute the *in vitro* or animal predictions, because the experimental designs in the these two models suffer from many drawbacks (Pal and Mitra, 2006; Venkataramanan *et al.*, 2006; Skalli *et al.*, 2007; Markowitz *et al.*, 2008; Gurley *et al.*, 2008b; Hermann and von Richter, 2012). Probe cocktails, a collection of relatively safe drug probes inactivated or eliminated primarily by a single metabolic process or transporter, and positive controls may be employed in

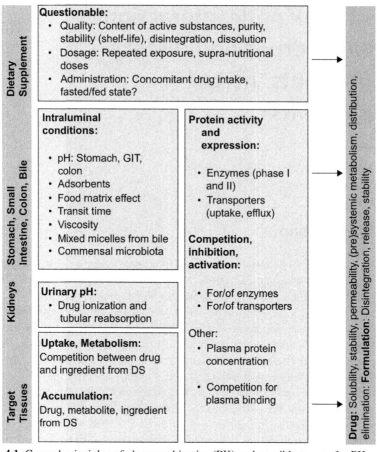

Figure 4.1 General principles of pharmacokinetics (PK) and possible targets for PK drug–dietary supplement interactions.

clinical trials to screen for possible changes in drug (pre-systemic) metabolism and excretion as a response to short-term or continued exposure to the DS (Tirona and Bailey, 2006). However, when considering DS–drug PK interactions, a number of other potential PK targets should also be explored, such as DS affecting *in vivo* drug/formulation performance by changing intraluminal conditions, which results in altered kinetics of drug release, drug stability, solubility, and/or permeability. Modification of drug distribution and tissue accumulation by DS may also be encountered.

Depending on the formulation, manufacturing process and physicochemical properties of allegedly active ingredients, the number of DSs available for consideration is prohibitive (MacDonald *et al.*, 2009). Although <1% of all drug–DS interactions is actually reported (Chavez *et al.*, 2006), dramatic case reports of possible interactions or exaggerated promotion of *in vitro* research may trump a well-controlled human trial with actual PK data showing no interaction and unnecessarily alarm the consumers, causing a lack of compliance with prescribed therapy, or diversion from methods and means of scientific medicine. Health-care providers should therefore stay alert and offer clear-cut and useful guidance bearing clinical relevance in the case of drug–DS PK interactions.

4.2 Herbals: introduction

Herbal supplements are highly concentrated, complex mixtures of potentially active compounds with inherent pharmacological and/or toxicological properties (Venkataramanan *et al.*, 2006). To avoid fluctuations in the content of the presumably active principles caused by growing, harvesting, and processing/manufacturing conditions, herbal supplements may be standardized; i.e. the quantity of marker compounds that occur naturally in the plant is standardized to ensure batch-to-batch consistency (Cupp, 1999). However, measurement and manipulation of marker compounds will not grant quality of the finished products, because many issues including adulteration, misidentification and contamination of the raw material continue to be a concern, while the production of a consistent product also entails routine evaluation of the finished product (impurities, solvent residues, dissolution/disintegration properties, labelling, storage and distribution conditions, stability testing, etc.) (Dog *et al.*, 2010; Block, 2012).

With the widespread use of herbal supplements, PK herb–drug interactions seem inevitable, and a considerable body of work has been published in this regard. Unfortunately, the scientific literature has also become a reservoir of poorly-designed *in vitro* studies applying exaggerated, non-physiological concentrations of DS in their tests that bear little or no resemblance to actual plasma levels of the corresponding species. The reliability of *in vitro* results can also be undermined by the presence of compounds that play no part in PK interactions *in vivo* owing to their limited systemic bioavailability (for instance, unabsorbable tannins precipitate proteins *in vitro*, fluorescent substances may interfere with the analytics).

Many papers also disregard the fact that species potentially responsible for PK interactions may not be phytochemicals accountable for pharmacological activity (i.e. standardized markers). A well-executed *in vitro* study should thus acknowledge PK limitations of plant polyphenols, believed to be the carriers of health-beneficial effects and culprits of PK interactions (Figure 4.2), and strive to comply with the proposed guidelines for *in vitro* settings. Because the main players involved in PK interaction are not only phytochemicals but also their metabolites, further scientific scrutiny should be endorsed (Butterweck *et al.*, 2004; Zhang *et al.*, 2009).

It has been estimated that >150 herbs may be involved in drug interactions, while only 34 drugs were identified as the most likely candidates whose PKs could be affected by herbal DSs. The majority of the identified drugs includes CYP3A4, CYP2C9 (82.4%), Pgp (29.4%) or dual CYP3A4 and Pgp substrates (23.5%), drugs

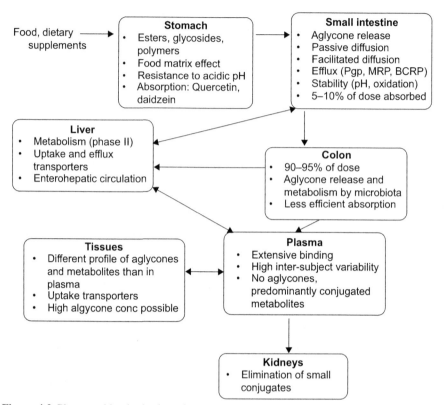

Figure 4.2 Pharmacokinetic destiny of polyphenols in humans.

intended for long-term use or substances with narrow therapeutic indices (Zhou et al., 2007; Sood et al., 2008).

Limited by the lack of data pertaining to the quality, identity and PK destiny of herbal products (i.e. phytoequivalence) and a wide variety of available brands, not even clinical trials may definitely answer whether a hidden risk of drug interactions exist in the case of herbal DSs (Pal and Mitra, 2006; Venkataramanan et al., 2006; Skalli et al., 2007; MacDonald et al., 2009).

Herbs containing mucilage polysaccharides (i.e. aloe, rhubarb, butternut, Iceland moss, European buckthorn, cascara, flax seeds, fenugreek, plantain, psyllium seed, etc.) are theoretically apt to bind simultaneously consumed drugs. Some may act as stool-softening and laxative agents, decreasing drug residence time at the absorption site. Salicylate rich botanicals (meadowsweet, black willow) may temporarily displace highly protein-bound drugs such as warfarin and sulfasalazine from plasma proteins, potentiating their pharmacological activities (Kuhn, 2002; Abebe, 2003; Bressler, 2005; Nutescu et al., 2006; van den Bout-van den Beukel et al., 2006; Zadoyan and Fuhr, 2012).

Clinical trials addressing PK drug–herb interactions for top-selling botanic products over the last decade are summarized in Table 4.1. Where none have been performed, *in vitro* data have been reviewed.

4.3 *Hypericum perforatum* (St John's Wort (SJW))

Besides quercetin, biapigenin, and hypericin, hyperforin is the main substance believed to affect drug PKs (Zhou et al., 2003; Pal and Mitra, 2006). Depending on the dosage and duration of use, no changes (i.e. midazolam) or increased exposure to prescribed drugs due to the inhibition of intestinal Pgp/CYP3A4 (i.e. voriconazole, fexofenadine) were observed in trials lasting up to 3 days (Izzo, 2005; Izzo and Ernst, 2009). Long-term SJW administration of more than 10 days causes a significant induction of hepatic CYPs (2C19, 2C8, 2E1), and CYP3A4 and Pgp in the liver and gut. No effect on CYP2D6, UGT1A1, and UGT1A9 expression or activity have been reported, while data on CYP1A2, CYP2C9 are controversial (Sparreboom et al., 2004; Tirona and Bailey, 2006; Venkataramanan et al., 2006; Nowack, 2008; Gurley et al., 2008a; Borrelli and Izzo, 2009; Rowe and Baker, 2009). More pronounced effects are expected with products richer in hyperforin (>10 mg/day) (Gurley et al., 2008a). After induction, CYP3A activity returns to basal levels progressively in approximately 1 week after cessation of SJW (Izzo and Ernst, 2009). Human trials evaluating 4–10-day exposure are lacking (Borrelli and Izzo, 2009).

Concomitant intake with drugs exerting extensive (pre)-systemic metabolism and/or narrow therapeutic indices is ill-advised. HIV patients on protease inhibitors (PI) or non-nucleoside reverse transcriptase inhibitors (NNRTI) should avoid SJW products (van den Bout-van den Beukel et al., 2006). For some drugs, monitoring and dose adjustments are necessary. Therapeutic manifestations triggered by SJW–drug PK interactions and possible therapeutic failure remains undetermined for alprazolam, chlorzoxazone, erythromycin, gliclazide, midazolam, nevirapine, simvastatin, tacrolimus, and verapamil. Paclitaxel, sirolimus, etoposide, doxorubicin and cyclophosphamide are also suspected to interact with SJW.

4.4 *Allium sativum* (garlic)

Clinical trials have failed to corroborate *in vitro/in vivo* animal PK predictions reporting significant modulation of PK targets by garlic products or organosulphur compounds (Zou et al., 2002; Izzo, 2005; Hu et al., 2005). Although a modest CYP2E1 inhibition was observed (Hermann and von Richter, 2012; Zadoyan and Fuhr, 2012), no notable or clinically relevant metabolism-based interactions are expected for CYP2E1 substrates, because except for chlorzoxazone, systemic clearance for other drugs does not rely solely on this isoform. Human trials seem to nullify any significant influence of garlic on drug PKs, but several PK targets (i.e. CYP2B1, 2B2, UGTs, GSTs, and transporters) have been identified to respond to garlic interventions *in vitro* and have not yet been explored *in vivo* (Hermann and von Richter, 2012).

Therefore, while the induction potential of garlic products seems clinically irrelevant, health-care providers should advise vigilance to patients on antiretrovirals and CYP2E1 substrates, because *in vitro* studies have highlighted important changes in the composition of different garlic DSs, which may explain perplexity pertaining to the potential for PK interactions (Borrelli et al., 2007).

Table 4.1 Human trials addressing pharmacokinetic herb–drug interactions for best-selling herbal DSs

Drug/probe	SJW	AS	GB	PG	PM	SR	EP
Alprazolam	IND³ᴬ⁴, ᴾᵍᵖ	N	N		? INH³ᴬ⁴	N	
Aminopyrine							
Amitryptiline	IND³ᴬ⁴ ⁽ᴳ⁺ᴸ⁾, 2C19, Pgp						
Amoxicillin							
Anticonvulsants	#IND³ᴬ⁴⁽ᴳ⁺ᴸ⁾						
Antipyrine			N				
Antiretrovirals	#$IND³ᴬ⁴, INH³ᴬ⁴, ᴾᵍᵖ	?	IND³ᴬ⁴				
Atorvastatin	*#IND³ᴬ⁴, ᴾᵍᵖ						
Bupropion			N				
Buspiron							
Caffeine	N	N	N	N	N	N	INH¹ᴬ²
Carbamazepine	N						
Cefaclor							
Chlorzoxazone	IND²ᴱ¹	IND²ᴱ¹	N	N	N, INH²ᴱ¹	N	N
Clopidogrel	IND³ᴬ⁴						
Cortisol	IND³ᴬ⁴		N	N			
Coumarin							
Cyclophosphamide	?						
Cyclosporin A	*#IND³ᴬ⁴, ᴾᵍᵖ, INHᴾᵍᵖ	N					
Dapsone			INDᴺ⁻ᴬᶜ⁻ᵀ				
Darunavir							IND³ᴬ⁴⁽ᴸ⁾
Debrisoquine	N	N	N	N	N	N	N
Desogestrel	INH²ᶜ⁹/²ᶜ¹⁹ and/or IND³ᴬ⁴						
Dextromethorphan	N	N	N			N	N
Diazepam			ᵅN				
Diclofenac			N				
Diltiazem			INH³ᴬ⁴				
Digoxin	$INDᴾᵍᵖ⁽ᴳ⁺ᴸ⁾		ᵅN		INH³ᴬ⁴⁽ᴳ⁾	N	N
Docetaxel		N	N				
Donepezil							
Doxorubicin							
Erythromycin	IND³ᴬ⁴						
Ethinylestradiol	IND³ᴬ⁴						
Etoposide							
Fexofenadine	*INDᴾᵍᵖ		N				
Flurbiprofen			N				

WM	SM	HC	VO	CR	GM	CS	VV	CL
			N, INH^{3A4}			N		
	N							
N								
						N	INH^{3A4}	
	N	N	N	N	INH^{1A2}, IND^{2A6}	N	IND^{1A2}	INH^{1A2}, IND^{2A6}
N								
	N	N	N	N				
	N				N			
N	N	INH^{3A4}					?	
	N	N, INH^{2D6}	N	N				
		INH^{2D6}	N			N	INH^{2D6}	
N								
	N	INH$^{Pgp(G)}$		N				
	N							
N								

Continued

Table 4.1 Continued

Drug/probe	SJW	AS	GB	PG	PM	SR	EP
Gliclazide	α?2C9						
Imatinib	*#IND$^{3A4, Pgp}$						
Indinavir	#IND$^{3A4, Pgp}$						
Irinotecan	#IND$^{3A4, Pgp(?)}$						
Iron							
Ivabradine	IND$^{3A4(G+L)}$						
Ketodesogestrel	IND^{3A4}						
Levothyroxine							
Lidocaine	IND^{3A4}						
Lopinavir	?		N				N
Losartan							
Mephenytoin	IND$^{2C19(wild\ type)}$		N				
Methadone	IND$^{3A4, Pgp}$						
Metronidazole							
Midazolam	IND$^{3A4(G+(L?))}$, Pgp	N	αN, INH^{3A4}	N	N	N	INH$^{3AG(G)}$, IND$^{3A4(L)}$
Mycophenolic acid	N						
Nelfinavir	IND^{3A4}						
Nevirapine	IND$^{3A4, 2B6(?)}$, Pgp						
Nifedipine	IND^{3A4}		αN	INH$^{3A4(G)}$			
Norethindrone	IND^{3A4}						
Nortriptyline	IND$^{2D6(?)}$						
Omeprazole	IND$^{3A4, 2C19}$		αIND(?)$^{2C19, 3A4}$				
Oral contraceptives	#IND$^{3A4(G+L)}$						
Oxycodon	INH^{3A4}						
Paracetamol		N					
Paclitaxel							
Phenprocoumon	IND$^{3A4>2C9}$						
Phenylbutazone							
Phenytoin			N				
Pravastatin	N						
Prednisone	N						
Quazepam	IND$^{3A4, 2C19, Pgp}$						
Ranitidine							
Ritonavir	IND$^{3A4, Pgp}$	?	?				N
Rosiglitazone	IND^{2C8}						
Rosuvastatin							
Saquinavir	?	?					
Simvastatin	IND$^{3A4, Pgp}$						
Sirolimus							
Statins	α#IND$^{3A4(G+L)}$, Pgp, INH^{Pgp}						
Tacrolimus	*IND$^{3A4, Pgp}$						
Talinolol	IND^{Pgp}						

WM	SM	HC	VO	CR	GM	CS	VV	CL
	N							
	N	N						
					INH^{Abs}			
					INH^{Abs}			
	N	INH^{2C9}			N	N	IND^{2C9}	
	N							
	IND$^{3A4,Pgp(G)}$							
N	N	N, INH^{3A4}	N	N			N	
	N							
		N						
	N							
	N							
	N							
	N							

Continued

Table 4.1 **Continued**

Drug/probe	SJW	AS	GB	PG	PM	SR	EP
Theophylline	#N, IND$^{3A4(G+L), 2E1}$						
Tibolone	?						
Ticlopidin			N				
Tizanidine							
Tolbutamide	N		N, INH^{2C9}				N
Trazodone			?IND^{3A4}				
Verapamil	*#IND$^{3A4(G+L)}$, Pgp						
Vinblastine	?						
Voriconazole	IND$^{2C19, 3A4, Pgp}$		N				
Warfarin	#IND$^{3A4(G+L), 2C19, 1A2(?)}$	N	N		#αIND$^{2C9(?)}$		N

IND – induction; INH – inhibition; N – no effect; G – gut; L – liver; 1A2 – CYP1A2; 2C9 – CYP2C9; 2C19 – CYP2C19; 2E1 – CYP2E1; 3A4 – CYP3A4; 2D6 – CYP2D6; Pgp – P-glycoprotein; OATP – Organic Anion Transporting Protein; Abs – absorption;? – unknown/speculated; N-Ac-T – N-acetyl transferase; > – the predominant/main interaction mechanism; * – adjust dose; # – avoid combination; $ – combination is contraindicated; α – close monitoring advised.
SJW – *Hypericum perforatum;* AS – *Allium sativum;* GB – *Ginkgo biloba;* PG – *Panax ginseng;* PN – *Piper methysticum;* SR – *Serenoa repens;* EP – *Echinacea purpurea;* VM – *Vaccinium macrocarpon;* HC – *Hydrastis canadensis;* VO – *Valeriana officinalis;* CR – *Cimicifuga racemosa;* GM – *Glycine max;* CS – *Camelia sinensis;* VV – *Vitis vinifera;* CL – *Curcuma longa.*

4.5 *Ginkgo biloba* (ginkgo)

In vitro studies identified ginkgolic acid I and II as potent CYP inhibitors. Other ginkgo constituents with even higher systemic bioavailability than ginkgolic acid (F_{abs} > 70%), showed moderate effects on CYPs bearing no *in vivo* relevance (Zou et al., 2002; Zhang et al., 2010). Although ginkgo–drug interactions seem unlikely at recommended doses (no effect on CYPs, OATPs, OCTs, OCTNs, MATEs), co-administration with CYP2C19 substrates should be avoided by poor CYP2C19 metabolizers (Izzo and Ernst, 2009; Zuo et al., 2010).

Owing to significant changes in gene expression observed in mice for phase I (CYP), II (glutathione-S-transferase, sulfotransferase), and III (solute carrier proteins, ATP-binding cassette proteins) proteins after 2-year exposure to ginkgo (Markowitz et al., 2003; Guo et al., 2010; Kim et al., 2010) accompanied by a lack of agreement regarding ginkgo impact on CYP3A4, 2C9 and 2C19 (Yoshioka et al., 2004), this herb may interfere with PKs of anticancer drugs, anticonvulsants, and UGT and CYP2C19 substrates (Sparreboom et al., 2004; Izzo and Ernst, 2009; Hermann and von Richter, 2012). Exercising self-administration of ginkgo products should thus be discouraged in elderly or in patients using prescribed drugs with narrow therapeutic indices (Uchida et al., 2006).

WM	SM	HC	VO	CR	GM	CS	VV	CL
					INH^{1A2}	INH^{1A2}		
N								
#INH$^{2C9(?)}$					?INH^{Pgp,} OATP (?)			

4.6 *Panax ginseng* (ginseng), *Piper methysticum* (kava kava) and *Serenoa repens* (saw palmetto)

Although no significant impact on CYP expression/activity was observed, a brand-specific impact on CYP3A4 substrates may be anticipated as demonstrated for digoxin and nifedipine (Sparreboom et al., 2004; Zadoyan and Fuhr, 2012). Slight inhibition of CYP2D6 was observed in elderly (Izzo and Ernst, 2009), while studies with warfarin are inconclusive. Siberian ginseng (*Eleutherococcus senticosus*) has no impact on CYP3A4, and 2D6, while American ginseng (*Panax quinquefolius*) does not influence UGT2B7. Siberian ginseng should be avoided during antiretroviral therapy, while its effect on warfarin is inconclusive (Zadoyan and Fuhr, 2012).

In the case of *Piper methysticum* (kava kava), clinical recommendations regarding the PK interaction of kava administration with drugs are mainly based on theoretical considerations. Patients taking anticancer, hepatotoxic drugs, and CYP2E1 and 3A4 substrates should be routinely monitored (Anke and Ramzan, 2004; Sparreboom et al., 2004; Gurley et al., 2005; Zadoyan and Fuhr, 2012). Case reports regarding kava-associated hepatotoxicity resulted in product withdrawal from the US and EU market in 2002 (Sarris et al., 2009; Rowe et al., 2011). Later publications revealed that patients with CYP2D6 polymorphism (poor metabolizers) are at higher risk of adverse reactions due to insufficient kavalactone metabolism (i.e. detoxification), while for most kava consumers, kava products do not raise safety issues (Rowe et al., 2011).

Saw palmetto extract at generally recommended doses poses minimal risk for drug disposition dependent on CYP3A4 and 2D6 pathways. Unfortunately, other potential targets for PK interactions (enzymes/transporters) have not been evaluated; therefore these findings cannot be extended to other supplements or drugs (Gordon and

Shaughnessy, 2003; Gurley et al., 2004; Chavez et al., 2006; van den Bout-van den Beukel et al., 2006; Nowack, 2008; Izzo and Ernst, 2009; Zadoyan and Fuhr, 2012).

4.7 Echinacea purpurea (purple coneflower), Vaccinium macrocarpon (cranberry) and Silybum marianum (milk thistle)

The probability of *Echinacea* triggering worrisome metabolism-/transporter-based interactions involving CYP1A2, 2C9, 2D6, 2E1 and Pgp in the general population is small (Gurley et al., 2004; Izzo and Ernst, 2009; Hermann and von Richter, 2012). However, seemingly minor changes in the activity of CYP1A2 and 3A4 merit further studies; therefore concomitant use with the corresponding substrates should be discouraged. *Echinacea* selectively inhibits intestinal and induces hepatic CYP3A4, thus creating two counteracting mechanisms in terms of net effect on systemic drug bioavailability (Gurley et al., 2008a; Nowack, 2008), which ultimately may lead to clinically relevant decrease in exposure to poorly bioavailable CYP3A4 substrates. In the case of antiretrovirals, low capacity of altering ritonavir-boosted PI PKs has been demonstrated (Hermann and von Richter, 2012). Case-by-case recommendations are needed for cancer and asthma patients.

In the case of cranberry (*Vaccinium macrocarpon*), based on little available data, no significant interactions may be expected with CYP3A4, 1A2, 2C9 and PepT1, PepT2 substrates with daily consumption not exceeding one glass of cranberry juice (Sparreboom et al., 2004; Li et al., 2009; Zadoyan and Fuhr, 2012). In general, rapid absorption and urinary elimination result in tissue bioavailability and low plasma levels of anthocyanins (bioavailability is <1% of dose; plasma levels 0.56–4.64 nM). However, plasma anthocyanin levels may not correctly reflect anthocyanin activity, because tissue accumulation and thus gene expression changes are possible during prolonged consumption (Milbury et al., 2010). Caution should be advised for patients on antiretrovirals, warfarin and other CYP3A4 and 2C9 substrates, because anthocyanins are potent *in vitro* inhibitors of both isoenzymes (Nutescu et al., 2006; van den Bout-van den Beukel et al., 2006; Greenblatt et al., 2006; Uesawa and Mohri, 2006; Gohil and Patel, 2007; Nowack, 2008). Salicylates in cranberry juice may displace warfarin from plasma proteins (Duthie et al., 2005).

In the case of milk thistle (*Silybum marianum*), no clinically relevant interactions through CYPs, UGT1A1, breast cancer resistance protein (BCRP) or OATP1B1 are expected even at supra-therapeutical doses because plasma levels of free and conjugated silymarin species (reported range 0.024–1.3 µg/mL) are significantly below IC_{50} (25–250 µM) values owing to insufficient solubility and dissolution kinetics of milk thistle DS, and high inter-subject variability (Gurley et al., 2004; Venkataramanan et al., 2006; Mohamed and Frye, 2011; Hermann and von Richter, 2012; Zadoyan and Fuhr, 2012). Although there are indications of decreased systemic exposure to CYP3A4 and Pgp substrates (i.e. indinavir), clinical trials do not support the premises of altered CYP3A4/Pgp expression/activity (Hermann and von Richter, 2012). As a precaution, concomitant medication with CYP3A4/Pgp substrates exerting low systemic bioavailability and milk thistle DS should be avoided (Gurley et al., 2006b; Zadoyan and Fuhr, 2012). An increased intra-luminal concentration of milk thistle flavolignans (40–1200 μg/mL predicted) reaching IC_{50} values may be expected during the use milk thistle DS formulated with dissolution enhancer phosphatidylcholine, which, combined with extensive enterohepatic circulation of these phytochemicals, raises the probability of intraluminal PK interactions (Gurley et al., 2004; De Smet, 2007; Mohamed and Frye, 2011).

4.8 Hydrastis canadensis (goldenseal), Valeriana officinalis (valerian) and Cimicifuga racemosa (black cohosh)

Goldenseal extract is a mild to moderate CYP3A4, 3A5, 2D6 and Pgp inhibitor; therefore patients should refrain from its concomitant use with prescription medications with narrow therapeutic indices, or drugs which rely extensively on these isoenzymes for systemic clearance (Fuchikami et al., 2006; Zadoyan and Fuhr, 2012; Hermann and von Richter, 2012). Mixed results may be found regarding clinical relevance of goldenseal-CYP3A4 substrates interactions; no effect on indinavir PKs has been reported, while cyclosporine A plasma levels increased (Gurley et al., 2005; Nowack, 2008). No trials were found regarding goldenseal impact on CYP2C9 and 2C19.

Pharmacologically active valepotriates, valerenic acid and alkaloids do not affect CYP activities or expression in humans even after multiple dosing (Sparreboom et al., 2004; Nowack, 2008), most probably due to lower quantities of these active principles resulting from high variability in DS composition and high instability of marker phytochemicals (Heiligenstein and Guenther, 1998). Additionally, valerenic acid attains significantly lower plasma levels (0.9–2.3 ng/mL) than necessary for modulation of CYPs (IC_{50} 5–10 μM) (Anderson et al., 2005). Interactions in intestinal lining were suggested, because a 500–1000 mg of valerian extract could yield sufficiently high intraluminal concentration to inhibit UGTs (Mohamed and Frye, 2011).

Pharmacologically active phyto-constituents in black cohosh have not yet been identified (Sparreboom et al., 2004). While in vivo evidence seems to render black cohosh an unlikely source of clinically relevant interactions through CYP1A2, 2D6, 3A4, 2E1 or Pgp, concomitant administration with atorvastatin is not recommended due to suspected CYP3A4 inhibition (Gurley et al., 2006a; Dog et al., 2010; Zadoyan and Fuhr, 2012).

4.9 Glycine max (soy), Camellia sinensis (green tea) and Zingiber officinale (ginger)

Isoflavonoids (daidzein, genistein, glycitein) inhibit CYP1A2, 2E1, GLUT1,4 and induce CYP1A2, 1A1, and 2A6. Their pro-catabolic effect on sex hormones was mediated through CYP1A1 and 1A2 induction (Nakajima et al., 2006, Wood et al., 2007). Soy isoflavonoids exert rapid absorption, BCRP-limited distribution to brain, testes, and foetus, and rapid elimination (Roberts et al., 2004; Enokizono et al., 2007; Burnett et al., 2011). More than 95% of plasma isoflavonoids is glucuronated and exhibits extensive enterohepatic circulation (Burnett et al., 2011). Daidzein, genistein and glycetin plasma levels (5 μM) are in the range of determined K_i or IC_{50} values, thus CYP2A6*1 (0.7–6 μM) or UGT2B17 (4.6 μg/mL) inhibition is possible (Nakajima et al., 2006; Mohamed and Frye, 2011). The safety of soy consumption has been questioned during concomitant medication with CYP1A2, and 3A4 substrates (PIs, NNRTIs) and in infants with congenital hypothyroidism, where decreased levothyroxine absorption was noticed (Conrad et al., 2004; Zadoyan and Fuhr, 2012).

In the case of green tea (camellia sinensis), repeated catechin ingestion is unlikely to result in modified drug disposition by CYPs (van den Bout-van den Beukel et al., 2006, Nowack, 2008; Zadoyan and Fuhr, 2012), while a decreased drug and calcium absorption may occur (Kuhn, 2002; Abebe, 2003). Data from in vitro and in vivo rodent studies indicate inhibition of intestinal UGT1A1, which could affect raloxifene and ezetimibe PKs (Mohamed and Frye, 2011). Gallated polyphenols were also shown to inhibit OATP1B1, 1B3 and 2B1 with IC_{50} values (7–10 μM) attainable in vivo with 1600 mg dose of epigallocatechingallate. Interactions outside the gut are unlikely due to extensive intestinal phase I, II, and III metabolism of green tea phytochemicals (metabolism is saturable at doses higher than 1600 mg) (Cai et al., 2002; Roth et al., 2011). Inhibition of MCT, SGLT1 and Pgp by tea polyphenols has also been communicated in the literature (Konishi et al., 2003) but no clinically relevant interactions have been reported.

Caution is advised when ginger is taken concomitantly with anticoagulants, whose metabolism depends on CYP3A4 and 2C9 (Zuo et al., 2010). No interactions with drugs are known (Akram et al., 2011), probably because only pharmacologically inert conjugates of ginger constituents have been detected in plasma (0.01–1.2 μg/mL range) (Yu et al., 2011). 6-gingerol is the only phytochemical exerting measurable absorption that could trigger PK interactions (Zick et al., 2008). In vivo animal research reported significantly decreased cyclosporine A and increased metronidazole bioavailability due to CYP-mediated interaction (Okonta et al., 2008).

4.10 Morinda citrifolia (noni), Aloe vera (aloe), Vitis vinifera (grape seed) and Curcuma longa (turmeric)

Rapid absorption, rapid elimination and uricosuric effect of scopoletin (purportedly active phytochemical in noni) were noticed in animal studies (Wang et al., 2002). Noni juice affected gastric transit time, interacted with Cyp3A in disease- and age-specific manner, increased GST activity after single dose and inhibited UGTs during chronic administration with no Pgp effect in rodent studies (Engdal and Nilsen, 2008; Mohamed and Frye, 2011). No interactions with drugs have been published. A complete list of ingredients may be found in (Pawlus and Kinghorn, 2007).

In the case of aloe vera, significantly increased vitamin C and E absorption were observed during concomitant ingestion, making aloe DS a potential adjunct for people taking vitamin supplements. Since glucuronidation of anthaquinones from aloe presents the main elimination pathway, interactions with extensively glucuronated drugs zidovudine and lamotrigine should be explored.

In the case of grape seed (*Vitis vinifera*), CYP2C9 and 2D6 inhibition, CYP1A2 induction and mixed reports about CYP3A4 effect may be found in the literature, suggesting caution for cancer patients on high-dose grape seed extracts (Sparreboom *et al.*, 2004). Resveratrol and ε-viniferin are potent CYPs, Pgp, OATP-B, and xanthine oxidase inhibitors *in vitro* (Piver *et al.*, 2003, Nabekura *et al.*, 2005; Etheridge *et al.*, 2007; Zadoyan and Fuhr, 2012). Plasma (ng/mL levels) and tissue accumulation of resveratrol and its conjugates may be expected after multiple daily administrations (Chow *et al.*, 2010).

Instability, rapid absorption and extensive pre-systemic metabolism hinder curcumin systemic bioavailability (plasma levels are in nM range), which may at least partially be overcome by formulating curcumin with dissolution/permeation enhancers (i.e. piperine) (Oetari *et al.*, 1996; Thapliyal *et al.*, 2002; Sharma *et al.*, 2005). *In vitro* curcumin potential to modify several CYPs, UGTs, GSTs has been established (Firozi *et al.*, 1996; Nowack, 2008; Nayak and Sashidhar, 2010). Based on IC_{50} values, interactions in the intestine seem possible (CYP2C9; IC_{50} 4.3 μM). Saturation of human pre-systemic metabolism may be achieved at supra-doses of 8–12 g/day, which could lead to erratic blood levels of CYP substrates *in vivo* (Sharma *et al.*, 2005).

4.11 *Stevia rebaudiana* (stevia), *Lepidium meyenii* (maca) and *Garcinia mangostana* (mangosteen)

Stevia is a high-potency bio-sweetener (Das *et al.*, 2005). Competition between aglycone steviol released by commensal microbiota in colon and drugs for transporters in intestine is questionable. Steviol showed significant accumulation in rodent liver, kidney and intestine. In humans, steviol and its glucuronides plasma levels are low; 121 ng/mL and 1.89 μg/mL, respectively. Urinary elimination is the predominant excretion pathway, and it includes active tubular secretion with OATs, OCTs or OATP4C1 as possible candidates. Since the accepted daily intake of 5 mg/kg does not assure plasma levels close to IC_{50}, steviol should not influence renal drug elimination (Srimaroeng *et al.*, 2005; Chatsudthipong and Muanprasat, 2009).

Ingestion of cooked maca (lepidium meyenii) significantly increased total plasma proteins and albumins, changing progesterone and testosterone plasma levels in mice, which was not corroborated in postmenopausal women (Brooks *et al.*, 2008; Coates, 2010). No drug interactions have been reported.

Although pure mangosteen juice contains c.5 mM xanthones, maximal plasma levels after 60 mL of juice ingestion were highly variable and only 0.1 μM for α-mangostin (levels of other species were even lower). Fed conditions aided absorption through lymph (F_{abs} = 2% of dose). Prolonged exposure to α-mangostin significantly increased its tumour concentrations in mice, while *in vitro* studies indicated CYP2C9 inhibition (Hidaka *et al.*, 2008; Chitchumroonchokchai *et al.*, 2013). No interactions with drugs have been reported.

4.12 Summary

Key points to note are:

- Numerous brands of herbal supplements available in different dosage forms exist. Human trials have indicated that a clinically significant interaction may occur during concomitant use with drugs depending on drug-, patient-, and herb-associated factors. Compared to the number of potential PK targets and available quantity of herbal DS (c.150) the number of identified and clinically relevant interactions is low (<10).
- Because the complete composition is usually unknown, no clinical study can prove phytoequivalence. Thus, results from one study may not be generalized for all DSs of the same herb.

References

(CDER), U. S. D. O. H. A. H. S. F. A. D. A. C. F. D. E. A. R. (2012). Guidance for industry: drug interaction studies – study design, data analysis, implications for dosing, and labeling recommendations.

Abebe, W. (2003). An overview of herbal supplement utilization with particular emphasis on possible interactions with dental drugs and oral manifestations. *J Dent Hyg*, 77, 37–46.

Akram, M., Shah, M. I., Usmanghan, K., Mohiuddin, E., Sami, A., Asif, M., Shah, S. A., Ahmed, K. and Shaheen, G. (2011). Zingiber officinale roscoe (A medicinal plant). *Pak. J. Nutr*, 10, 399–400.

Anderson, G. D., Elmer, G. W., Kantor, E. D., Templeton, I. E. and Vitiello, M. V. (2005). Pharmacokinetics of valerenic acid after administration of valerian in healthy subjects. *Phytother Res*, 19, 801–803.

Anke, J. and Ramzan, I. (2004). Pharmacokinetic and pharmacodynamic drug interactions with Kava (Piper methysticum Forst. f.). *J Ethnopharmacol*, 93, 153–160.

Block, K. I. (2012). Integrative cancer therapies. *Integr Cancer Ther*, 11, 3–4.

Borrelli, F., Capasso, R. and Izzo, A. A. (2007). Garlic (Allium sativum L.): Adverse effects and drug interactions in humans. *Mole Nutr Food Res*, 51, 1386–1397.

Borrelli, F. and Izzo, A. A. (2009). Herb-drug interactions with St John's wort (Hypericum perforatum): an update on clinical observations. *AAPS J*, 11, 710–727.

Bressler, R. (2005). Herb-drug interactions – Interactions between ginkgo biloba and prescription medications. *Geriatrics*, 60, 30–33.

Brooks, N. A., Wilcox, G., Walker, K. Z., Ashton, J. F., Cox, M. B. and Stojanovska, L. (2008). Beneficial effects of Lepidium meyenii (Maca) on psychological symptoms and measures of sexual dysfunction in postmenopausal women are not related to estrogen or androgen content. *Menopause*, 15, 1157–1162.

Burnett, B. P., Pillai, L., Bitto, A., Squadrito, F. and Levy, R. M. (2011). Evaluation of CYP450 inhibitory effects and steady-state pharmacokinetics of genistein in combination with cholecalciferol and citrated zinc bisglycinate in postmenopausal women. *Int J Womens Health,* 3, 139–150.

Butterweck, V., Derendorf, H., Gaus, W., Nahrstedt, A., Schulz, V. and Unger, M. (2004). Pharmacokinetic herb-drug interactions: are preventive screenings necessary and appropriate? *Planta Medica,* 70, 784–791.

Cai, Y., Anavy, N. D. and Chow, H. H. (2002). Contribution of presystemic hepatic extraction to the low oral bioavailability of green tea catechins in rats. *Drug Metab Dispos,* 30, 1246–1249.

Chatsudthipong, V. and Muanprasat, C. (2009). Stevioside and related compounds: therapeutic benefits beyond sweetness. *Pharmacol Ther,* 121, 41–54.

Chavez, M. L., Jordan, M. A. and Chavez, P. I. (2006). Evidence-based drug – herbal interactions. *Life Sci,* 78, 2146–2157.

Chitchumroonchokchai, C., Thomas-Ahner, J. M., Li, J., Riedl, K. M., Nontakham, J., Suksumrarn, S., Clinton, S. K., Kinghorn, A. D. and Failla, M. L. (2013). Antitumorigenicity of dietary α-mangostin in an HT-29 colon cell xenograft model and the tissue distribution of xanthones and their phase II metabolites. *Mol Nutr Food Res,* 57(2), doi:10.1002/mnfr.201200539.

Chow, H. H., Garland, L. L., Hsu, C. H., Vining, D. R., Chew, W. M., Miller, J. A., Perloff, M., Crowell, J. A. and Alberts, D. S. (2010). Resveratrol modulates drug- and carcinogen-metabolizing enzymes in a healthy volunteer study. *Cancer Prev Res (Phila),* 3, 1168–1175.

Coates, P. M. (2010). Encyclopedia of dietary supplements. 2nd edn. New York: Informa Healthcare.

Conrad, S. C., Chiu, H. and Silverman, B. L. (2004). Soy formula complicates management of congenital hypothyroidism. *Arch Dis Child,* 89, 37–40.

Cupp, M. J. (1999). Herbal remedies: adverse effects and drug interactions. *Am Fam Physician,* 59, 1239–1245.

Das, K., Dang, R., Shivananda, T. and Sur, P. (2005). Interaction effect between phosphorus and zinc on their availability in soil in relation to their contents in stevia (Stevia rebaudiana). *Scientific World J,* 5, 490–495.

De Smet, P. A. (2007). Clinical risk management of herb-drug interactions. *Br J Clin Pharmacol,* 63, 258–267.

Dog, T. L., Marles, R., Mahady, G., Gardiner, P., Ko, R., Barnes, J., Chavez, M. L., Griffiths, J., Giancaspro, G. and Sarma, N. D. (2010). Assessing safety of herbal products for menopausal complaints: an international perspective. *Maturitas,* 66, 355–362.

Duthie, G. G., Kyle, J. A., Jenkinson, A. M., Duthie, S. J., Baxter, G. J. and Paterson, J. R. (2005). Increased salicylate concentrations in urine of human volunteers after consumption of cranberry juice. *J Agric Food Chem,* 53, 2897–900.

Engdal, S. and Nilsen, O. G. (2008). Inhibition of P-glycoprotein in Caco-2 cells: Effects of herbal remedies frequently used by cancer patients. *Xenobiotica,* 38, 559–573.

Enokizono, J., Kusuhara, H. and Sugiyama, Y. (2007). Effect of breast cancer resistance protein (Bcrp/Abcg2) on the disposition of phytoestrogens. *Mole Pharmacol,* 72, 967–975.

Etheridge, A. S., Black, S. R., Patel, P. R., So, J. and Mathews, J. M. (2007). An in vitro evaluation of cytochrome P450 inhibition and P-glycoprotein interaction with goldenseal, ginkgo biloba, grape seed, milk thistle, and ginseng extracts and their constituents. *Planta Medica,* 73, 731–741.

Firozi, P., Aboobaker, V. and Bhattacharya, R. (1996). Action of curcumin on the cytochrome P450-system catalyzing the activation of aflatoxin B1. *Chem-Biol Interact,* 100, 41–51.

Fuchikami, H., Satoh, H., Tsujimoto, M., Ohdo, S., Ohtani, H. and Sawada, Y. (2006). Effects of herbal extracts on the function of human organic anion-transporting polypeptide OATP-B. *Drug Metab Dispos,* 34, 577–582.

Gohil, K. J. and Patel, J. A. (2007). Herb-drug interactions: A review and study based on assessment of clinical case reports in literature. *Indian J Pharmacol,* 39, 129–139.

Gordon, A. E. and Shaughnessy, A. F. (2003). Saw palmetto for prostate disorders. *Am Fam Physician,* 67, 1281–1283.

Greenblatt, D. J., Von Moltke, L. L., Perloff, E. S., Luo, Y., Harmatz, J. S. and Zinny, M. A. (2006). Interaction of flurbiprofen with cranberry juice, grape juice, tea, and fluconazole: in vitro and clinical studies. *Clin Pharmacol Ther,* 79, 125–133.

Guo, L., Mei, N., Liao, W., Chan, P. C. and Fu, P. P. (2010). Ginkgo biloba extract induces gene expression changes in xenobiotics metabolism and the myc-centered network. *Omics-a J Integr Biol,* 14, 75–90.

Gurley, B., Hubbard, M. A., Williams, D. K., Thaden, J., Tong, Y., Gentry, W. B., Breen, P., Carrier, D. J. and Cheboyina, S. (2006a). Assessing the clinical significance of botanical supplementation on human cytochrome P450 3A activity: comparison of a milk thistle and black cohosh product to rifampin and clarithromycin. *J Clin Pharmacol,* 46, 201–213.

Gurley, B., Hubbard, M. A., Williams, D. K., Thaden, J., Tong, Y. D., Gentry, W. B., Breen, P., Carrier, D. J. and Cheboyina, S. (2006b). Assessing the clinical significance of botanical supplementation on human cytochrome P450 3A activity: Comparison of a milk thistle and black cohosh product to rifampin and clarithromycin. *J Clin Pharmacol,* 46, 201–213.

Gurley, B. J., Gardner, S. F., Hubbard, M. A., Williams, D. K., Gentry, W. B., Carrier, J., Khan, I. A., Edwards, D. J. and Shah, A. (2004). In vivo assessment of botanical supplementation on human cytochrome P450 phenotypes: citrus aurantium, echinacea purpurea, milk thistle, and saw palmetto. *Clin Pharmacol Ther,* 76, 428–440.

Gurley, B. J., Gardner, S. F., Hubbard, M. A., Williams, D. K., Gentry, W. B., Khan, I. A. and Shah, A. (2005). In vivo effects of goldenseal, kava kava, black cohosh, and valerian on human cytochrome P450 1A2, 2D6, 2E1, and 3A4/5 phenotypes. *Clin Pharmacol Ther,* 77, 415–426.

Gurley, B. J., Swain, A., Hubbard, M. A., Williams, D. K., Barone, G., Hartsfield, F., Tong, Y., Carrier, D. J., Cheboyina, S. and Battu, S. K. (2008a). Clinical assessment of CYP2D6-mediated herb-drug interactions in humans: effects of milk thistle, black cohosh, Goldenseal, kava kava, St. John's Wort, and echinacea. *Mol Nutr Food Res,* 52, 755–763.

Gurley, B. J., Swain, A., Williams, D. K., Barone, G. and Battu, S. K. (2008b). Gauging the clinical significance of P-glycoprotein-mediated herb-drug interactions: comparative effects of St. John's Wort, echinacea, clarithromycin, and rifampin on digoxin pharmacokinetics. *Mol Nutr Food Res,* 52, 772–779.

Hanhineva, K., Torronen, R., Bondia-Pons, I., Pekkinen, J., Kolehmainen, M., Mykkanen, H. and Poutanen, K. (2010). Impact of dietary polyphenols on carbohydrate metabolism. *Int J Mol Sci,* 11, 1365–1402.

Harrison, E. H. and Hussain, M. M. (2001). Mechanisms involved in the intestinal digestion and absorption of dietary vitamin A. *J Nutr,* 131, 1405–1408.

Heiligenstein, E. and Guenther, G. (1998). Over-the-counter psychotropics: a review of melatonin, St John's Wort, valerian, and kava-kava. *J Am Coll Health,* 46, 271–276.

Henderson, L., Yue, Q. Y., Bergquist, C., Gerden, B. and Arlett, P. (2002). St John's Wort (Hypericum perforatum): drug interactions and clinical outcomes. *Br J Clin Pharmacol,* 54, 349–356.

Hermann, R. and Von Richter, O. (2012). Clinical Evidence of Herbal Drugs As Perpetrators of Pharmacokinetic Drug Interactions. *Planta Medica*, 78, 1458–1477.

Hidaka, M., Nagata, M., Kawano, Y., Sekiya, H., Kai, H., Yamasaki, K., Okumura, M. and Arimori, K. (2008). Inhibitory effects of fruit juices on cytochrome P450 2C9 activity in vitro. *Biosci Biotechnol Biochem*, 72, 406–411.

Hu, Z., Yang, X., Ho, P. C., Chan, S. Y., Heng, P. W., Chan, E., Duan, W., Koh, H. L. and Zhou, S. (2005). Herb-drug interactions: a literature review. *Drugs*, 65, 1239–1282.

Hulmi, J. J., Volek, J. S., Selanne, H. and Mero, A. A. (2005). Protein ingestion prior to strength exercise affects blood hormones and metabolism. *Med Sci Sports Exerc*, 37, 1990–19907.

Izzo, A. A. (2005). Herb-drug interactions: an overview of the clinical evidence. *Fundam Clin Pharmacol*, 19, 1–16.

Izzo, A. A. and Ernst, E. (2009). Interactions between herbal medicines and prescribed drugs: an updated systematic review. *Drugs*, 69, 1777–1798.

Kim, B. H., Kim, K. P., Lim, K. S., Kim, J. R., Yoon, S. H., Cho, J. Y., Lee, Y. O., Lee, K. H., Jang, I. J., Shin, S. G. and Yu, K. S. (2010). Influence of ginkgo biloba extract on the pharmacodynamic effects and pharmacokinetic properties of ticlopidine: an open-Label, randomized, two-period, two-treatment, two-sequence, single-dose crossover study in healthy Korean male volunteers. *Clin Ther*, 32, 380–390.

Konishi, Y., Kobayashi, S. and Shimizu, M. (2003). Tea polyphenols inhibit the transport of dietary phenolic acids mediated by the monocarboxylic acid transporter (MCT) in intestinal Caco-2 cell monolayers. *J Agric Food Chem*, 51, 7296–7302.

Kuhn, M. A. (2002). Herbal remedies: drug-herb interactions. *Crit Care Nurse*, 22, 22–28, 30, 32; quiz 34–35.

Li, M., Andrew, M. A., Wang, J., Salinger, D. H., Vicini, P., Grady, R. W., Phillips, B., Shen, D. D. and Anderson, G. D. (2009). Effects of cranberry juice on pharmacokinetics of beta-lactam antibiotics following oral administration. *Antimicrob Agents Chemother*, 53, 2725–2732.

Macdonald, L., Foster, B. C. and Akhtar, H. (2009). Food and therapeutic product interactions – a therapeutic perspective. *J Pharm Pharm Sci*, 12, 367–377.

Mallet, L., Spinewine, A. and Huang, A. (2007). The challenge of managing drug interactions in elderly people. *Lancet*, 370, 185–191.

Markowitz, J. S., Donovan, J. L., Devane, L., Sipkes, L. and Chavin, K. D. (2003). Multiple-dose administration of ginkgo biloba did not affect cytochrome P-450 2D6 or 3A4 activity in normal volunteers. *J Clin Psychopharmacol*, 23, 576–581.

Markowitz, J. S., Von Moltke, L. L. and Donovan, J. L. (2008). Predicting interactions between conventional medications and botanical products on the basis of in vitro investigations. *Mol Nut Food Res*, 52, 747–754.

Mckenna, A. A., Ilich, J. Z., Andon, M. B., Wang, C. and Matkovic, V. (1997). Zinc balance in adolescent females consuming a low-or high-calcium diet. *Am J Clin Nutr*, 65, 1460–1464.

Milbury, P. E., Vita, J. A. and Blumbergs, J. B. (2010). Anthocyanins are bioavailable in humans following an acute dose of cranberry juice. *J Nutr*, 140, 1099–1104.

Mohamed, M. E. and Frye, R. F. (2011). Effects of herbal supplements on drug glucuronidation. Review of Clinical, Animal, and in vitro studies. *Planta Medica*, 77, 311–321.

Nabekura, T., Kamiyama, S. and Kitagawa, S. (2005). Effects of dietary chemopreventive phytochemicals on P-glycoprotein function. *Biochem Biophys Res Commun*, 327, 866–870.

Nabokina, S. M., Kashyap, M. L. and Said, H. M. (2005). Mechanism and regulation of human intestinal niacin uptake. *Am J Physiol Cell Physiol*, 289, C97–C103.

Nakajima, M., Itoh, M., Yamanaka, H., Fukami, T., Tokudome, S., Yamamoto, Y., Yamamoto, H. and Yokoi, T. (2006). Isoflavones inhibit nicotine C-oxidation catalyzed by human CYP2A6. *J Clin Pharmacol,* 46, 337–344.

Nayak, S. and Sashidhar, R. B. (2010). Metabolic intervention of aflatoxin B1 toxicity by curcumin. *J Ethnopharmacol,* 127, 641–644.

Nowack, R. (2008). Review article: cytochrome P450 Enzyme, and transport protein mediated herb-drug interactions in renal transplant patients: grapefruit juice, St John's Wort – and beyond! *Nephrology (Carlton),* 13, 337–347.

Nutescu, E. A., Shapiro, N. L., Ibrahim, S. and West, P. (2006). Warfarin and its interactions with foods, herbs and other dietary supplements. *Expert Opin Drug Saf,* 5, 433–451.

Oetari, S., Sudibyo, M., Commandeur, J. N., Samhoedi, R. and Vermeulen, N. P. (1996). Effects of curcumin on cytochrome P450 and glutathione S-transferase activities in rat liver. *Biochem Pharmacol,* 51, 39–45.

Okonta, J. M., Uboh, M. and Obonga, W. O. (2008). Herb-drug interaction: a case study of effect of ginger on the pharmacokinetic of metronidazole in rabbit. *Indian J Pharm Sci,* 70, 230–232.

Pal, D. and Mitra, A. K. (2006). MDR- and CYP3A4-mediated drug-herbal interactions. *Life Sci,* 78, 2131–2145.

Pawlus, A. D. and Kinghorn, D. A. (2007). Review of the ethnobotany, chemistry, biological activity and safety of the botanical dietary supplement morinda citrifolia (noni). *J Pharm Pharmacol,* 59, 1587–1609.

Piver, B., Berthou, F., Dreano, Y. and Lucas, D. (2003). Differential inhibition of human cytochrome P450 enzymes by epsilon-viniferin, the dimer of resveratrol: comparison with resveratrol and polyphenols from alcoholized beverages. *Life Sci,* 73, 1199–1213.

Pouton, C. W. (2006). Formulation of poorly water-soluble drugs for oral administration: physicochemical and physiological issues and the lipid formulation classification system. *Eur J Pharm Sci,* 29, 278–287.

Roth, M., Timmermann, B. N. and Hagenbuch, B. (2011). Interactions of green tea catechins with organic anion-transporting polypeptides. *Drug Metab Dispos,* 39, 920–926.

Rowe, A., Zhang, L. Y. and Ramzan, I. (2011). Toxicokinetics of kava. *Adv Pharmacol Sci,* 2011, 326724.

Rowe, D. J. and Baker, A. C. (2009). Perioperative risks and benefits of herbal supplements in aesthetic surgery. *Aesthet Surg J,* 29, 150–157.

Saris, N.-E. L., Mervaala, E., Karppanen, H., Khawaja, J. A. and Lewenstam, A. (2000). Magnesium: an update on physiological, clinical and analytical aspects. *Clinica Chimica Acta,* 294, 1–26.

Sarris, J., Kavanagh, D. J., Adams, J., Bone, K. and Byrne, G. (2009). Kava Anxiety Depression Spectrum Study (KADSS): A mixed methods RCT using an aqueous extract of Piper methysticum. *Complement Ther Med,* 17, 176–178.

Sayed-Ahmed, M. M. (2010). Progression of cyclophosphamide-induced acute renal metabolic damage in carnitine-depleted rat model. *Clin Exp Nephrol,* 14, 418–426.

Sharma, R., Gescher, A. and Steward, W. (2005). Curcumin: the story so far. *Eur J Cancer,* 41, 1955–1968.

Skalli, S., Zaid, A. and Soulaymani, R. (2007). Drug interactions with herbal medicines. *Ther Drug Monit,* 29, 679–686.

Sood, A., Sood, R., Brinker, F. J., Mann, R., Loehrer, L. L. and Wahner-Roedler, D. L. (2008). Potential for interactions between dietary supplements and prescription medications. *Am J Med,* 121, 207–211.

Sparreboom, A., Cox, M. C., Acharya, M. R. and Figg, W. D. (2004). Herbal remedies in the United States: potential adverse interactions with anticancer agents. *J Clin Oncol,* 22, 2489–2503.

Srimaroeng, C., Jutabha, P., Pritchard, J. B., Endou, H. and Chatsudthipong, V. (2005). Interactions of stevioside and steviol with renal organic anion transporters in S2 cells and mouse renal cortical slices. *Pharm Res,* 22, 858–866.

Thapliyal, R., Deshpande, S. S. and Maru, G. B. (2002). Mechanism (s) of turmeric-mediated protective effects against benzo (a) pyrene-derived DNA adducts. *Cancer Lett,* 175, 79–88.

Tirona, R. G. and Bailey, D. G. (2006). Herbal product-drug interactions mediated by induction. *Br J Clin Pharmacol,* 61, 677–681.

Tomlinson, B., Hu, M. and Lee, V. W. (2008). In vivo assessment of herb-drug interactions: possible utility of a pharmacogenetic approach? *Mol Nutr Food Res,* 52, 799–809.

Uchida, S., Yamada, H., Li, X. D., Maruyama, S., Ohmori, Y., Oki, T., Watanabe, H., Umegaki, K., Ohashi, K. and Yamada, S. (2006). Effects of ginkgo biloba extract on pharmacokinetics and pharmacodynamics of tolbutamide and midazolam in healthy volunteers. *J Clin Pharmacol,* 46, 1290–1298.

Uesawa, Y. and Mohri, K. (2006). Effects of cranberry juice on nifedipine pharmacokinetics in rats. *J Pharm Pharmacol,* 58, 1067–1072.

Van den Bout-Van Den Beukel, C. J., Koopmans, P. P., Van der Ven, A. J., De Smet, P. A. and Burger, D. M. (2006). Possible drug-metabolism interactions of medicinal herbs with antiretroviral agents. *Drug Metab Rev,* 38, 477–514.

Venkataramanan, R., Komoroski, B. and Strom, S. (2006). In vitro and in vivo assessment of herb drug interactions. *Life Sci,* 78, 2105–2115.

Wang, M. Y., West, B. J., Jensen, C. J., Nowicki, D., Su, C., Palu, A. K. and Anderson, G. (2002). Morinda citrifolia (Noni): A literature review and recent advances in Noni research. *Acta Pharmacologica Sinica,* 23, 1127–1141.

Wolff, A. C., Donehower, R. C., Carducci, M. K., Carducci, M. A., Brahmer, J. R., Zabelina, Y., Bradley, M. O., Anthony, F. H., Swindell, C. S. and Witman, P. A. (2003). Phase I study of docosahexaenoic acid-paclitaxel a taxane-fatty acid conjugate with a unique pharmacology and toxicity profile. *Clin Cancer Res,* 9, 3589–3597.

Wood, C. E., Register, T. C. and Cline, J. M. (2007). Soy isoflavonoid effects on endogenous estrogen metabolism in postmenopausal female monkeys. *Carcinogenesis,* 28, 801–808.

Yoshioka, M., Ohnishi, N., Sone, N., Egami, S., Takara, K., Yokoyama, T. and Kuroda, K. (2004). Studies on interactions between functional foods or dietary supplements and medicines. III. Effects of ginkgo biloba leaf extract on the pharmaco kinetics of nifedipine in rats. *Biol Pharm Bulletin,* 27, 2042–2045.

Yu, Y., Zick, S., Li, X., Zou, P., Wright, B. and Sun, D. (2011). Examination of the pharmacokinetics of active ingredients of ginger in humans. *AAPS J,* 13, 417–426.

Zadoyan, G. and Fuhr, U. (2012). Phenotyping studies to assess the effects of phytopharmaceuticals on in vivo activity of main human cytochrome p450 enzymes. *Planta Medica,* 78, 1428–1457.

Zhang, J., Zhou, F., Wu, X., Gu, Y., Ai, H., Zheng, Y., Li, Y., Zhang, X., Hao, G., Sun, J., Peng, Y. and Wang, G. (2010). 20(S)-ginsenoside Rh2 noncompetitively inhibits P-glycoprotein in vitro and in vivo: a case for herb-drug interactions. *Drug Metab Dispos,* 38, 2179–2187.

Zhang, L., Zhang, Y. D., Zhao, P. and Huang, S. M. (2009). Predicting drug-drug interactions: an FDA perspective. *AAPS J,* 11, 300–306.

Zhou, S., Gao, Y., Jiang, W., Huang, M., Xu, A. and Paxton, J. W. (2003). Interactions of herbs with cytochrome P450. *Drug Metab Rev,* 35, 35–98.

Zhou, S. F., Zhou, Z. W., Li, C. G., Chen, X., Yu, X. Y., Xue, C. C. and Herington, A. (2007). Identification of drugs that interact with herbs in drug development. *Drug Dis Today,* 12, 664–673.

Zick, S. M., Djuric, Z., Ruffin, M. T., Litzinger, A. J., Normolle, D. P., Alrawi, S., Feng, M. R. and Brenner, D. E. (2008). Pharmacokinetics of 6-gingerol, 8-gingerol, 10-gingerol, and 6-shogaol and conjugate metabolites in healthy human subjects. *Cancer Epidemiol Biomarkers Prev,* 17, 1930–1936.

Zou, L., Harkey, M. R. and Henderson, G. L. (2002). Effects of herbal components on cDNA-expressed cytochrome P450 enzyme catalytic activity. *Life Sci,* 71, 1579–1589.

Zuo, X. C., Zhang, B. K., Jia, S. J., Liu, S. K., Zhou, L. Y., Li, J., Zhang, J., Dai, L. L., Chen, B. M., Yang, G. P. and Yuan, H. (2010). Effects of ginkgo biloba extracts on diazepam metabolism: a pharmacokinetic study in healthy Chinese male subjects. *Eur J Clin Pharmacol,* 66, 503–509.

Pharmacokinetic interactions between drugs and dietary supplements: probiotic and lipid supplements

5

K. Berginc
Lek Pharmaceuticals d.d., Ljubljana, Slovenia

5.1 Introduction

Chapter 4 summarizes some of the factors affecting pharmacokinetic (PK) interactions, as well as methods for evaluating those interactions. This chapter reviews available clinical studies of PK interactions between drugs, probiotic and lipid supplements.

5.2 Probiotics and drug delivery in the colon

Colon physiology (i.e. slower propulsion, neutral pH, lower mixing rate) allows colonization by more than 500 bacterial species with preferentially anaerobic demands (Das, 2008; Amdekar and Singh, 2012). Compelling clinical evidence testify to their health-promoting effects, consequent on their widespread use (Jia *et al.*, 2008; Collado *et al.*, 2009). Based on growing scientific evidence, the importance of commensal microbiota surpasses just the nutritional advantages. An intimate association has been demonstrated between complex eukaryotic–prokaryotic (i.e. host–microbe) cell interactions and local and systemic immunological, respiratory, and digestive health benefits (Sinha and Kumria, 2003; Possemiers *et al.*, 2011).

Owing to the marketing hype in probiotics (Hütt, 2012; Lidder and Sonnino, 2012), there is a high probability of simultaneous consumption with prescribed therapy, which could have deleterious implications for drug effectiveness and safety (Sousa *et al.*, 2008; Rabot *et al.*, 2010). Therefore, probiotics, although exerting rather simple PKs (i.e. microbiota release in the lumen and faecal elimination), could influence several relevant PK targets (Figure 5.1).

The small intestine is the preferred absorption site for the majority of orally administered drugs. However, insufficient absorption due to the biopharmaceutical issues (i.e. stability, pre-systemic metabolism, hydrophilicity, proteolytic cleavage, etc.) (Jain *et al.*, 2007; Ravi *et al.*, 2009), intentional disease-directed drug delivery, and delayed drug release necessitate drug delivery to the more distal parts, such as the colon, where less pronounced proteolytic activity, neutral pH, longer transit time

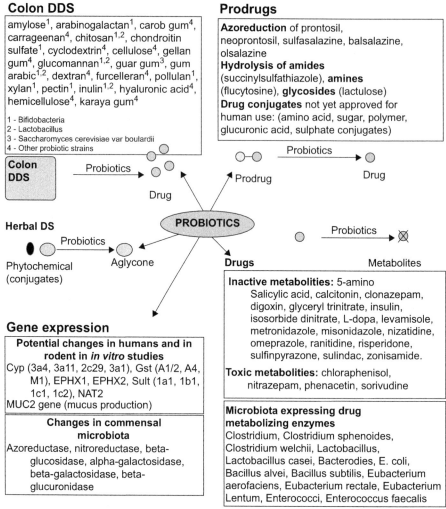

Figure 5.1 Potential PK targets influenced by probiotics and commensal microbiota. Sources: LINES and MICROSCOPY, 2010; Nicholson et al., 2005; Brown et al., 1998; Claus et al., 2011; Gibson et al., 2004; Matuskova et al., 2009; Matuskova et al., 2010; Vernazza et al., 2005; Chávarri et al., 2010; Van Laere et al., 2000; Fitzpatrick et al., 2004; Brown et al., 1997; Connolly et al., 2010; Badia et al., 2012a; Badia et al., 2012b; Fooks and Gibson, 2006; Šimáneka et al., 2005; Fanaro et al., 2005; Singh et al., 2008; Ferguson and Jones, 2000; Mozafari, 2006; Figueroa – González et al., 2011; Chen et al., 2007; Calame et al., 2008; Al – Ghazzewi et al., 2007; Huang et al., 2003; Cole et al., 1989; Goossens et al., 2003; Pérez Chaia et al., 1999; Tannock et al., 2000; Blaut, 2002; Kolida et al., 2002; Kajander et al., 2007; Macfarlane and Cummings, 1999; Timmerman et al., 2004; Burns and Rowland, 2000; Rada et al., 2006; Cardona, 2002; Mountzouris et al., 2007; Laparra and Sanz, 2010; Wollowski et al., 2001; Brady et al., 2000.

and better mucosal responsiveness to permeation enhancers favour the absorption of high-molecular weight substances susceptible to enzymatic degradation (Kosaraju, 2005; Possemiers *et al.*, 2011).

Drug release in the colon can be triggered by pH change during passage from small to large intestine (i.e. pH-sensitive systems) or time, which has purportedly elapsed from formulation administration to the supposed arrival to the colon (i.e. time-release systems). Unfortunately, the usefulness of such products has been limited by significant inter-subject variability, which fails to satisfy the criteria of predictable and reproducible drug release. The focus has thus turned to the residing bacteria, whose density in the colon profoundly outnumbers the content elsewhere in the gut (10^{13}–10^{14} in the colon versus 10^{3}–10^{4} in the small intestine) (Possemiers *et al.*, 2011).

Colon drug delivery systems may therefore be composed of non-digestible, natural polysaccharides acting as drug carriers, matrices or as coating films, to be fermented in the colon by the heterogeneous myriad of bacterial enzymes devoid elsewhere in the gut (Jain *et al.*, 2007; Ravi *et al.*, 2009). Because biodegradable polysaccharides do not always exhibit desirable formulation characteristics pertaining to the solubility, film-forming behaviour, swelling properties and degradability, they are often synthetically derivatized but, as such, can only be used in *in vitro* and *in vivo* animal studies before attaining Generally Regarded As Safe (GRAS) status. Figure 5.1 summarizes natural polysaccharides (prebiotics), amenable for colon drug delivery systems, which may be fermented by certain probiotic strains.

Various approaches have been adopted to design probiotic formulations as colon delivery systems with the aim of protecting microbiota from detrimental intestinal conditions (gastric pH, bile acids). Since this approach consumes monetary resources, probiotics usually exert simpler composition allowing immediate release. Simultaneous application of immediate-release probiotics with colon drug delivery systems could, however, culminate in the failure of therapeutic systems. Namely, during the passage of medicine and probiotics through proximal alimentary canal, the fermentation of polysaccharides in the dosage form could have already begun by the released probiotic strains. The effort to formulate reliable colon drug delivery systems in such cases may be futile, because dumping the drug in the proximal parts of the small intestine could result either in drug ineffectiveness or unwanted systemic effects and toxicities (Sousa *et al.*, 2008).

5.2.1 Interactions between drugs, prodrugs and plant polyphenols

Prodrugs are pharmacologically inert adducts prepared to mask undesirable drug properties. For the management of local, colonic diseases, preparation of prodrugs targeting colonic mucosa involves non-specific chemical drug derivatization to unabsorbable complexes, which, upon arrival into the colon, intentionally exploit reductive and hydrolytic enzymatic activities of the resident microbiota to release the active moiety (Sousa *et al.*, 2008). Because the microbiota species and/or enzymes involved in prodrug activation are mostly unknown, simultaneous administration of such medications and probiotics could result in the release of active moiety outside the designated absorption site and therapeutic failure.

In many *in vitro* and *in vivo* animal studies addressing targeted drug delivery to the colon, non-absorbable complexes have been prepared by conjugating drugs to amino acids, saccharides, polymers, glucuronic acid, sulphate, dextran or cyclodextrin, in order to tailor drug release by microbial enzymatic transformation – Figure 5.1 (Possemiers et al., 2011). Because such adducts represent new chemical moieties, they await clinical trials to confirm their effectiveness and safety.

Food borne polyphenols and polyphenol dietary supplements (DS) exploit bacterial and human metabolic apparatuses to yield highly permeable aglycones (see previous section). By releasing the bioactive aglycones, gut microbiota affects the ultimate human exposure to these species and corresponding metabolites and thus plays a crucial role in the PK and pharmacodynamics of plant polyphenols. Furthermore, polyphenol bioactivation by commensal bacteria depends also on the presence of prebiotics (fructooligosaccharides, inulin-type fructans, and inulin), whose addition to the polyphenol-rich diet or polyphenol DS yields higher aglycone and metabolite plasma levels compared to prebiotic-free regimens, therefore potentiating the expected polyphenol bioefficacy.

The beneficial interactions between microbiota and polyphenols has been successfully exploited by manufacturers, who consciously combine probiotic strains and phytochemicals or drugs into one formulation to boost phytochemical/drug medicinal effects and accelerate its onset. Manipulating *in vivo* luminal conditions in the duodenum by probiotic strains thus enables aglycone release directly above the most permeable mucosa and provides additional β-glucuronidase supply, which enables more efficient enterohepatic aglycone cycling to prolong polyphenol activity (Reddy et al., 2000).

5.2.2 Interactions between drugs and probiotics

With 2–4 million genes encompassed in the intestinal bacteria genomes, their bioactivation and detoxification potential is estimated to exceed the metabolic capacity of the human liver by a factor of 100, which leads to the conclusion that microbial machinery may be regarded as a separate organ within the human host (Hütt, 2012). While bacterial catalytic potential beneficially affects PKs of prodrug and phytochemicals, profound colonic bacterial degradation of drugs to inactive or even toxic species has been noted. Unfortunately, the research regarding the identification of bacterial enzymes and strains potentially involved in drug inactivation is scarce (Figure 5.1).

The probability of drugs being subjected to bacterial degradation in the colon depends on their physicochemical properties and formulation release kinetics. While the absorption of highly permeable compounds applied in immediate-release formulations proceeds in the proximal intestine with low probability of confrontation with bacterial enzymes, this is not true for modified-release systems, where a considerable portion of the dose is deposited in the distal small intestine and colon, exposing it to potential bacterial degradation. On the other hand, a substantial fraction of the administered dose of low permeable compounds in immediate-release products is always exposed to bacteria in the ileum and colon (Possemiers *et al.*, 2011).

During drug enterohepatic cycling, intestinal microbial consortia may also restore the drug's activity and prolong its biological half-life, even if the administered drug itself may not be a substrate for bacterial metabolism per se. Following absorption, some xenobiotics (indomethacin, morphine, digitoxin, digoxin, glucocorticoids, sex hormones) undergo extensive hepatic conjugation to inactive and unabsorbable conjugates (glucuronides, sulphates), which are deconjugated to parent compounds by bacterial enzymes in the intestinal lumen after biliary elimination and ready for re-entry into systemic circulation (Grundmann, 2010).

Short-time and prolonged probiotic administration have also been found to significantly influence gene expression in commensal bacteria for key-point drug metabolizing enzymes (Figure 5.1). Because this field of endeavour is still in its infancy, hard data regarding the safety of probiotics for drug efficacy and safety in the long-run are lacking.

Drug–probiotic interactions may be everyday occurrences, which can become clinically important if they involve potent drugs with narrow therapeutic indices. Owing to the combinatory chemistry, we are witnessing an increasing number of new, potent chemical entities with poor drug-like properties coming on to the market as immediate- and modified-release formulations, with the latter ones receiving considerably higher attention. In this regard, the impact of probiotics/commensal microbiota on drug stability will have to be addressed more systematically and with the highest possible confidence to improve the de-risking process before undertaking human clinical studies with new chemical entities.

In vivo animal studies addressing the question, whether commensal microbiota influences human gene expression, have just begun. The preliminary data on germ-free and inoculated animals with human faecal microbiota or individual probiotic strains have indicated subtle host–microorganism interactions involving nuclear receptors (CAR, FXR) and changed lipid profile in the enterohepatic circuit during transient composition modifications of intestinal habitat that have led to changed expression of several key-player enzymes important for drug PKs (Figure 5.1) (Björkholm *et al.*, 2009). Despite the animal origin of these data, alterations in rat CYP3A11 expression warrant further investigation, because this gene corresponds to the human CYP3A4 gene, which tailors the metabolism of at least half of the prescribed drugs.

5.3 Probiotics: summary

Key points to note are:

- Probiotics should not be taken simultaneously with immediate- or modified-release drug delivery systems, or formulations targeting the colon to provide reliable and predictable drug release at the designated delivery site.

- Probiotics may boost the effect of polyphenols and accelerate the onset of polyphenol health-beneficial effects.
- Probiotic administration influences gene expression in the host (hepatic and intestinal genes) and in commensal microbiota. Clinical relevance of these data is awaited in future studies.

5.4 Lipids and drug delivery

Lipids represent small hydrophobic or amphiphilic molecules, whose structural heterogeneities precondition their epidemiologically and experimentally confirmed health consequences. Because of enzymatic restraints, the synthesis of essential fatty acids (linoleic, α-linolenic) is absent or limited, so they must be provided with diet (marine products, vegetables) and DS.

The recommendations regarding dietary intake of different types of fat are set and regularly revised (Burlingame et al., 2009); however, the endorsement of lipid intake from marine sources is a complex risk message to deliver in an effective, responsible and comprehensive manner based on methylmercury (and other pollutants) contamination data in fish and shellfish. To avoid compromising nutritional benefits from consumption of marine products and DSs, guidelines were set for high-risk populations (pregnant women, infants, children) to avoid certain fish/shellfish, to consume varied protein sources avoiding toxin overexposure, and to prudently choose lipid DSs (Mahaffey, 2004; Agriculture, 2011; Aspenström-Fagerlund, 2012). A summary of relevant nutritional studies and PK details are outlined in Figure 5.2.

Unfortunately, there are no studies specifically addressing lipid–drug PK interactions, but the beneficial impact of dietary fat on drug dissolution (increased solubility of lipidic drugs by incorporation into mixed micelles), absorption (increased drug absorption through lymph), and an unfavourable complexation of some basic drugs with bile salts have been thoroughly characterized.

Studies evaluating the impact of low/high-fat diets on gene expression mainly in rodents confirmed changed gene expression of CYPs, caused (in) directly through the impact on transcription factors or formation of reactive oxygen species (Berger et al., 2002). However, fat content applied in animal studies was significantly lower compared to normal fat intake in humans. Thus, potential alterations in gene expression as a result of lipid DS consumption may be vastly underestimated in humans (Aspenström-Fagerlund, 2012).

5.5 Lipidic excipients and drug release

Marketed for over two decades, lipid-drug delivery systems (LDDS) comprise 2–4% of the commercial products, which aim to overcome unacceptable drug absorption due to poor drug-like properties when drug bioavailability is formulation dependent. In spite of the reluctance to develop LDDSs, their current resurgence has effectively resolved delivery of many drugs previously perceived as problematic from a

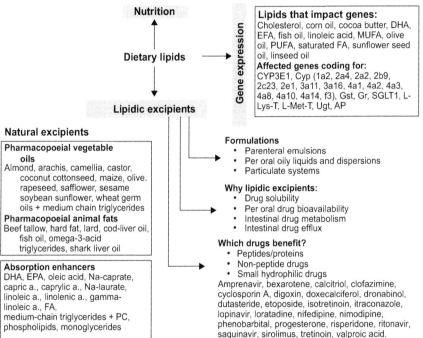

Figure 5.2 PKs of dietary lipids, their role in pharmaceutical formulations as lipidic excipients and impact on gene expression and/or enzymatic activities.
Sources: Burlingame et al., 2009; Agriculture, 2011; Aspenström-Fagerlund, 2012; Ilbäck et al., 2004; Berger et al., 2002; Hwang et al., 2011; Mahaffey, 2004; Strickley, 2004; Hauss, 2007; Sparreboom et al., 2003; Rao et al., 2010; Charman, 2000; Tompkins et al., 2010; Wasan, 2001; Jump et al., 1999; Chen et al., 2003; Mathias and Li, 2010; Belhaj et al., 2012; Clamp et al., 1997; Ferrer et al., 2003; Harris, 2004; Namal Senanayake and Shahidi, 2000.

biopharmaceutical viewpoint (Figure 5.2). The formulation approach to managing insufficient drug solubility, extensive pre-systemic luminal metabolism, and poor intestinal permeability with lipidic excipient, aids systemic drug delivery by improving drug solubilization or by delivering already dissolved dose. Certain lipids may also bind Ca^{2+}, restrict enzyme-transporter alliance, or change the composition of the apical enterocytic membrane, which temporarily and reversibly compromises tight junction integrity, increases membrane fluidity, and decreases the extent of pre-systemic metabolism. Overall, by acting as absorption enhancers, lipids favour drug absorption (Strickley, 2004; Pouton, 2006; Hauss, 2007).

During normal digestion of dietary fat to numerous surface active lipids (fatty acids, and mono/di/triglycerides) superficial, transient damage of enterocytic membranes and tight junctions were also observed reflecting a remarkable capacity of gut mucosa to adopt its structure and function in response to dietary fat. This postprandial effect of lipids serves to increase uptake of water soluble nutrients in the same manner as lipidic excipients improve drug absorption (Ilbäck *et al.*, 2004). Namely, the composition of dietary fat (mainly saturated and mono-unsaturated fatty acids), will eventually be reflected in the composition and physicochemical properties of cell membrane, which in turn will affect transporter/enzyme activities (Ferrer *et al.*, 2003; Hwang *et al.*, 2011). Many of the health-beneficial lipids found in DSs may be considered to act as lipidic excipients; therefore, a similar impact on drug absorption may be anticipated during their concomitant use. Total amounts of lipidic excipients in single dose formulations were estimated in the 0.5–5 g (soft capsules) or 0.1–20 mL (oily liquids) range (Hauss, 2007), which also corresponds to the amounts of lipids formulated in DSs.

5.6 Summary: pharmacokinetic drug–lipid interactions

These interactions can be summarized under three main headings:

- Absorption.
- Hepatic metabolism.
- Plasma distribution.

These are reviewed below:

- Absorption:
  - Oral cyclosporine A bioavailability in rats significantly increased after application with docosahexaenoic acid DHA due to inhibition of gut Cyp3A (Hirunpanich *et al.*, 2006).
  - Decreased rate and extent of absorption (i.e. a laxative effect) was reported in studies with flaxseed oil (Kris-Etherton *et al.*, 2003). Also, decreased intestinal permeability to furosemide, ketoprofen (Laitinen *et al.*, 2004), and metoprolol were published.
  - Orlistat reduced absorption of fat by inhibiting their luminal hydrolysis in rats (Porsgaard *et al.*, 2003).
  - Castrol oil may decrease warfarin absorption (Nutescu *et al.*, 2006).
  - Loose stools were reported as a side effect of palm kernel oil consumption, which could influence drug transit time in the intestine (Wardlaw *et al.*, 1995).
- Hepatic metabolism:
  - Linoleic acid and primrose oil extracts (rich in linoleic, stearic, oleic, palmitinic, gamma-linoleic acids) mildly inhibited CYP1A2, 2C9, 2C19, 2D6, and 3A4 enzymes *in vitro*, which raises possibility for *in vivo* modification of CYP3A4-dependent metabolism of drugs (Nowack, 2008). Because these lipids are highly bound to plasma albumin, a possibility of competition with i.v. administered drugs highly bound to plasma protein exists. Close monitoring is thus advised for patients undergoing chemotherapy during concurrent consumption of evening primrose DS (Sparreboom *et al.*, 2004).

- Fish oil supplements inhibited CYP2C19, 2D6 and 3A4 *in vitro*, raising the possibility to increase bioavailability of CYP3A4 substrates *in vivo* (Nowack, 2008).
- Omega-3 fatty acids may increase warfarin plasma levels by inhibiting CYP2C9 (MacDonald *et al.*, 2009).

- Plasma distribution:
  - Two-week supplementation with safflower oil to paediatric patients increased plasma levels of albumin, which could influence drug plasma binding (Coran *et al.*, 1982).
  - Caprylic acid affects drug binding to albumin (Olsen *et al.*, 2004).
- **Key points to note are:**
- Ingestion of lipidic DS may transiently increase permeability of gut mucosa to nutrients, drugs and allergens.
- Lipids may significantly affect enzymatic gene expression. Human data are warranted.

References

Agriculture, D. (2011). *Report of the Dietary Guidelines Advisory Committee on the Dietary Guidelines for Americans 2010*, Northern House Media, LLC.

AL – Ghazzewi, F. H., Khanna, S., Tester, R. F. and Piggott, J. (2007). The potential use of hydrolysed konjac glucomannan as a prebiotic. *Journal of the Science of Food and Agriculture*, 87, 1758–1766.

Amdekar, S. and Singh V. (2012) "Probiotics: for stomach disorders-an evidence based review." *American Journal of Pharmatech and Research*, 3, 4.

Aspenström-Fagerlund, B. (2012). Dietary fatty acids increase the absorption of toxic substances and drugs by modifying different absorption pathways in the intestinal epithelium. http://pub.epsilon.slu.se/9226/1/aspenstrom_fagerlund_b_121109.pdf.

Badia, R., Brufau, M. T., Guerrero-Zamora, A. M., Lizardo, R., Dobrescu, I., Martin-Venegas, R., Ferrer, R., Salmon, H., Martínez, P. and Brufau, J. (2012a). β-galactomannan and Saccharomyces Cerevisiae var. Boulardii modulate the immune response against salmonella enterica serovar typhimurium in porcine intestinal epithelial and dendritic cells. *Clinical and Vaccine Immunology*, 19, 368–376.

Badia, R., Zanello, G., Chevaleyre, C., Lizardo, R., Meurens, F., Martínez, P., Brufau, J. and Salmon, H. (2012b). Effect of Saccharomyces cerevisiae var. Boulardii and b-galactomannan oligosaccharide on porcine intestinal epithelial and dendritic cells challenged in vitro with Escherichia coli F4 (K88), *Veterinary Research*, 43, 4–15.

Belhaj, N., Dupuis, F., Arab-Tehrany, E., Denis, F. M., Paris, C., Lartaud, I. and Linder, M. (2012). Formulation, characterization and pharmacokinetic studies of coenzyme Q_{10} PUFA's nanoemulsions. *European Journal of Pharmaceutical Sciences*, 47(2), 305–312.

Berger, A., Mutch, D. M., German, J. B. and Roberts, M. A. (2002). Dietary effects of arachidonate-rich fungal oil and fish oil on murine hepatic and hippocampal gene expression. *Lipids Health Disease*, 1, 8.5.

Björkholm, B., Bok, C. M., Lundin, A., Rafter, J., Hibberd, M. L. and Pettersson, S. (2009). Intestinal microbiota regulate xenobiotic metabolism in the liver. *PLoS One*, 4, e6958.

Blaut, M. (2002). Relationship of prebiotics and food to intestinal microflora. *European Journal of Nutrition*, 41(1), i11–i16.

Brady, L. J., Gallaher, D. D. and Busta, F. F. (2000). The role of probiotic cultures in the prevention of colon cancer. *The Journal of Nutrition*, 130, 410S–414S.

Brown, I., Wang, X., Topping, D., Playne, M. and Conway, P. (1998). High amylose maize starch as a versatile prebiotic for use with probiotic bacteria. *Food Australia,* 50, 603–613.

Brown, I., Warhurst, M., Arcot, J., Playne, M., Illman, R. J. and Topping, D. L. (1997). Fecal numbers of bifidobacteria are higher in pigs fed Bifidobacterium longum with a high amylose cornstarch than with a low amylose cornstarch. *The Journal of Nutrition,* 127, 1822–1827.

Burlingame, B., Nishida, C., Uauy, R. and Weisell, R. (2009). *Fats and Fatty Acids in Human Nutrition: Joint FAO/WHO Expert Consultation, 10–14 November, 2008, Geneva, Switzerland,* S Karger Ag.

Burns, A. and Rowland, I. (2000). Anti-carcinogenicity of probiotics and prebiotics. *Current Issues in Intestinal Microbiology,* 1, 13–24.

Calame, W., Weseler, A. R., Viebke, C., Flynn, C. and Siemensma, A. D. (2008). Gum arabic establishes prebiotic functionality in healthy human volunteers in a dose-dependent manner. *British Journal of Nutrition,* 100, 1269–1275.

Cardona, M. E. (2002). Effect of probiotics on five biochemical microflora-associated Characteristics, in vitro and in vivo. *Food and Nutrition Research,* 46, 73–79.

Charman, W. N. (2000). Lipids, lipophilic drugs, and oral drug delivery – some emerging concepts. *Journal of Pharmaceutical Sciences,* 89, 967–978.

Chávarri, M., Marañón, I., Ares, R., Ibáñez, F. C., Marzo, F. and Villarán, M. D. C. (2010). Microencapsulation of a probiotic and prebiotic in alginate-chitosan capsules improves survival in simulated gastro-intestinal conditions. *International Journal of Food Microbiology,* 142, 185–189.

Chavez, M. L., Jordan, M. A. and Chavez, P. I. (2006). Evidence-based drug – herbal interactions. *Life Science,* 78, 2146–2157.

Chen, H.-W., Tsai, C.-W., Yang, J.-J., Liu, C.-T., Kuo, W.-W. and Lii, C.-K. (2003). The combined effects of garlic oil and fish oil on the hepatic antioxidant and drug-metabolizing enzymes of rats. *British Journal of Nutrition,* 89, 189–200.

Chen, M. J., Chen, K. N. and Kuo, Y. T. (2007). Optimal thermotolerance of Bifidobacterium bifidum in gellan–alginate microparticles. *Biotechnology and Bioengineering,* 98, 411–419.

Chitchumroonchokchai, C., Thomas-Ahner, J. M., Li, J., Riedl, K. M., Nontakham, J., Suksumrarn, S., Clinton, S. K., Kinghorn, A. D. and Failla, M. L. (2013). Antitumorigenicity of dietary α-mangostin in an HT-29 colon cell xenograft model and the tissue distribution of xanthones and their phase II metabolites. *Molecular Nutrition & Food Research,* 57(2), 203–211.

Clamp, A., Ladha, S., Clark, D., Grimble, R. and Lund, E. (1997). The influence of dietary lipids on the composition and membrane fluidity of rat hepatocyte plasma membrane. *Lipids,* 32, 179–184.

Claus, S. P., Ellero, S. L., Berger, B., Krause, L., Bruttin, A., Molina, J., Paris, A., Want, E. J., DE Waziers, I. and Cloarec, O. (2011). Colonization-induced host-gut microbial metabolic interaction. *Mbio,* 2.

Cole, C., Fuller, R. and Carter, S. (1989). Effect of Probiotic Supplements of Lactobacillus acidophilus and Bifidobacterium adolescentis 2204 on β-glueosidase and β-glueuronidase Activity in the Lower Gut of Rats Associated with a Human Faecal Flora. *Microbial Ecology in Health and Disease,* 2, 223–225.

Collado, M. C., Isolauri, E., Salminen, S. and Sanz, Y. (2009). The impact of probiotic on gut health. *Current Drug Metabolism,* 10, 68–78.

Connolly, M. L., Lovegrove, J. A. and Tuohy, K. M. (2010). Konjac glucomannan hydrolysate beneficially modulates bacterial composition and activity within the faecal microbiota. *Journal of Functional Foods,* 2, 219–224.

Coran, A. G., Drongowski, R., Sarahan, T. M. and Wesley, J. R. (1982). Studies on the efficacy of a new 20% fat emulsion in pediatric parenteral nutrition. *Journal of Parenteral and Enteral Nutrition,* 6, 222–225.

Das, A. (2008). *Effect of Red Wine and Grape Juice Against Foodborne Pathogens and Probiotics.* University of Missouri.

Fanaro, S., Jelinek, J., Stahl, B., Boehm, G., Kock, R. and Vigi, V. (2005). Acidic oligosaccharides from pectin hydrolysate as new component for infant formulae: effect on intestinal Flora, stool characteristics, and pH. *Journal of Pediatric Gastroenterology and Nutrition,* 41, 186–190.

Ferguson, M. J. and Jones, G. P. (2000). Production of short – chain fatty acids following in vitro fermentation of Saccharides, Saccharide Esters, fructo – Oligosaccharides, Starches, modified starches and non – starch polysaccharides. *Journal of the Science of Food and Agriculture,* 80, 166–170.

Ferrer, C., Pedragosa, E., Torras-Llort, M., Parcerisa, X., Rafecas, M., Ferrer, R., Amat, C. and Moretó, M. (2003). Dietary lipids modify brush border membrane composition and nutrient transport in chicken small intestine. *The Journal of Nutrition,* 133, 1147–1153.

Fitzpatrick, A., Roberts, A. and Witherly, S. (2004). Larch arabinogalactan: A novel and multifunctional natural product. *Agro Food Industry HI Tech,* 15, 30–32.

Fleisher, D., Li, C., Zhou, Y., Pao, L. H. and Karim, A. (1999). Drug, meal and formulation interactions influencing drug absorption after oral administration. Clinical implications. *Clinical Pharmacokinetics,* 36, 233–254.

Fooks, L. J. and Gibson, G. R. (2006). In vitro investigations of the effect of probiotics and prebiotics on selected human intestinal pathogens. *FEMS Microbiology Ecology,* 39, 67–75.

Gibson, G. R., Probert, H. M., Van Loo, J., Rastall, R. A. and Roberfroid, M. B. (2004). Dietary modulation of the human colonic microbiota: updating the concept of prebiotics. *Nutrition Research Reviews,* 17, 259–275.

Goossens, D., Jonkers, D., Russel, M., Stobberingh, E., Van den Bogaard, A. and Stockbrügger, R. (2003). The effect of Lactobacillus plantarum 299v on the bacterial composition and metabolic activity in faeces of healthy volunteers: a placebo-controlled study on the onset and duration of effects. *Alimentary pharmacology and Therapeutics,* 18, 495–505.

Grundmann, O. (2010). The gut microbiome and pre-systemic metabolism: current state and evolving research. *Journal of Drug Metabolism and Toxicology,* 1, 105. doi:10.4172/2157-7609.1000104.

Harris, W. S. (2004). Fish oil supplementation: evidence for health benefits. *Cleveland Clinic Journal of Medicine,* 71, 208–210.

Hauss, D. J. (2007). Oral lipid-based formulations. *Advanced drug delivery Reviews,* 59, 667–676.

Hirunpanich, V., Katagi, J., Sethabouppha, B. and Sato, H. (2006). Demonstration of docosahexaenoic acid as a bioavailability enhancer for CYP3A substrates: in vitro and in vivo evidence using cyclosporin in rats. *Drug metabolism and Disposition,* 34, 305–310.

Huang, Y., Kotula, L. and Adams, M. C. (2003). The in vivo assessment of safety and gastrointestinal survival of an orally administered novel Probiotic, Propionibacterium jensenii 702, in a male Wistar rat model. *Food and chemical Toxicology,* 41, 1781–1787.

Hütt, P. (2012). *Functional Properties, Persistence, Safety and Efficacy of Potential Probiotic Lactobacilli*, PhD dissertation, 2012. http://dspace.utlib.ee/dspace/bitstream/handle/10062/25608/hytt_pirje.pdf.

Hwang, J., Chang, Y.-H., Park, J. H., Kim, S. Y., Chung, H., Shim, E. and Hwang, H. J. (2011). Dietary saturated and monounsaturated fats protect against acute acetaminophen hepatotoxicity by altering fatty acid composition of liver microsomal membrane in rats. *Lipids in health and Disease*, 10, 184.

Ilbäck, N.-G., Nyblom, M., Carlfors, J., Fagerlund-Aspenström, B., Tavelin, S. and Glynn, A. (2004). Do surface-active lipids in food increase the intestinal permeability to toxic substances and allergenic agents? *Medical Hypotheses*, 63, 724–730.

Jain, A., Gupta, Y. and Jain, S. K. (2007). Perspectives of biodegradable natural polysaccharides for site-specific drug delivery to the colon. *Journal of Pharmacy and Pharmaceutical Sciences*, 10, 86–128.

Jia, W., Li, H., Zhao, L. and Nicholson, J. K. (2008). Gut microbiota: a potential new territory for drug targeting. *Nature Review Drug Discovery*, 7, 123–129.

Jump, D. B., Thelen, A. and Mater, M. (1999). Dietary polyunsaturated fatty acids and hepatic gene expression. *Lipids*, 34, 209–212.

Kajander, K., Krogius – Kurikka, L., Rinttilä, T., Karjalainen, H., Palva, A. and Korpela, R. (2007). Effects of multispecies probiotic supplementation on intestinal microbiota in irritable bowel syndrome. *Alimentary Pharmacology and Therapeutics*, 26, 463–473.

Kolida, S., Tuohy, K. and Gibson, G. (2002). Prebiotic effects of inulin and oligofructose. *British Journal of Nutrition*, 87, S193–S197.

Kosaraju, S. L. (2005). Colon targeted delivery systems: review of polysaccharides for encapsulation and delivery. *Critical Reviews in Food Science and Nutrition*, 45, 251–258.

Kris-Etherton, P. M., Harris, W. S. and Appel, L. J. (2003). Omega-3 fatty acids and cardiovascular disease new recommendations from the American Heart Association. *Arteriosclerosis, Thrombosis, and Vascular Biology*, 23, 151–152.

Kuhn, M. A. (2002). Herbal remedies: drug-herb interactions. *Critical Care Nurse*, 22, 22–8, 30, 32; quiz 34–35.

Laitinen, L. A., Tammela, P. X. E., Sm, I., Galkin, A., Vuorela, H. J., Marvola, M. L. and Vuorela, P. M. (2004). Effects of extracts of commonly consumed food supplements and food fractions on the permeability of drugs across Caco-2 cell monolayers. *Pharmaceutical Research*, 21, 1904–1916.

Laparra, J. M. and Sanz, Y. (2010). Interactions of gut microbiota with functional food components and nutraceuticals, *Pharmacological Research*, 61(3), 219–225.

Lidder, P. and Sonnino, A. (2012). Biotechnologies for the management of genetic resources for food and agriculture. *Advances in Genetics*, 78, 1–167.

Lines, A. F. C. and Microscopy, A. F. (2010). The molecular mechanisms of selected pathological processes in the cell. *Biomed Pap Med Fac Univ Palacky Olomouc Czech Repub*, 154, S1–S8.

Macdonald, L., Foster, B. C. and Akhtar, H. (2009). Food and therapeutic product interactions – a therapeutic perspective. *Journal of Pharmacy and Pharmaceutical Sciences*, 12, 367–377.

Macfarlane, G. T. and Cummings, J. H. (1999). Probiotics and prebiotics: can regulating the activities of intestinal bacteria benefit health? *BMJ*, 318, 999–1003.

Mahaffey, K. R. (2004). Fish and shellfish as dietary sources of methylmercury and the ω-3 fatty Acids, eicosahexaenoic acid and docosahexaenoic acid: risks and benefits. *Environmental Research*, 95, 414–428.

Mathias, N. R. and Li, L. (2010). Composition for enhancing absorption of a drug and method. Google Patents.

Matuskova, Z., Tunkova, A., Anzenbacherova, E., Vecera, R., Siller, M., Tlaskalova-Hogenova, H., Zidek, Z. and Anzenbacher, P. (2010). Effects of probiotic Escherichia coli Nissle 1917 on expression of cytochromes P450 along the gastrointestinal tract of male rats. *Neuroendocrinology Letters*, 31, 46–50.

Matuskova, Z., Tunkova, A., Anzenbacherova, E., Zidek, Z., Tlaskalova-Hogenova, H. and Anzenbacher, P. (2009). Influence of probiotics on rat liver biotransformation enzymes. *Neuro endocrinology Letters*, 30, 41.

Mountzouris, K., Tsirtsikos, P., Kalamara, E., Nitsch, S., Schatzmayr, G. and Fegeros, K. (2007). Evaluation of the efficacy of a probiotic containing Lactobacillus, Bifidobacterium, Enterococcus, and Pediococcus strains in promoting broiler performance and modulating cecal microflora composition and metabolic activities. *Poultry Science*, 86, 309–317.

Mozafari, M. R. (2006). *Nanocarrier Technologies: Frontiers of Nanotherapy*, Springer Dordrecht, The Netherlands.

Nabokina, S. M., Kashyap, M. L. and Said, H. M. (2005). Mechanism and regulation of human intestinal niacin uptake. *American Journal of Physiology Cell Physiology*, 289, C97–C103.

Namal Senanayake, S. P. and Shahidi, F. (2000). Lipid components of borage (Borago officinalis L.) seeds and their changes during germination. *Journal of the American Oil Chemists' Society*, 77, 55–61.

Nicholson, J. K., Holmes, E. and Wilson, I. D. (2005). Gut Microorganisms, mammalian metabolism and personalized health care. *Nature Reviews Microbiology*, 3, 431–438.

Nowack, R. (2008). Review article: cytochrome P450 Enzyme, and transport protein mediated herb-drug interactions in renal transplant patients: grapefruit juice, St John's Wort – and beyond! *Nephrology (Carlton)*, 13, 337–47.

Nutescu, E. A., Shapiro, N. L., Ibrahim, S. and West, P. (2006). Warfarin and its interactions with foods, herbs and other dietary supplements. *Expert Opinion on Drug Safety*, 5, 433–451.

Pérez Chaia, A., Zarate, G. and Oliver, G. (1999). The probiotic properties of propionibacteria. *Le Lait*, 79, 175–185.

Porsgaard, T., Straarup, E. M., Mu, H. and Høy, C.-E. (2003). Effect of orlistat on fat absorption in rats: A comparison of normal rats and rats with diverted bile and pancreatic juice. *Lipids*, 38, 1039–1043.

Possemiers, S., Bolca, S., Verstraete, W. and Heyerick, A. (2011). The intestinal microbiome: A separate organ inside the body with the metabolic potential to influence the bioactivity of botanicals. *Fitoterapia*, 82, 53–66.

Pouton, C. W. (2006). Formulation of poorly water-soluble drugs for oral administration: physicochemical and physiological issues and the lipid formulation classification system. *European Journal of Pharmaceutical Sciences*, 29, 278–287.

Rabot, S., Rafter, J., Rijkers, G. T., Watzl, B. and Antoine, J.-M. (2010). Guidance for substantiating the evidence for beneficial effects of probiotics: impact of probiotics on digestive system metabolism. *The Journal of Nutrition*, 140, 677S–689S.

Rada, V., Vlková, E., Nevoral, J. and Trojanová, I. (2006). Comparison of bacterial flora and enzymatic activity in faeces of infants and calves. *FEMS Microbiology Letters*, 258, 25–28.

Rao, Z., Si, L., Guan, Y., Pan, H., Qiu, J. and Li, G. (2010). Inhibitive effect of cremophor RH40 or tween 80-based self-microemulsiflying drug delivery system on cytochrome

P450 3A enzymes in murine hepatocytes. *Journal of Huazhong University of Science and Technology – Medical Sciences,* 30, 562–568.

Ravi, K., Patil, B., Patil, S. and Paschapur, M. (2009). Polysaccharides based colon specific drug delivery: A review. *International Journal of PharmTech Research,* 1, 334–346.

Ravi Kumar, M. N. (2000). A review of chitin and chitosan applications. *Reactive and Functional Polymers,* 46, 1–27.

Reddy, M. S., Reddy, D. R. K. and Prasad, N. A. (2000). Herbal and pharmaceutical drugs enhanced with probiotics. Google Patents.

Saris, N.-E. L., Mervaala, E., Karppanen, H., Khawaja, J. A. and Lewenstam, A. (2000). Magnesium: an update on physiological, clinical and analytical aspects. *Clinica Chimica Acta,* 294, 1–26.

Singh, R. S., Saini, G. K. and Kennedy, J. F. (2008). Pullulan: microbial sources, production and applications. *Carbohydrate Polymers,* 73, 515–531.

Sinha, V. R. and Kumria, R. (2003). Microbially triggered drug delivery to the colon. *European Journal of Pharmaceutical Science,* 18, 3–18.

Sousa, T., Paterson, R., Moore, V., Carlsson, A., Abrahamsson, B. and Basit, A. W. (2008). The gastrointestinal microbiota as a site for the biotransformation of drugs. *International Journal of Pharmaceutics,* 363, 1–25.

Sparreboom, A., Cox, M. C., Acharya, M. R. and Figg, W. D. (2004). Herbal remedies in the United States: potential adverse interactions with anticancer agents. *Journal of Clinical Oncology,* 22, 2489–503.

Sparreboom, A., Wolff, A. C., Verweij, J., Zabelina, Y., Van Zomeren, D. M., Mcintire, G. L., Swindell, C. S., Donehower, R. C. and Baker, S. D. (2003). Disposition of docosahexaenoic acid-paclitaxel, a novel taxane, in blood in vitro and clinical pharmacokinetic studies. *Clinical Cancer Research,* 9, 151–159.

Strickley, R. G. (2004). Solubilizing excipients in oral and injectable formulations. *Pharmaceutical Research,* 21, 201–230.

Tannock, G., Munro, K., Harmsen, H., Welling, G., Smart, J. and Gopal, P. (2000). Analysis of the fecal microflora of human subjects consuming a probiotic product containing Lactobacillus rhamnosusDR20. *Applied and Environmental Microbiology,* 66, 2578–2588.

Timmerman, H., Koning, C., Mulder, L., Rombouts, F. and Beynen, A. (2004). Monostrain, multistrain and multispecies probiotics – a comparison of functionality and efficacy. *International Journal of Food Microbiology,* 96, 219–233.

Tompkins, L., Lynch, C., Haidar, S., Polli, J. and Wang, H. (2010). Effects of commonly used excipients on the expression of CYP3A4 in colon and liver cells. *Pharmaceutical Research,* 27, 1703–1712.

Van Laere, K. M., Hartemink, R., Bosveld, M., Schols, H. A. and Voragen, A. G. (2000). Fermentation of plant cell wall derived polysaccharides and their corresponding oligosaccharides by intestinal bacteria. *Journal of Agricultural and Food Chemistry,* 48, 1644–1652.

Vernazza, C., Gibson, G. and Rastall, R. (2005). In vitro fermentation of chitosan derivatives by mixed cultures of human faecal bacteria. *Carbohydrate Polymers,* 60, 539–545.

Wardlaw, G. M., Snook, J. T., Park, S., Patel, P. K., Pendley, F. C., Lee, M.-S. and Jandacek, R. J. (1995). Relative effects on serum lipids and apolipoproteins of a caprenin-rich diet compared with diets rich in palm oil/palm-kernel oil or butter. *The American Journal of Clinical Nutrition,* 61, 535–542.

Wasan, K. M. (2001). Formulation and physiological and biopharmaceutical issues in the development of oral lipid-based drug delivery systems. *Drug development and industrial Pharmacy,* 27, 267–276.

Wollowski, I., Rechkemmer, G. and Pool-Zobel, B. L. (2001). Protective role of probiotics and prebiotics in colon cancer. *The American Journal of Clinical Nutrition,* 73, 451s–455s.

Pharmacokinetic interactions between drugs and dietary supplements: carbohydrate, protein, vitamin and mineral supplements

K. Berginc
Lek Pharmaceuticals d.d., Ljubljana, Slovenia

6.1 Introduction

This chapter reviews available clinical studies of pharmacokinetic (PK) interactions between drugs, carbohydrate, protein, vitamin and mineral supplements.

6.2 Carbohydrates as dietary supplements

Despite the overwhelming epidemic of all-cause mortalities related to poor food choices, dietary fibre remains under-consumed, while the intake of added sugars in processed and prepared foods is rising (Hite *et al.*, 2010; Welsh *et al.*, 2010). Clinical data show that fibre DSs are more efficacious in increasing total fibre intake than high-fibre foods, due to better adherence to DS use than to the substantial improvements in dietary practices one should make (Anderson *et al.*, 2009).

To serve as food additives, carbohydrates must undergo a scrutinizing assessment of scientific data by authorizing agencies before being added to foodstuffs in limited amounts according to good manufacturing practice to satisfy a specific technological need (palatability, texture, organoleptic properties, etc.). Excessive use of artificial sweeteners (sucralose, maltitol, mannitol, lactitol, xylitol, sorbitol, and isomalt) may provoke gastrointestinal distress, similarly to osmotic laxatives, which may affect the residence time of the bolus and drug formulations in the small intestine.

After consumption, carbohydrates may either be digested to monosaccharides or fermented in the colon, depending on their solubility, digestibility, and fermentability (Figure 6.1). Ingesting fibre as part of a well-balanced diet or as a DS induces gastric distension, changes secretion of saliva and gastric juices, and increases viscosity of the luminal content, which results in retarded or reduced rates of nutrient/drug absorption. On the other hand, accelerated GIT motility and transit time may be encountered during excessive consumption of artificial sweeteners welcomed by so many weight-conscious, calorie-counting individuals (Howarth *et al.*, 2001; Ismail, 2009).

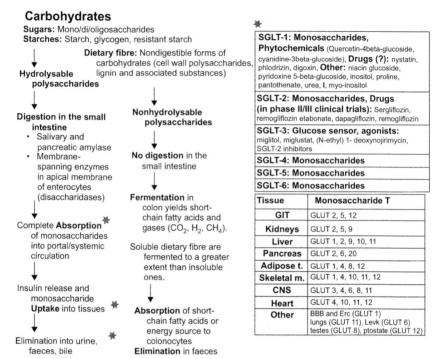

Figure 6.1 Carbohydrate PK and transporters involved in sugar transport/uptake.
Note: T refers to transporter.
Sources: Ross *et al.*, 1983; Phillips, 1998; Walgren *et al.*, 2000; Ravi Kumar, 2000; Howarth *et al.*, 2001; Wood and Trayhurn, 2003; Steffansen *et al.*, 2004b; Puntheeranurak *et al.*, 2007; Voss *et al.*, 2007; Jabbour and Goldstein, 2008; Goodman, 2010; Hanhineva *et al.*, 2010; Hite *et al.*, 2010; Isaji, 2011.

Carbohydrate DSs have been advocated for weight control, support of the immune, skeletal and cardiovascular systems, and they have also been advertised in sports nutrition as promoters of muscle growth/retention and endurance. In the case of weight control, appetite suppression and control of food/hunger, craving is triggered by swelling of the satiety-promoting carbohydrates into thick viscous gels, which causes distension of the gastric wall, delays gastric emptying, adsorbs macro/micro-nutrient and limits a compound's diffusion to the absorptive surface, thus eliciting the feeling of fullness. However, given the totality of scientific evidence and the lack of high quality long-term clinical trials, the safety and effectiveness of carbohydrate anti-obesity/fat-reducing agents have not been convincingly demonstrated (Robert *et al.*, 2004) except for the weight-controlling effect of glucomannan.

Over-the-counter supplements for obesity control usually encompass more than ten compounds with varying mechanisms of action. Owing to diverse composition and high commercial interest (15% of adult USA population; 11% of 11–19 year-old adolescents) the probability of interactions among the ingredients in DS or with the prescribed medications is high (Table 6.1).

Table 6.1 Carbohydrates – the (alleged) active substances in dietary supplements and their impact on drug PK

Carbohydrate	Drug–carbohydrate interactions
Agar[DS-WLM, EX]	• May influence drug release in general • May decrease warfarin absorption
Arabinogalactan[P]	May decrease warfarin absorption
Arabinoxylan[P]	Increased expression of ZO-1 proteins improve gating function of tight junctions and may decrease paracellular permeability
β- and α-glucans[DS-SIS]	Interactions unknown
Calcium polycarbophil[DS-WLM, EX]	• May act as adsorbent for drugs • Bioadhesive polymer, which may obstruct alimentary canal
Carrageenan[DS-SIS, DS-OBE, EX]	• Induces local inflammation in the gut and changes activity and expression of Pgp, MPR2 transporters in rat studies • Decreased intestinal digoxin and amiodarone permeability in rats observed (drugs adsorb to carrageenan) • May decrease warfarin absorption
Cellulose[DS-WLM, DS-OBE, EX]	• Laxative effect expected in excessive doses • Drug adsorption to cellulose possible
Chitosan[DS-WLM, DS-OBE, EX]	• Reduced absorption rate of oral contraceptives, fat-soluble vitamins (vitamin K), indomethacin, and piroxicam due to drug adsorption • Increased binding of bile surfactants to chitosan may reduce drug solubilization in fed conditions (no effect on water-soluble drugs) • Ca^{2+}, Mg^{2+} malabsorption during long-term use • Metal complexation ($Cu^{2+} > Zn^{2+} > Ni^{2+} > Co^{2+} > Ca^{2+} > Cr^{3+}$) • Opens tight junctions – possible increase in paracellular drug absorption • Permeability enhancer for small polar molecules, peptides, proteins (insulin, calcitonin, busereline)
Chondroitin sulphate[DS-SN, DS-O]	Interactions unknown
Cyclodextrin[EX]	• increased dissolution rate of griseofulvin, spironolactone • increased chlorpromazine hydrochloride, tacrolimus, and coenzyme Q10 bioavailability • possible Pgp and MRP2 inhibition
Dextrin[DS-SN, DS-WLM, DS-OBE, EX]	Adsorption of drugs to dextrin possible
Eritrol[DS-WLM, EX]	No laxative effect
Fructooligosaccharides[P]	Laxative effect expected in excessive doses
Fructose[DS-SN, EX]	Can react with amines, amino acids, peptides and proteins into inactive and coloured adducts

Continued

Table 6.1 Continued

Carbohydrate	Drug–carbohydrate interactions
Fucoidans[DS-SIS]	May be contaminated with arsenic
Galactose[DS-SIS]	Relatively new supplement, no studies available
Galactooligosaccharides[P]	• Laxative effect expected in excessive doses
	• Increased Ca^{2+} absorption
Glucosamine[DS-O]	• Increased tetracycline absorption
	• Reduced absorption of penicillins
Glucose[DS-SN, EX]	Increased MRP2 mediated *in vitro* fluorescein, ketoprofen, ibuprofen, amoxicillin efflux (animal studies)
Glucomannan[DS-WLM]	• May modify drug bioavailability
	• Reduced glibenclamide, and vitamin E absorption
	• May decrease warfarin absorption
	• Laxative effect expected in excessive doses
	• Modifies enzymatic faecal content of commensal microbiota
	• It may block the passage through the alimentary canal (it swells up to 17-times its original volume)
Guar gum[DS-WLM, EX]	• Slower absorption rate of metformin, digoxin (clinical study), bumetanide
	• Reduced Ca^{2+}, glibenclamide, metformin, penicillin V absorption
	• Increased Na^+, K^+, Mg^{2+} renal clearance
	• Decreased bioavailability and increased renal clearance of oestrogen
	• Decreased plasma vitamin A and E levels
	• Increased Zn^{2+} plasma levels
	• Decreased plasma levels of proline, serine, tryptophan
Gum Arabic[P, EX, FA]	• Decreased amoxicillin, metformin, glibenclamide absorption
	• Decreased rate of absorption of digoxin, acetaminophene, bumetanide
	• Increased absorption of anticancer drugs due to Pgp inhibition
	• Increased glutamate absorption rate
	• Increased absorption of water and electrolytes due to morphological changes in intestinal villi (used in rehydration therapy): Na^+, K^+, Zn^{2+}
	• Increased renal elimination of Ca^{2+}, Mg^{2+} in mice
	• Decreased renal elimination of inorganic P in mice
	• Decreased plasma levels of 1,25-dihydroxyl vitamin D_3 in mice
Hemicellulose[DS-WLM]	Increased faecal elimination of Zn^{2+}, Cu^+, Mg^{2+}
Hyaluronic acid[DS-WLM, DS-O, EX]	Interactions unknown
Inulin[P, EX]	Increased Ca^{2+} absorption
Isomalt[DS-WLM, P, EX, FA]	Laxative effect expected in excessive doses
Lactitol[P, DS-WLM, D, EX]	Laxative effect expected in excessive doses

Table 6.1 Continued

Carbohydrate	Drug–carbohydrate interactions
Lactulose[D, DS-WLM]	• Laxative effect expected in excessive doses • Increased plasma levels of phenytoin observed when lactulose was used as excipient in drug delivery systems
Maltitol[DS-WLM, EX, FA]	Laxative effect expected in excessive doses
Maltodextrin[DS-SN]	
Maltose[DS-SN, EX]	Maillard reactions with amines possible (see fructose)
Mannitol[DS-WLM, EX]	• Laxative effect in large doses • Decreased cimetidine bioavailability • Competition with drugs for paracellular absorption (nitroglycerin, isosorbide dinitrate, loperamide) • Increased *in vitro* absorptive permeability of ketoprofen and ibuprofen through rat jejunum
Methylcellulose[DS-WLM, EX]	• Laxative effect expected in large doses
Pectin[DS-WLM, EX]	• Binds Ca^{2+} and opens tight junctions – increased paracellular drug absorption possible • Delayed acetaminophen absorption • Binds and traps lovastatin • Adsorbs digoxin, acetaminophene
Polydextrose[DS-WLM, P, DS-SN, EX]	Laxative effect expected in excessive doses
Psyllium[DS-WLM, EX]	• Psyllium traps lithium and carbamazepine in the gut, lowers absorption and decrease Li^+ plasma levels • Psyllium may decrease warfarin and carbamazepine absorption • A minimum of 2 h window between application of other drugs to allow drug absorption
Starch[DS-SN, EX] (see waxy maize)	May influence drug release
Sorbitol[FA, EX]	• Inhibits vitamin B_{12} absorption in man, but rat studies indicate higher plasma vitamin B_{12} levels due to stimulation of B_{12} synthesis by the commensal bacteria • Increased absorption of Fe^{2+}, and Ca^{2+} • Increased renal clearance of citric acid • Laxative effect
Tragacanth[FA, EX]	• Reduced absorption of oral drugs possible (caution with warfarin)
Trehalose[DS-SN, EX]	
Xanthan gum[DS-WLM, EX]	Incompatible with verapamil, tamoxifen, amitriptyline
Xylitol[DS-WLM, EX]	• Laxative effect expected in large doses • Affects plasma Li^+ levels
Waxy maize (amylopectin)[DS-SN]	May influence drug release (gelation, dissolution in stomach)
Wheat bran[DS]	Decreased plasma levels of oestrogens due to laxative effect

DS – dietary supplement, WLM – for weight-loss management, SIS – for stimulation of the immune system; OBE – with other beneficial effects, SN – for sport nutrition, O – for osteoarthritis, EX – excipient, P – prebiotic, FA – food additive, D – drug.

Based on their mechanism of action, non-specific adsorption, limited diffusion (i.e. budisomide, furosemide, chlorothiazide, lovastatin, digoxin, metformin), or delayed absorption (i.e. disopyramide, bumetanide, clindamycin, paracetamol) of solubilized drugs represent the predominant events that may decrease per-oral drug bioavailability (Goole et al., 2010).

Highly concentrated carbohydrate sports drinks and juices, with up to 75–90 g/L sugar content, are designed for ingestion before, during and after exercise to support the performances of competitive athletes engaged in intense moderate to high volume training (Kreider et al., 2004). To ensure faster monosaccharide digestion, absorption and sustenance of increased energy demands, different monosaccharides, referred to as "multiple transportable carbohydrates," are combined (i.e. glucose and fructose) exploiting different intestinal transporters (i.e. facilitated diffusion by GLUT-2 and GLUT-5, active uptake by SGLT-1; Figure 6.1) for the absorption, which ensures high delivery rate to systemic circulation and muscles.

However, high-capacity and low-affinity SGLT-1 transporters are also targeted by many oral drugs, which by themselves exert poor intestinal permeability but formulated as glycoside prodrugs, may attain therapeutic plasma levels. Similarly, SGLT-1 proteins participate in the uptake of many polyphenolic glycosides (i.e. quercetin). Simultaneous consumption would thus result in competitive inhibition between drug/phytochemicals and monosaccharides.

6.3 Carbohydrates as pharmaceutical excipients and prodrugs

Carbohydrates have found their role as excipients in pharmaceutical, food, and dietary supplement industry owing to their abundance, favourable physicochemical (biocompatibility, potential biodegradability, amenable for chemical modifications) and physiological properties (non-toxic), and economically justifiable use (Vitaglione et al., 2008).

Application of conventional drug delivery systems for immediate drug release may provoke wide swings in serum drug concentration, with steep rises followed by sharp declines, which may result in unacceptable side effects and/or inadequate therapy (Ravi Kumar, 2000). Thus, inclusion of carbohydrates to tailor drug release, improve formulation stability, overcome biopharmaceutical barriers, and mask unpleasant taste seems a reasonable approach (Beneke et al., 2009; Goole et al., 2010).

However, some carbohydrate excipients may, contrary to the general belief of their inert character, impact:

- chemical drug stability (i.e. fructose may react with amines and peptides to inactive, coloured adducts),
- physiological parameters at the site of absorption (i.e. carrageenan, chitosan, pectin, and mannitol increase paracellular permeability; cyclodextrin, guar gum, and glucose affect the activity of efflux transporters; sugar alcohols may decrease residence time in the small intestine; chitosan adsorbs bile acids and decreases solubility capacity for lipophilic drugs),

- luminal drug diffusion through thick viscous carbohydrate gels,
- non-specific adsorption of the actives (Table 6.1).

The extent to which drug bioavailability is affected depends on many factors, and is drug-specific (Panakanti and Narang, 2012). These excipients are also frequently applied in DSs available as tablets or capsules, which could hamper release, dissolution and/or permeability of concomitantly applied drugs and/or (allegedly) active compounds from DS.

Carbohydrates can also be used as (pro)drugs. Lactitol and lactulose are registered drugs indicated for the relief of obstipation. Lactulose is used also for the treatment of hepatic encephalopathy. Recently, attention has been focused on SGLT transporters as potential targets for antidiabetic drugs, acting as SGLT-2 inhibitors in kidneys, which decrease plasma glucose levels by preventing renal glucose reabsorption (Steffansen *et al.*, 2004a). Also, SGLT proteins have been exploited for improving oral drug bioavailability by formulating drug candidates as glycosides (SGLT-1 substrates/inhibitors nystatin, digoxin, streptozocin). No clinically relevant pharmacokinetic carbohydrate–drug interactions have been reported.

6.4 Carbohydrates: summary

Key points to note are:

- The main concern regarding the consumption of carbohydrate DSs pertains to the possibility of carbohydrates influencing gastrointestinal residence time (i.e. laxative effect) and drug diffusibility (i.e. increased intraluminal viscosity), which could affect the fraction of the absorbed drug.
- More PK drug–carbohydrate interactions may arise in the future with new therapeutic drug classes targeting sugar transporters as a means to increase drug oral bioavailability or to exert the desired pharmacological activity.

6.5 Proteins, peptides, and amino acids

Insulinotropic and ergogenic effects can result in exponential increase in the use of protein supplements among athletes as a means to increase athletic ability and performance (Schaafsma, 2009). The necessity of additional dietary supplementation beyond dietary intake in healthy adults undertaking resistance or endurance exercise, however, is highly questionable in spite of c.150–200% higher needs for amino acid nutrients in the active population compared to sedentary people (0.8 g/kg/day for adults; 1.2–1.8 g/kg/day for athletes, up to 2.8 g/kg/day reserved for well-trained, strength athletes) (Halestrap and Meredith, 2004; Williams, 2005).

Because poor nutritional status, malnutrition, and impaired immune response may result in certain disease states, protein DSs enjoy popularity among elderly, people in recovery, those unable to ingest solid foods, patients exhibiting neurological, muscular and neuromuscular conditions, patients prescribed drugs with the impact on nutritional status, and HIV patients (Sahai *et al.*, 1992; Fleisher *et al.*, 1999; Persky *et al.*, 2003; White, 2010). Consumption of protein DSs is also a popular avenue for people striving to lose weight and improve the appearance of skin, hair, and nails.

The perception that proteins, protein hydrolysates and fractions thereof are natural and, by extension, safe is not unequivocally supported by published data. In view of the lack of safe upper limits for daily intake of amino acids, extreme commercial popularity among polypharmaceutical patients and athletes, and potential impact on PK targets (Table 6.2), certain populations should avoid or be closely monitored for possible adverse effects or therapy failure during concomitant administration with drugs (Schaafsma, 2009; White, 2010).

Physically active populations represent the main consumers of protein products. It has been demonstrated that changes in drug PKs in this population may not originate only from proteins affecting PK targets, but may also be elicited by exercise, which shunts blood supply away from central organs toward the working muscles. During and shortly after the exercise, blood redistribution, changes in cell osmolality and hydrostatic pressure accompanied by fluid loss could alter drug binding to plasma proteins, volume of distribution and the delivery to target tissues. Exercise may also significantly attenuate hepatic metabolism and renal elimination of drugs with high hepatic extraction or depending on glomerular filtration, respectively. Overall, increased plasma levels of atenolol, propranolol, doxycycline, theophylline and decreased digoxin concentrations have been demonstrated during increased physical activity (Lenz *et al.*, 2004; Williams, 2005). Exaggerated protein intake may also predispose diabetic individuals and those prone to kidney stones to unnecessary complications.

6.6 The impact of proteins on drug pharmacokinetics and their use as prodrugs

Before gaining systemic and tissue access, proteins must be digested with the help of diverse transporters and enzymatic machinery (Figure 6.2). During protein digestion, altered gastric pH, delayed gastric emptying, and non-specific drug binding (complexation, chelation) leading to detrimental effects on drug stability and the rate and extent of absorption may be expected (Table 6.2). Protein supplementation also affects gene expression of key enzymes (hepatic mixed-function oxidase system, individual CYPs) involved in pro-carcinogen activation (Juan *et al.*, 1986; Robertson *et al.*, 1991; Gidal *et al.*, 1996; Walter *et al.*, 1996; Fleisher *et al.*, 1999). Theoretically, competition between drugs and peptides/amino acids for uptake transporters of amino acids and peptides is possible, although no clinically significant effects have been substantiated (with the exception of levodopa).

Proteins have been proposed as prodrugs. A molecular mass of 1200 g/mol has been suggested as a cut-off value, above which the systemic peptide absorption from intestine becomes negligible. Identification of uptake transporters for peptides and amino acids, coupled with the availability of therapeutic proteins on a commercial scale, has thus prompted biotechnological research and receptor-based screening assays to tailor chemical structures of peptides and prodrugs to feature the essential molecular components necessary for transporter-targeted uptake. In the case

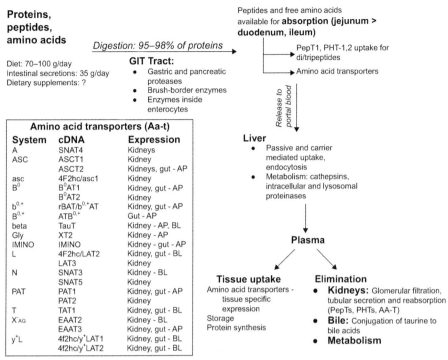

Figure 6.2 PK of proteins, peptides, amino acids, and prodrugs that exploit peptide/amino acid transporters.

of attaching amino acids residues on synthetic drugs, additional benefits besides improved intestinal permeability could be expected, such as shielding prodrugs from efflux transporters (i.e. saquinavir), and improving solubility and/or stability. ACE inhibitors, β-lactams, renin inhibitors, etc. are examples of prodrugs targeting peptide transporters, while fewer drugs rely on amino acid transporters (i.e. cycloserine, levodopa) for systemic and tissue access (Table 6.2). For most of these prodrugs, no clinically relevant food–drug interactions were found (based on drug SmPCs), indicating that protein–drug interactions in the intestine are most probably insignificant. This premise is additionally corroborated by *in vitro* and *in vivo* mechanistic studies, showing that simultaneous exposure of drug and peptides/amino acids to peptide/amino acid transporters does not yield competition but rather trans-stimulation of transporters (i.e. concomitant activation of multiple transporters), leading to improved or not significantly changed drug absorption (Amidon and Lee, 1994; Cao et al., 2012).

6.7 Proteins: summary

No clinically significant drug–protein, drug–peptide or drug–amino acid PK interactions have been reported; however, caution should be exercised during concomitant consumption with levodopa, or in diabetic and kidney patients.

Table 6.2 **Pharmacokinetic drug interactions with proteins, peptides and amino acids**

Protein, peptide, amino acid or derivatives thereof	Drug interactions
L-creatine	↓c_p of L-creatine: anticonvulsants[a] (phenobarbital, phenytoin, valproic acid, carbamazepine) questionable quality of DS reported (residues from chemical synthesis)
L-carnitine	↓c_p of L-carnitine: cephalosporin[a], pivampicillin[a], adefovir dipivoxil[a], anticonvulsants
	↑Cl_R of L-carnitine: cisplatin[a], ifosfamide[a], oxaliplatin, carboplatin, penicillin derivatives
	drugs that displace L-carnitine from OCTN1,2,3 determined only *in vitro* (verapamil, mildronate, spironolactone, sulpiride, pyrilamin, quinidine, valproate, procainamide, lidocain, imatinib, β-lactams, levofloxacin, grepafloxacin, oxaliplatin, metaproterenol, isoproterenol, pamidronic acid, miglitol, alendronate, tebutaline, triethanolamine, acyclovir, decitabine, cidofovir, levodopa, tizanidine, emtricitabine, lamivudine, gemcitabine, pregabalin, ethambutol)
	OCTNs targeted to improve drug systemic availability after per-oral administration: prodrug approach
β-alanine	May compete with betaine[a], D-cycloserine[a], taurine, D-serine, proline, alanine, pipecolic acid, azetidine-2-carboxylic acid for absorptive transporters
L-tryptophan	May compete with L-DOPA[a], gabapentin[a], tyrosine[a], triiodothyroxine[a], melphalan[a] for uptake with LAT1 (also TAT1 for L-DOPA)
5-hydroxy tryptophan	May alter concentration of CYPs
Branched chain amino acids	Drug A: L-DOPA[a], gabapentin[a], tyrosine[a], triiodothyroxine[a], melphalan[a] possible competition for uptake with LAT1
Glutamine	Decreases intestinal permeability to drugs (i.e. indomethacin)
	Increases absorption of water, electrolytes and fructose
Lysine	May increase Ca absorption from intestines
	binds to Zn and increases its Cl_R
	may inhibit tubular reabsorption of peptides
Alanine	May compete with betaine[a], D-cycloserinea, taurine, D-serine, proline, glycine, pipecolic acid, azetidine-2-carboxylic acid for intestinal uptake transporters
L-tyrosine	May compete with L-DOPA[a] for TAT1
	L-DOPA[a], gabapentin[a], tyrosine[a], triiodothyroxine[a], melphalan[a] may compete for LAT1

Table 6.2 Continued

Protein, peptide, amino acid or derivatives thereof	Drug interactions
Glycine	May compete with betaine[a], D-cycloserine[a], taurine, D-serine, proline, alanine, pipecolic acid, azetidine-2-carboxylic acid for PAT1
Taurine	May compete with betaine[a], D-cycloserine[a], D-serine, glycine, alanine, proline, pipecolic acid, azetidine-2-carboxylic acid for uptake transporters May increase absorption of fat and iron and reduce elimination of fatty acids May $\downarrow c_p$ of tyrosine and $\uparrow c_p$ of prealbumin
Proline	May compete with betaine[a], D-cycloserine[a], taurine, D-serine, glycine, alanine, pipecolic acid, azetidine-2-carboxylic acid for uptake transporters
Whey proteins	Decreases absorption of levodopa, alendronate, quinolone antibiotics and tetracycline (whey proteins contain Ca^{2+}) binds diclofenac, prednisolone, propranolol, warfarin $\downarrow c_p$ of estradiol and testosterone $\downarrow$ mRNA of Cyp1A1 observed in animals *in vitro* changes of albendazole metabolism observed
High-protein diet/mix	Excess quantities may interfere with protein metabolism Possible competition for amino acid transporters (melphalan, capropril) or trans-stimulation of amino acid transporters (increasing drug absorption) $\downarrow$ Metabolism of perindopril to active compound delayed gastric emptying increases levodopa[b] metabolism in stomach and caused multiple peaks in its PKs profile; $\downarrow$AUC, $\downarrow c_{max}$, $\uparrow t_{max}$ mixed reports regarding the effect on L-DOPA absorption $\downarrow$ Absorption of methyldopa $\uparrow$ Extent and rate of gabapentin absorption $\downarrow$ Rate but not extent of zidovudine A $\uparrow$ Theophylline Cl_R in high-protein diet mixed effects reported on hepatic N-demethylase enzyme and $t_{1/2}$ (metabolism of antypirine, caffeine and theophylline) $\uparrow$M of propranolol, theophylline, estradiol by CYPs. In rats no effect on CYPs buffers gastric HCl and $\downarrow$gastric emptying; may precipitate basic drugs (i.e. indinavir) possible drug binding to proteins – phenytoin, indinavir amino acids ($D > 2$ g/kg) and levodopa compete for amino acid transporters and entry to central nervous system no impact on cefdinir increases water absorption via aquaporin-2 water channels in kidneys

Continued

Table 6.2 **Continued**

Protein, peptide, amino acid or derivatives thereof	Drug interactions
β-hydroxy-β-methyl butyrate Di/tripeptides	↓c_p of cortisol PepT substrates: β-lactam antibiotics, ACE inhibitors, renin inhibitors, bestatin, thrombin inhibitors, valganciclovir, valacyclovir, sulpiride, L-DOPA and its prodrugs, pamidronate prodrugs, prodrugs of tetrahydrofuranyl carbapenems, hydroxyprolyserine, PD 158473, L-Val zidovudine, oseltamivir, 5-aminolevulinic acid, arphamenine-A, LY 354740, midodrine, Pro-Phe-alendronate, 5′-L-Val-cytarabine, 5′-O-L-Val-didanosine, ethylene glycol-linked amino acid ester of oleanoic acid – no significant impact of food on absorption; no clinical significance. PepT1 expression may be changed by chronic intake of insulin, thyroid hormones, 5-fluorouracil, clonidine, pentazocin, cyclosporin A, tacrolimus
L-phenylalanine	May compete with L-DOPA[a] for intestinal uptake May interact with CYPs Theoretically may decrease baclofen absorption
Glutamine	Decreased intestinal permeability to indomethacin Increased fructose absorption

c_p – decreased plasma levels; Cl_R – renal clearance; DS – dietary supplement; D – dose; a – clinical significance not determined; b – not clinically relevant; HMG-CoA – 3-hydroxy-3-methylglutaryl-coenzyme A; A – absorption; EAAT – excitatory amino acid transporter; TAT1 – ; M – metabolism; AP – apical; BL – basolateral; PAT – proton-coupled amino acid transporter.
Sources: Sachan, 1975; Kappas *et al.*, 1983; Belli *et al.*, 1987; Atkinson and Begg, 1988; Zlotkin and Buchanan, 1988; Holme *et al.*, 1989; Tyson *et al.*, 1989; Hug *et al.*, 1991; Robertson *et al.*, 1991; ten Dam *et al.*, 1991; Wang and Liaw, 1991; Rustom *et al.*, 1992; Sahai *et al.*, 1992; Civitelli, 1993; Shimizu *et al.*, 1993; Semino-Mora *et al.*, 1994; Abrahamsson *et al.*, 1995; Alvarez *et al.*, 1996; Hoekstra and van den Aker, 1996; Barditch-Crovo *et al.*, 1997; Heuberger et al., 1998; Fleisher *et al.*, 1999; Marthaler *et al.*, 1999; Persky and Brazeau, 2001; Yanagida *et al.*, 2001; Yoshida *et al.*, 2001; Brodin *et al.*, 2002; Schmidt and Dalhoff, 2002; Sirdah *et al.*, 2002; Uchino *et al.*, 2002; Anderson *et al.*, 2004; Halestrap and Meredith, 2004; Quan *et al.*, 2004; Hulmi *et al.*, 2005; Williams, 2005; Fujita *et al.*, 2007; Fukumori *et al.*, 2008; Hirano *et al.*, 2008; Nagaoka *et al.*, 2009; Ma, 2010; Sayed-Ahmed, 2010; Indiveri *et al.*, 2010; White, 2010; Diao and Polli, 2011; Cao *et al.*, 2012; El-Kattan and Varma, 2012; Ekins *et al.*, 2012.

6.8 Vitamins

Misguided by numerous market drivers and accompanied by other personal and epidemiological factors, the majority of interviewed DS users admitted regular consumption of vitamin/multivitamin preparations (Younis, 2003; Sundlof and Kellermann, 2009; Stoimenova, 2010), even though vitamin supplementation is justified and medically indicated only in conditions associated with vitamin deficiency (Rogovik *et al.*, 2010). Recent analysis has revealed that the subpopulation with adequate vitamin status and polypharmaceutical patients (especially elderly) represents cohorts with the highest daily vitamin/multivitamin overall consumption (as well-balanced health foods, fortified foods and dietary supplements). In the effort to exploit a diverse range of (dishonestly) publicized vitamin pharmacological activities, excess vitamin dosing, adverse effects, toxicities and vitamin – drug interactions may be encountered (Table 6.3) (Ohnishi and Yokoyama, 2004; Rogovik *et al.*, 2010). The main PK steps after oral vitamin DS intake are depicted in Figure 6.3, which is complemented by PK details in Table 6.4.

As well as complex PKs, the performance of vitamin DSs could also be hindered by stability issues (protection from environmental insults – light, atmosphere, metals etc.). While stability guidelines are strictly followed during production of vitamin solutions intended for parenteral application, registered as drugs, permissive legislation for DSs allows market overflow with poor quality vitamin DSs, containing significantly less vitamin than labelled. It can be said that pharmaceutical companies usually provide DSs of higher quality, because they are familiar with drug legislation and it is not difficult for the manufacturers to abide by different standard operating procedures, guidelines, and to enusre proper working conditions. These companies also tend to test the effectiveness and quality of their products more, in order to gain consumer trust and market advantage over other suppliers.

Besides stability, DSs must also exert suitable *in vivo* behaviour: ensuring the release of as much of the vitamin as possible at the exact time when the formulation is supposed to reside at the site of absorption, mostly the small intestine. Therefore, the residence time is limited to 3–4 h (unless sustained release is desired, such as in the case of niacin – vitamin B_3). Based on *in vitro* dissolution tests of commercially available vitamin B_9 DS for pregnant and lactating women, which showed poor or no release in the designated time-frame, it became obvious that many of products available, not just the ones with folates, most probably do not live up to consumer expectations. Since vitamin B_9 is essential to prevent neural tube defects in the foetus, guidelines for *in vitro* evaluation of vitamin/multivitamin supplements were included in the USP pharmacopoeia. USP 28 recommends the quality of oral dosage forms designed as vitamin supplements to be assessed on the basis of the outcome of four tests (Löbenberg and Steinke, 2006; Maswadeh and Al-Jarbou, 2011): tablet friability, weight variation, manufacturing practices of DSs, and disintegration and dissolution of DSs.

Table 6.3 provides a comprehensive overview of (potential) drug–vitamin PK interactions, occurring especially at high vitamin intakes or during chronic medication that depletes vitamin body stores due to increased vitamin catabolism or increased renal elimination. Because clinical significance of drug–vitamin PK interactions has not been established for all *in vivo/in vitro* identified interactions, Table 6.3 is designed to help health-care professionals to improve the quality of patient care and, hopefully, to convey the message and raise patient/consumer awareness about the importance of intelligent vitamin use and potential vitamin safety issues.

6.9 Vitamins: summary

Key points to note are:

- People with adequate vitamin intake and polypharmaceutical patients represent the main consumers of multivitamin products.

Table 6.3 **Pharmacokinetic vitamin–drug interactions**

Vitamin	PK interactions
A	↓VIT A: neomycin, bile acid sequestrants, omeprazole (reduces β-carotene abs.), laxatives and mineral oils ↑VIT A: in the presence of sufficient zinc plasma levels ↓DRUG M: warfarin (vitamin inhibits CYP 2C19; avoid concomitant use of high vitamin A doses with anticoagulants or inhibitors of platelet aggregation). ↑VIT PLASMA LEVELS: antipsoriatics, retinoid derivatives (acitretin, etretinate, isotretinoin, tretinoin), betaxarotene (excessive exposure to the vitamin and possible vitamin A intoxication), oral contraceptives (mobilize hepatic vitamin stores in healthy women), statins (exacerbate vitamin's A hepatotoxicity and may increase vitamin A plasma levels). ↓VIT PLASMA LEVELS: medroxyprogesterone (increases plasma levels of retinol binding protein by improving appetite and protein intake in cancer patients). ↓DRUG A: paracetamol in some reports.
B_1	↑VIT M + ↑CL^R: oral contraceptives (induce hepatic CYPs expression, increased vitamin catabolism, and increase CLR of vitamin metabolites). Additional vitamin supplementation to women on contraceptives is indicated only when a pre-existent vitamin deficiency or other diseases have been confirmed. ↑DRUG CL^R: loop diuretics (deficiency most pronounced in patients on furosemide). ↓VIT A: prolonged antacid ingestion (vitamin instability at higher pH – avoid antacid intake with meals), chronic alcoholism (alcohol damages intestinal mucosa). ↓VIT UPTAKE INTO TISSUES: digoxin, phenytoin (uptake into central nervous system). ↑VIT M theophylline
B_2	↓A + ↑M + ↑CL$_r$ DRUGS: quinacrine ↑DRUG M: anticancer drugs ↓DRUG UPTAKE INTO CELLS: methotrexate uptake into cancerous cells DRUG COMPLEXATION INTO INACTIVE ADDUCTS: methotrexate, doxorubicin C INH VIT CONVERSION TO ACTIVE COFACTORS: doxorubicin ↑VIT M + ↑ VIT CL^R: oral contraceptives ↓VIT A + ↑VIT CL^R + DEPLETION OF BODY STORES: antipsychotics and tricyclic antidepressants (chlorpromazine, amitryptiline and imipramine), tetracyclines.
B_3	↓PLASMA VIT LEVELS + IMPAIRED VIT UTILIZATION: anti-tuberculosis drugs WORSENED GOUT MANAGEMENT: Vitamin decreases CLR of uric acid (increase dosages of allopurinol, probenecid and sulfinpyrazine). ↓VIT M + ↓ VIT CL^R: primidone ↓VIT A: ibuprofen, naproxen (competition for intestinal uptake transporter and mucosal damage)

Table 6.3 **Continued**

Vitamin	PK interactions
B_5	↑VIT PLASMA LEVELS: acetylsalicylic acid (competition for hepatic conjugation with glycine) ↓VIT PLASMA LEVELS: oral contraceptives, valproic acid INH OF VIT TRANSPORT ACROSS PLACENTA: carbamazepine, primidone (competition for SMVT transporters).
B_6	INACTIVE VIT – DRUG COMPLEXES: hydralazine ↑VIT M + ↑VIT CL^R: oral contraceptives ↑VIT M: phenytoin, carbamazepine, primidone, topiramate, phenobarbital ↓VIT A: corticosteroids ↓PLASMA VIT LEVELS: theophylline, steroids ↑DRUG M: L-dopa, phenytoin
B_7	↓VIT A: chronic alcoholism or alcohol damage to intestinal mucosa ↓VIT A + VIT DISPLACEMENT FROM PLASMA PROTEIN + ↑VIT M + ↑CL^R: carbamazepine, topiramate, zonisidine, primidone, phenobarbital, carbamazepine, phenytoin
B_9	↓VIT A + ↓ERYTHROCYTE UPTAKE: isoniazid ↓VIT A: bile acid sequestrants, antipsychotics (valproic acid), corticosteroids, sulfasalazine, mesalazine, ranitidine and omeprazole, pancreatic enzymes, aminosalicylic acid, metformin ↓DRUG A: methotrexate, H2-antagonists (precipitation and decreased facilitated diffusion), ibuprofen, supra-nutritional doses of green/black tea catechins ↓DRUG M: clobazam ↓VIT INTRACELLULAR CYCLING: methotrexate, triamterene, sulfasalazine, mesalamine, non-steroid anti-inflammatory drugs, colchicine. ↑VIT M + ↑CL^R: oral contraceptives, acetylsalicylic acid (chronic use) ↑DRUG CL^R: diuretics, antihypertensives, metformin (long-term treatment, > 5 years)
B_{12}	↑VIT A: metronidazole (reduces the number of bacteria, decreased probability of vitamin binding), prednisolone (increased HCl secretion, intrinsic factor) ↓VIT A: cimetidine, omeprazolr, neomycin, bile acid sequestrants, ethanol, aminosalicylic acid, vitamin C, colchicine, anticonvulsants, metformin ↓VIT BODY STORES + ↓ PLASMA LEVELS: azithromycin, zidovudine, steroids ↑VIT M + ↑VIT CL^R: oral contraceptives ↑VIT CL^R: metformin. ↓VIT DISSOCIATION FROM FOOD MATRIX: H2-antagonists, inhibitors of proton pump DEPLETION OF BODY STORES: phenytoin, carbamazepine, primidone, oxacarbazepine, levetiracetam, valproic acid, chemotherapeutics
C	↓VIT PLASMA LEVELS + ↑DRUG PLASMA LEVELS: tetracyclines ↓VIT PLASMA LEVELS: fluphenazine, corticosteroids, protein pump inhibitors ↑VIT M + ↑CL^R: oral contraceptives ↓DRUG A: β-blockers, indinavir ↑DRUG A: iron, aluminium, lutein, chromium, aluminium ↓VIT A: hydrocortisone

Continued

Table 6.3 **Continued**

Vitamin	PK interactions
D	↑VIT CL^R: diuretics ↑DRUG CL^R: antidepressants (acidic urine prevents passive drug reabsorption), amphetamines ↓DRUG CL^R: acetylsalicylic acid, paracetamol ↑PROBABILITY OF UNWANTED EFFECTS, IF TAKEN WITH DRUG: acetazolamide (kidney stones during excessive vitamin intake) ↑DRUG PLASMA LEVELS: ethinyl estradiol ↑DRUG M: indinavir, vitamin B$_{12}$ ↓ACTIVATION OF VIT TO ACTIVE FORMS: anti-tuberculosis, cimetidine, anticonvulsants (tissue and kidney hydroxylation), corticosteroids. ↑VIT PLASMA LEVELS: calpotriene (simultaneous use, topical application and systemic absorption) ↓VIT A: bile acid sequestrants, laxatives and mineral oils, anticonvulsants, steroids ↓DRUG A: bisphosphonates ↑CALCIUM A DURING CONCOMITANT USE: digoxin (foetal cardiac arrhythmias) ↑DRUG A: magnesium.
E	↑VIT M: anticonvulsants, orlistat, theophylline ↓VIT A: bile acid sequestrants, statins, laxatives and mineral oils, anticonvulsants ↑VIT A: cyclosporin ↓DRUG A: propranolol ↑DRUG A: cyclosporin COMPETITION WITH THE DRUG FOR METABOLIZING ENZYMES: statins DEPLETION OF VIT BODY STORES: gemfibrozil, chlorpromazine, desimipramine, orlistat, olestra, anticonvulsants
K	↓VIT CYCLING IN CELLS: cephalosporins, warfarin, coumarin (K-epoxide reductase) ↓VIT A: bile acid sequestrants, laxatives, mineral oils, orlistat, colchicine ↑VIT CATABOLISM: anticonvulsants, barbiturates
All vitamins	long-term treatment with aminoglycosides, cephalosporines, fluoroquinolones, sulfonamides, tetracyclines reduces the number of colon bacteria, which leads to a declined synthesis of bacterially produced vitamins GIT symptoms induced by chemotherapy (i.e. nausea, vomiting, and diarrhoea) reduce overall dietary vitamin intake.

A – absorption, M – metabolism, CL$_R$ – renal elimination, INH – inhibition
Sources: Rogovik et al., 2010; Yetley, 2007; Ohnishi and Yokoyama, 2004; Cannell and Hollis, 2008; Marcuard et al., 1994; Barrowma et al., 1973; Pinto and Rivlin, 1987; Thurnham, 2004; Nutescu et al., 2006; Katz et al., 1999; Thorp, 1980; Meletis and Zabriskie, 2007; Trovato et al., 1991; Russell et al., 1988; Zangen et al., 1998; Botez and Young, 1991; Christian and West, 1998; Nutescu et al., 2006; Jeffries et al., 1966; Thomas and Burns, 1998; Selhub et al., 1978; Boullata and Armenti, 2009; Goldman et al., 2008; Augustin et al., 2009.

Table 6.4 **Pharmacokinetic details for vitamins**

PK process	Details
Food matrix effect Luminal stability F_{abs}	Vit A: no food matrix effect; F_{abs} (β-carotene) = 14–22%; F_{abs} (retinyl esters) = 79–99%. Vit D: $BU_{p.o.}$ = 56–60% Vit E: significant food matrix effect (i.e. quality and quantity of dietary fat); F_{abs} (α-tocopherol) = F_{abs} (γ-tocopherol) = 21–29%; F_{abs} (synthetic all-rac tocophetol) = 10–15% Vit K: food matrix significant effect (thylakoid membranes in plant lower F_{abs}); dietary fat, surface acting excipients in dietary supplements improve vit K_1 F_{abs}; F_{abs} (K_1 dietary supplements) = 2–80%; F_{abs} (K_1 fatty diet) = 24%; F_{abs} (K_1 vegetables) = 0.1–10%; no data for menaquinones produced by colonic bacteria. Vit B_1: no food matrix effect; GIT phosphatases release B_1 from dietary di/monophosphate vitamers. Vit B_2: HCl, GIT proteases, alkaline phosphatases and FAD/FMN phosphatases release B_2 from food matrix; plant sources of vit are not absorbed (covalently bound to macromolecules); F_{abs} =74.6% (D: 20 mg); 43.3% (D: 40 mg); 36.4% (D: 60 mg); F_{abs} higher from animal than plant sources. Vit B_3: F_{abs} = 100%; NAD(H), NADP(H) digested in by NADP-glycohydrolase to NAD, which is digested by gut flora to NMN and nicotinamide riboside. The rate of B_3 release affects plasma levels, metabolism and adverse side effects ($\uparrow$ release rate – flushing (immediate release formulations); $\downarrow$ release – hepatotoxicity (extended release formulations)). Vit B_5: 4-phospho-pantetheine released from dietary sources and hydrolysed to pantetheine, which is converted by intestinal pantotheinase to pantothenic acid; $BU_{p.o.}$ 40–61%. Vit B_6: phosphorylated vitamers hydrolized by GIT phosphatases or released from glycosides by glucosidases; peptide adducts not absorbed. $BU_{p.o.}$ 70–100% (mixed diet 50%; glycosides 60%; peptide adducts 0%). Vit B_7: Biocytin (biotinyl-L-lysine) and biotin-containing short peptides released from proteins by intestinal proteases, and peptidases; biotinidase (from pancreatic secretions) releases free biotin. $BU_{p.o.}$ 5–100% (diet); 100% (DS); F_{abs} from colon 25% of F_{abs} in jejunum. Vit B_9: Monoglutamates of 5-methyl THF released from polyglutamates from food with folyl poly-gamma-glutamate carboxypeptidase (may be inhibited by citrate, maleate, phytate, ascorbate, orange juice, cabbage, yeast, EtOH, beans …); F_{abs} (polyglutamates) = 60–80%; F_{abs} (folic a./5-methyl/10-formyl THF) = 100% Vit B_{12}: food matrix can diminish F_{abs}; F_{abs} (meal) < 50%; F_{abs} (fortified foods) = 85%; F_{abs} (dairy products) = 65%; F_{abs} (bread) = 55%; F_{abs} (DS) = 100% Vit C: contradictory reports: equally bioavailable from fruits, vegetables and DS or BU from citrus extract higher (35% increase); BU (D < 200 mg) = 90%; BU (D = 500 mg) = 73%; BU (D = 1250 mg) = 49%

Continued

Table 6.4 Continued

PK process	Details
Absorption (transporters, enzymes)	Vit A: • Enzymes (pancreatic triacyl lipase, phospholipases B and E) release retinol from retinyl esters in micelles and vesicles • Retinoic acid and β-carotene passive diffusion; retinol passive and facilitated diffusion (by CD36, FABP,FATP) Vit D: rapid and complete absorption by passive diffusion (it is BCS II compounds) Vit E: Tocopherols absorbed by passive and facilitated (by SR-BI Rec) diffusion after release from vesicles/micelles by pancreatic lipases and intestinal enzymes. Vit K: passive diffusion of K_1 and K_2 vitamers Vit B_1: A in proximal GIT (jejunum > duodenum > ileum) by facilitated uptake (THTR-1 (AP, BL), THRT-2 (AP)) at conc. < 2 uM; by passive diffusion at D > 2.5 mg. Vit B_2: free B_2 absorbed in proximal GIT. Absorption higher in fed state (slower gastric emptying and transit time); facilitated uptake by RFT1, 2; BCRP efflux; esterified inside enterocytes. Vit B_3: along entire small intestine (BCS I); facilitated diffusion at ↓ conc by MCT1, OAT-10 and SLC5A8 transporters; passive diffusion at ↑ conc; BL transporter not identified. Vit B_5: along entire small intestine; facilitated diffusion by SMVT and SGLT1 at ↓conc and passive diffusion at ↑conc; BL transporter not identified; esterification of pantothenic acid inside enterocytes. Vit B_6: rapid facilitated diffusion at ↓ conc and passive diffusion at ↑conc; pyridoxin and pyridoxamine oxidized to pyridoxal inside enterocytes. Vit B_7: proximal small intestine and colon; facilitated (↓ conc; by SMVT (AP membrane) and MCT1 (AP and BL membrane)) and passive diiffusion (↑conc). Vit B_9: passive (↑conc) and facilitated diffusion (↓conc) of folic a., 5-methyl-, 10-formyl-THF or monoglutamates by RFC, PCFT and α-folate Rec; active transport to portal blood by MRP3; efflux by BCRP, MRP1-5, 8. Vit B_{12}: vit binds to R-proteins from saliva (haptocorrin – TC I) in acidic gastric environment and is then released in duodenum by HCl and pepsine. Free B_{12} binds to IF in proximal ileum and is absorbed in distal ileum as B_{12}-IF complex by B_{12}-IF Rec and endocytosis; passive diffusion not efficient unless very high doses (500 μg). Vit C: facilitated diffusion of AA by SVCT-1, 2 (AP and BL membrane) and of DHAA by GLUT 1,3, 4 and SGLT-1.; passive diffusion at ↑conc; inside enterocyte DHAA rapidly reduced to AA by DHAA reductase and GSH
Blood transport	Vit A: bound to albumin or on RBP Vit D: bound to DBP Vit B_1: free, bound to albumin, or as phosphates Vit B_2: free B_2 (50%), FAD (22%), FMN (28%); bound to albumin, α- and β-globulins, immunoglobulins, fibrinogen.

Table 6.4 Continued

PK process	Details
	Vit B_3: NAD, nicotinamide, nicotinic acid (1/3 bound to albumin)
	Vit B_5: pantothenic acid
	Vit B_6: pyridoxal phosphate (portal blood); pyridoxal phosphate free or bound to albumin, haemoglobin in Erc.
	Vit B_7: biotin (80%); bound to α- and β-globulins (12%), covalently bound to other plasma proteins (10%).
	Vit B_9: monoglutamates (free or bound to FBP) or 5-methyl THF (free or bound to albumin).
	Vit B_{12}: free B_{12}, B_{12}-TC II (10–25% of total plasma B_{12}), B_{12}-TC I (80% of total plasma B_{12}).
	Vit C: free AA or bound to albumin (DHAA in plasma < 2% of total absorbed D).
Lymph transport	Vit A, D, E, K: as CHY
Liver (active	VitA:
uptake,	• Uptake of CHY and CHY remnants by LDL-Rec, CHY-remnant Rec and
M, efflux,	LPL; release of retinol from retinyl esters and transfer to RBP. Retinol-RBP
enterohepatic	may be stored in stellate cells, where retinol is re-esterified, and secreted
circulation)	into plasma at increased demands for Vit A. β-carotene secreted as VLDL.
	• M: retinol to retinal CYP 1A2, 1B1, 1A1, 3A4, 3A5, 2D6, alcohol dehydrogenase, or short-chain dehydrogenase. Retinal to retinoic acid CYP 1A1, 1A2, 1B1, 2C8, 2C9, 3A4, 3A7, aldehyde dehydrogenase.
	Retinoic acid: isomerization, decarboxylation, glucuronidation.
	Vit D:
	• Uptake of CHY, CHY remnants and metabolism of D_3 to 25-OHvitD_3, which binds to DBP and is released into plasma. 25-OHvitD_3 – DBP complex enters kidneys, where 1,25-diOHvitD_3 is synthesized.
	• M: D_3 to 25-OHvitD_3 CYP 3A4, 2J3, 2R1, 27A1 (liver); 25-OHvitD_3 to 1,25-diOHvitD_3 CYP 27B1 (kidney, extrahepatic tissues); 1,25-diOHvitD_3 to 25,26-diOHvitD_3 CYP 27A1, 24; 1,25-diOHvitD_3 to 24,25-diOHvitD_3, 25-OHvitD3-26,23-lactone, calcitroic acid CYP 24A; conjugation.
	Vit E:
	• Uptake of CHY, CHY remnants and transfer of tocopherol to TTP (TTP affinity α-tocopherol > β-tocopherol > tocotrienols > synthetic all-rac tocopherol > γ- and δ-tocopherol).
	• M: α-tocopherol oxidation to hydroquinone, Simons metabolites (α-tocopheronic acid, α-tocopheronolactone), possible conjugation (glucuronides and sufphates); oxidation to α-CEHC by CYP 3A4, 4F2 (minor metabolite; only 1–3% of dose); γ-tocopherol oxidation to γ-CEHC.
	Vit K:
	• Uptake of CHY and CHY remnants by apoB Rec; K_1 transfer to VLDL, HDL and LDL; K_2 rapid uptake into liver but immediate biliary elimination and enterohepatic circulation; storage of K_2 as menaquinones 6–13; composition of gut flora determines the composition of body stores.

Continued

Table 6.4 **Continued**

PK process	Details
	• M: K_1 oxidation (to γ-methyl metabolites); β-oxidation; and conjugation of oxidative metabolites. Vit B_1: facilitated uptake and M: oxidation of side chain and ring cleavage; (de)phosphorylation Vit B_2: M: catabolism by CYP-hydroxylation to 7-alpha-/8-alpha-riboflavin, 10-hydroxyethylflavin, lumiflavin, 8-alpha sulphonyl riboflavin, etc. Vit B_3: extensive, saturable M; conjugation with glycine to nicotinuric a. (causes cutaneous flushing) not saturable; oxidation to N-methyl-2-pyridone 5-carboxamide (hepatotoxicity) saturable, methylation to trigonelline. Vit B_5: SMVT enables facilitated uptake; no M; 15% of absorbed D oxidized to CO_2. Vit B_6: passive diffusion and M; oxidation and phosphorylation to pyridoxal phosphate; oxidation to pyridoxic acid. Vit B_7: SMVT facilitated uptake of biotin; poor M (oxidation to biotin-L-sulfoxide, biotin-D-sulfoxide, and β-oxidation to bisnorbin). Vit B_9: • PCFT uptake of 5-methyl THF, THF and monoglutamates; M to polyglutamates for storage, biliary secretion by MRP-2 or released into circulation. • M only 0.5–1% of absorbed B_9 to p-acetoamidobenzoat, p-acetamidobenzoyl glutamate. Vit B_{12}: uptake of B_{12}-TC I complex and biliary secretion; B_{12}-TC II rapidly cleared from plasma (5–90 min $t_{1/2}$), because B_{12} is transferred from TC II to TC I, whose $t_{1/2}$ is 9–12 days; storage (50% of total body stores: 2–5 mg); no M. Vit C: facilitated uptake by SVCT 1 and M: reversible AA oxidation to DHAA or AA sulfatation to ascorbic a-2-sulphate; DHAA irreversible hydrolysis to 2,3-diketo-L- gulonic a; 2,3-diketo-L-gulonic a decarboxylated to CO_2 + xylose, xylonic a, lyxonic a; minor part (1.5% of D) oxidized to oxalic a and threonic a.
Tissue availability	Vit A: retinol uptake from retinol-RBP (by retinol-RBP-Rec), retinol-albumin or CHY (by LPL). Vit D: extrahepatic tissues receive D_3, 25-OHvitD_3, and 1,25-diOHvitD_3 from CHY or DBP. Tissues can synthetize 1,25-diOHvitD_3 from precursors (skin). Vit E: α- and γ-tocopherol from CHY by LPL; α-tocopherol from VLDL, HDL, and LDL by LDL-, VLDL-, and SR-BI-Rec; passive diffusion into erythrocytes. Body stores: liver, adipose tissue. Vit K: uptake from CHY by LPL; VLDL, HDL, LDL particles (by VLDL-, LDL-Rec, SR-BI); storage of K_1 in adipose tissue. Vit B_1: facilitative uptake into Erc (90% of all plasma B_1); THTR-1,2 uptake in other tissues; only free B_1 or B_1-phosphate cross membranes; no stores, max B1 quantities determined in skeletal muscles and liver. Vit B_2: FMN, FAD dephosphorylated to free B_2 that enters cells passively and by RFT and Rec-mediated endocytosis; inside re-phosphorylated; 1/3 of body B_2 stored in liver (high concentration found also in kidneys and heart).

Table 6.4 Continued

PK process	Details
	Vit B_3: passive and facilitated uptake into tissues.
	Vit B_5: facilitated uptake (SMVT, glucose transporters) and passive diffusion in Erc; immediate conversion to CoA by pantothenic acid kinase; the highest conc in liver (also adrenal glands, kidney, brain, heart, testes) in mitochondria.
	Vit B_6: Pyridoxal phosphate is released from plasma proteins, dehosphorylated by non-specific alkaline phosphatase and enters passively into tissues, where it is immediately rephosphorylated; stored as phosphates of pyridoxal and pyridoxamine in skeletal muscles, liver, kidney, spleen; interconversion of vitamers by pyridoxal kinase, alkaline phosphatase and transaminase.
	Vit B_7: SMVT uptake; poorly stored in liver; stored vit not mobilized when needed; intracellular biotin recycling by biotinidase.
	Vit B_9: uptake by RFC, PCFT and folate Rec; stored in liver; intracellular folate circulation and recycling by methionin synthase, 10-formyl THF synthetase, serine hydroxymethyl transferase, 5,10-methylene THF reductase, thymidalate synthetase, and dihydrofolate reductase.
	Vit B_{12}: Rec-mediated endocytosis of B12-TC II complex by TC II-Rec in the presence of Ca^{2+} ions; TC II degraded in lysosomes, B_{12} released and incorporated into coenzymes; 30% of body stores in skeletal muscles.
	Vit C: AA uptake into kidneys and epithelial cells by SVCT-1; uptake of AA into brain, lungs, heart, eye, neuroendocrine cells, exocrine tissues by SCVT-2; uptake of DHAA by GLUT-1,3,4 into Erc; neutrophiles, levkocytes and monocytes saturated at 100 mg D (1–4 mM intracellular AA conc); all cells accumulate AA; passive diffusion is negligible.
Elimination • Renal • Biliary	Vit A: Urinary and biliary elimination of retinol, retinal and metabolites. Retinol-RBP complex binds to prealbumin or transthyretin in plasma to prevent urinary filtration.
	Vit D: enterohepatic cycling lowers its bioavailability; urinary and biliary elimination of metabolites.
	Vit E: α- and γ-CEHC into urine; biliary elimination of metabolites, tocotrienols and tocopherols (except α-isoform).
	Vit K: biliary (35–50% of absorbed dose) and urinary (20% of absorbed dose) elimination of conjugates.
	Vit B_1: doses above body requirements excreted in urine (also sweat) as vit B_1, B_1-phosphate, B_1-pyrophosphate, thiochrome and other metabolites (> 20 metabolites – derivatives of pyrimidine and acetic acid).
	Vit B_2: biliary elimination < 5% of D, faeces mostly B_2 from bacteria; Cl_R more important than metabolism (GF+TS+TR); 60–70% eliminated as B_2, the rest as metabolites. At higher D TS and TR saturated thus increased Cl_R.
	Vit B_3: Cl_R (GF+TS+TR) of metabolites; at normal intake only metabolites but at higher 65–85% of D eliminated as NAD.
	Vit B_5: at physiological conc no Cl_R due to TR; at $\uparrow$D TS of pathothenic acid and 4-phospho pantethenate.
	Vit B_6: Cl_R of pyridoxic acid, lactone of pyridoxic acid, at $\uparrow$D pyridoxine, pyridoxal, pyridoxamine and their corresponding phosphates.

Continued

Table 6.4 **Continued**

PK process	Details
	Vit B_7: only <2% of D eliminated in bile; Cl_R 43–75% of absorbed D; GF+TR; 50% of biotin cleared as biotin, 50% cleared as metabolites. Vit B_9: biliary; faecal excretion of intact folates from bacterial production; Cl_R (GF+TR) = 0; TR by folate Rec, OAT-K1, OAT-K2 into kidney cells and by RFC to circulation (<1% eliminated at physiological D); eliminated as folates or metabolites (pteroylglutamic a., 5-methyl pteroylglutamic a., pteridine, acetaminobenzoylglutamic a.) Vit B_{12}: enterohepatic circulation (30–60% of D); 0.1% lost daily in GIT secretion (bacteria, desquamated cells); 65–75% of biliary secretion reabsorbed in ileum: Cl_R (GF) of B_{12}-TC I, which is then reabsorbed by Rec-mediated endocytosis with megalin-Rec (AP) and one not yet identified transporter on BL membrane; eliminated as cobolamin. Vit C: Cl_R not observed at D < 100 mg due to TR of filtered AA; at ↑D AA present in urine as AA and metabolites; D > 500 mg; everything above body stores (1.5–5 g) eliminated in urine.

A – acid; AA – ascorbic acid; AP – apical membrane; BCRP – breast cancer resistance protein; BL – basolateral membrane; BU – bioavailability; CEHC – 2,5,7,8-tetramethyl-2(29-carboxyethyl)-6-hydroxychroman; CHY – chylomicrons; Cl_R – renal clearance; CoA – coenzyme A; D – dose; DBP – vitamin D binding protein; DHAA – dehydro-L-acetic acid; DS – dietary supplement; Erc – erythrocytes; FABP – fatty acid binding protein; FATP – fatty acid transporting protein; FAD – flavin adenine dinucleotide; FBP – folate binding protein; FMN – flavin mononucleotide; GF – glomerular filtration; GLUT – glucose transporter; GSH – glutathione; IF – intrinsic factor; LPL – lipoprotein lipase; M – metabolism; NAD(H) – nicotinamide adenine dinucleotide; NADP(H) – nicotinamide adenine dinucleotide phosphate; NMN – nicotinamide mononucleotide; OAT – organic anion transporter; OAT-K – kidney organic anion transporter; PCFT – proton-coupled folate transporter; RFC – reduced folate carrier; RBP – retinol binding protein; Rec – receptor; RFT – riboflavin transporter; SMVT – sodium-dependent multivitamin transporter; SR-BI – scavenger receptors for cholesterol; SVCT – sodium-dependent vitamin C transporter; SGLT – sodium coupled glucose transporter; TC – transcobalamin; $t_{1/2}$ – elimination half-time; THF – tetrahydrofolate; THTR-1,2 – thiamine transporter; TS – tubular secretion; TR – tubular reabsorption; TTP – tocopherol transfer protein; Vit – vitamin.
Sources: Rogovik *et al.*, 2010; Debier and Larondelle, 2005; Wortsman *et al.*, 2000; Booth *et al.*, 2002; Preedy and Watson, 2007; Jones, 2008; Borel *et al.*, 2001; Harrison and Hussain, 2001; Lo *et al.*, 1985; Lamon-Fava *et al.*, 1998; Gijsbers *et al.*, 1996; Prosser and Jones, 2004; Said, 2004; Said, 2011; Gibney *et al.*, 2009; Yamamoto *et al.*, 2009; Nabokina *et al.*, 2005; Gropper and Smith, 2012; di Salvo *et al.*, 2011; Zhao *et al.*, 2009; Rumsey and Levine, 1998; Boudry *et al.*, 2010; Olson *et al.*, 2002; Kagan *et al.*, 2006; Menon *et al.*, 2007; Van den Berg, 1997; Zempleni, 2005; Said, 2009; Carmel, 2008; Blanchard *et al.*, 1997.

- Vitamin users are jeopardized by the excessive vitamin intake at pharmacological doses, which sets the stage for PK interactions with prescribed therapy (besides vitamin pharmacological and toxic effects).

6.10 Minerals and oligoelements

Considering their vital physiological functions, providing adequate mineral (macro- and micro-elements) intake with a well-balanced diet has become a challenge because

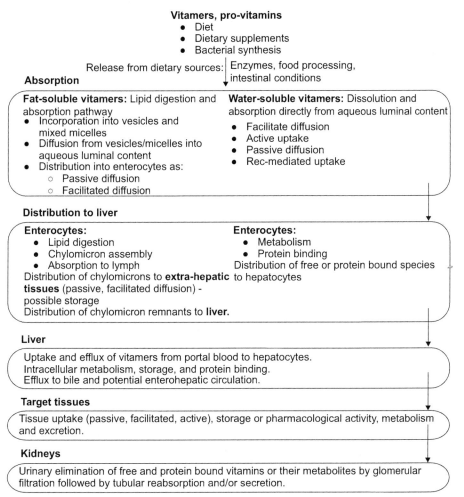

Figure 6.3 Vitamin PK.

of significant soil and crop mineral deprivation inflicted by aggressive agriculture striving for mass production (Lukaski, 2004). People with increased mineral demands (pregnancy, adolescence), compromised mineral metabolism (chronic patients), and populations with dietary restrictions (geriatric patients, vegetarians, low-calorie diets) are thus at high risk of mineral deficiency. Mineral DSs can help to meet daily mineral requirements but, owing to their pharmacokinetic (Table 6.5) and physicochemical (Table 6.6) properties, concomitant use with drugs may lead to interactions (Table 6.6), especially when minerals are consumed in high doses as mono-mineral products (i.e. OTC medications, DS). The concentration of minerals at the site of absorption may be lower due to the food matrix effect (i.e. binding of minerals to food components forming unabsorbable complexes) or because the mineral content in DSs is actually lower

Table 6.5 **Pharmacokinetic drug–mineral interactions and summary of the main pharmacokinetic mineral properties**

	Absorption	Plasma/tissues	"E"	Drug – mineral PK interactions
Ca	Sig food matrix effect 500–2000 mg/day possible GIT complaints. F_{abs} < 2% (duodenum); 25% (jejunum); 73% (ileum) A: • Uptake to Ent: • Active transcellular in proximal parts at ↓D (TRPV6/V5 and vit D dependant uptake); • Passive paracellular in distal parts at ↑D (Na$^+$·K$^+$·Cl$^-$ transporters, ROMK and CLCNKB); • Ca^{2+} diffusion through cytoplasm bound to calbindin D$_{9k}$ • Uptake to portal blood by NCX1 and PMCA1b.	50% as free 45% bound to albumin and organic anions 5% unidentified Hormonal regulation: parathyroid hormone, calcitonin, vitamin D, and others (FGF-23, sFRP-4, MEPE proteins)	Skin, hair, nails (minor) faeces: unabsorbed and Ca^{2+} from digestive juices Cl$_R$: • GF • TR: paracellular in PT, transcellular in DT	↓Ca solubility: H$_2$-blockers, proton pump inhibitors, antacids. ↓drug solubility by CaCO$_3$: cefpodoxime, itraconazole, atevirdine, delavirdine, mycophenolate, atazanivir, azithromycin, gabapentin, penicillamine, rosuvastatin, allopurinol phosphates ↑drug solubility: glipizide, glyburide ↓Ca absorption: anticonvulsants (↑ vit D catabolism changes gene expression for proteins involved in calcium absorption), aminoglycosides, phytic acid, green tea. ↑Ca absorption: estrogens, vit D ↑drug Cl$_R$: chronic CaCO$_3$ prevents TR of salicylate (pH changes)

Fe	Sig food matrix effect *Non-heme Fe*: F_{abs} 2–20%; reduction Fe^{3+} to Fe^{2+} by food components/duodenal reductase Cyp_b; active uptake by DMT1 *Heme Fe*: F_{abs} 5–40%; transporters for the uptake of hem complex *Ent*: Fe^{2+} release from hem by hemoxidase hephaestin, oxidation to Fe^{3+} (stored bound to ferritin) or transported on ferroportin as Fe^{2+} through BL membrane. *Blood*: Fe^{2+} oxidized by hephaestin to Fe^{3+} and bound to transferrin.	Tissues: uptake of Fe^{3+}-transferrin by transferrin Rec (vesicular endocytosis), release of Fe^{3+} and storage on ferritin, hemosiderin (liver, bone marrow, spleen, muscles). *Ery*: iron cycling	14 μg/kg/day NO active elimination Desquamation of cells in GIT, skin, urinary tract, airways (sweat – minor).	↓Ca Cl_R: thiazide diuretics (milk-alkali syndrome), estrogens ↑Ca Cl_R: Na, caffeine, proteins, high Ca-doses ↓absorption of other minerals: (non)heme iron (D_{Ca} > 300 mg), zinc (use zinc citrate at bedtime or between meals), magnesium, manganese, iodine (only animal data). ↑Cl_R of other minerals: Mg ↓drug BU: atenolol ↓drug effectiveness: sotalol, labetalol, captopril ↓Fe solubility: H_2-blockers, proton pump inhibitors, antacids. ↓Fe absorption: cholestyramine, tannic acid, Ca, Cr, Mg salts (Mg(OH)$_2$, MgCO$_3$, Mg-silicate – non-heme Fe) ↑Fe absorption: ethanol ↓absorption of other minerals by Fe^{2+}: Zn, Cu, Cr, Mg Nephrotoxic complexes: dimercaprol

Continued

Table 6.5 Continued

	Absorption	Plasma/tissues	"E"	Drug – mineral PK interactions
Mg	No food matrix effect F_{abs} 50–90% (breastfeeding); 25–75% (adults) A along entire GIT (jejunum, ileum and colon high F_{abs}). AP: passive diffusion (paracellular) and Active transport, vit D sensitive uptake (ion channel or carrier?). BL: active extrusion (Na/Mg-antiporter).	32% bound to albumin, globulin 55% free Mg: $MgHPO_4$ (3%), Mg-citrate (4%), other Mg-complexes (6%). Hormonal regulation	Enterohepatic circulation Cl_R • GF • TR in PT and ascending Henley loop	Insoluble Mg-drug complexes: trientine, nitrofurantion. ↓drug solubility by $MgCO_3$ and $Mg(OH)_2$: amprenavir, cefpodoxime, zalcitabine. ↓Mg absorption: folates, fibre, Ca ↑Mg absorption: doxercalciferol, vit B_6, Fe (high D), Zn ↓drug absorption: ACE inhibitors ↑Mg Cl_R: caffeine (>300 mg/day), diuretics of Henley loop, corticosteroids, thiazide diuretics, Ca, Na, ethanol, glucose, aminoglycosides, cyclosporin A, cisplatin. ↑drug Cl_R: chronic $Mg(OH)_2$ prevents TR of salicylate (pH changes) ↓Mg Cl_R: digoxin ↑Mg c_p: Mg-containing antacids and laxatives ↓absorption of other minerals: non-heme Fe, Mn

Zn	Sig food matrix effect • Uptake: DMT-1, DCT-1, Fe-independent transporters (?) • Efflux: ZnT-1 • Passive diffusion Ent: binding to metallothionein and CRIPs F_{abs} 60–70% (solution), less for solids (20–30%), depends on diet composition, sex, age	Bound to albumin and transferrin ZnT for tissue uptake	Cl_R Skin, semen, hair, sweat, menstrual cycle, GIT secretions, desquamated Ent	↓Zn absorption: folates, fibre, Ca (use Zn-citrate at bedtime or between meals), Fe (high D) ↑Zn Cl_R: thiazide diuretics, trauma, starvation ↓absorption of other minerals: Mg, Cr
Cu	Sig food matrix effect F_{abs} higher in W; in breastfed infants than those on milk formula. F_{abs} = 65–90% (infants); 30–40% (dietary Cu); 63–67% max reduction of Cu^{2+} in gut by membrane bound reductases: ↓A due to ↓solubility of Cu^+ A of Cu^+ along entire small intestine: diffusion (Cu^+), active uptake of Cu^+-ceruloplasmin by DMT-1, hCTR-1 with the help of Na-H-exchanger and Na-Ca-ATPase. Ent: Cu^+ binds to metallotionenin for storage or other copper chaperone proteins. BL efflux by Menkenson ATPase from vesicles.	Tissue uptake of Cu by CTR1 transporters; neuronal uptake by and prion proteins. Plasma: 70–95% bound to albumin, ceruloplasmin, transcupretin, histamine, other Cu binders	Desquamated Ent GIT secretions Bile (half of absorbed Cu as unabsorbable Cu-complexes) faeces (unabsorbed Cu) Sweat Urine	Insoluble Cu-drug complexes: trientine ↓Cu solubility: H2-blockers, proton pump inhibitors, antacids. ↓drug effectiveness: Cu binds to sodium polystyrene sulfonate, preventing potassium exchange. ↓Cu absorption: Fe (high D)

Continued

Table 6.5 Continued

	Absorption	Plasma/tissues	"E"	Drug – mineral PK interactions
I	Sig food matrix effect rapid and complete A organic I; F_{abs} 50% anorganic I; F_{abs} 100%	free I⁻ and bound to thyroid hormones Na-I-symporter for I⁻ uptake into thyroid	Cl_R>90% of D Sweat: conc equals 35% of plasma I⁻ conc GIT secretions Bile: glucuronides and sulphates of thyroide hormones faeces: anorganic I⁻ completely reabsorbed, sig elimination of organic I⁻.	↑I_{cp}: ACE inhibitors, antagonists of angiotensine II receptors, potassium sparring diuretics, expectorants, topical antiseptics, water purification tablets containing iodine ↓I absorption: Ca (only animal data) Changed drug PKs: radioiodides
Se	Sig food matrix effect F_{abs} (SeO_3^{2-}) > 80%, F_{abs} (SeO_4^{2-}) >90%, F_{abs} (Se-methionine) > 90%, F_{abs} (food) 50–80% A: efficient, no homeostatic control ↑F_{abs} for organic Se • passive diffusion: selenite • Sulphur absorption pathway: selenate • Se-methionine, Se-cysteine: uptake transporters for amino acids	bound to β-lipoproteins; VLDL, VDL, albumin, selenoprotein P ↑c_p sustained for longer period with organic Se	Cl_R: GF (anorganic Se) Faeces: unabsorbed dietary Se Enterohepatic circulation Dermal and respiratory elimination (?)	Insoluble Se-drug complexes: trientine ↓Se absorption: vit A ↓drug effectiveness: Se binds to sodium polystyrene sulfonate, preventing potassium exchange Nephrotoxic complexes: dimercaprol
Cr	Sig food matrix effect F_{abs} (picolinate) 2.8%; ($CrCl_3$) 0.5%; (Cr-acetate) < 1%; (anorganic salts) 0.4–3%	Tissue uptake by Rec-mediated endocytosis Plasma: bound to transferrin (newly absorbed Cr), albumin (binds the remaining Cr)	↑Cl_R by sugars, pregnancy, heavy exercise, infection, trauma, stress)	↑Cr absorption: vit C, nicotinic acid, acetylsalicylic acid, indomethacin.

Carbohydrate, protein, vitamin and mineral supplements

	Absorption	Transport	Elimination	Notes
	A: rapid, saturable, jejunum (less duodenum and ileum) • Passive diffusion • Facilitated diffusion (with proteins involved in iron absorption)	↑D also γ- and β-globulins and lipoproteins	Faeces (unabsorbed dietary Cr) sweat, hair, bile	↑Cr body demands: long-term corticosteroid use ↓absorption of other minerals: Fe ↓Cr absorption: Fe (high D), Zn
Mn	Only Mn^{2+} absorbed (not Mn^{4+}). Mn-contaminants may be absorbed through respiratory mucosa. F_{abs} 3–46%; ↑ in W A: Fe absorptive transporters – better iron storages/status in inhibits Mn A.	Bound to transfferin	Enterohepatic circulation GIT secretions Faeces (unabsorbed Mn) Kidneys quick elimination prevents neurotoxicity	↓Mn c_p; oral contraceptives ↓Mn absorption: Ca, Mg, P
Mo	Sig food matrix effect F_{abs} > 80% (20–95%, depending on the solubility of salts). A: fast from stomach and upper small intestine as passive diffusion (active transport questionable).	Bound to plasma proteins	Faeces (unabsorbed Mn) Kidneys Sweat quick elimination	
Co	Not common in DS. Abused by athletes (increased synthesis of haemoglobin) A: fast and incomplete with ↑D F_{abs} 73–97%	Bound to albumin, 5–12% as free Co^{2+} Ca-pump for tissue uptake	Kidney, faeces	
P	Phytate-associated P_i (F_{abs} < 50%) Animal P_i sources (F_{abs} 40–60%) Inorganic P_i (F_{abs} 100%) A: passive and facilitated diffusion;	Inorganic P: 10% protein bound 90% free as Ca/Mg salts (5%), Na-salts (30%), or free P_i (65% – HPO_4^{2-} $H_2PO_4^-$)	Cl_R: GF of free P_i; 85–90% reabsorbed in PT (60–75%), loop of Henley (15–20%) and DT (5–10%)	↑P absorption: vit D Insoluble complexes: calcium binds mono-, di-, tribasic salts (use $Ca_3(PO_4)_2$ to avoid hipophosphatemia),

Continued

Table 6.5 Continued

	Absorption	Plasma/tissues	"E"	Drug – mineral PK interactions
	AP: Na$^+$/P$_i$ contransporter, BL: Na$^+$/K$^+$-ATPase and unidentified P$_i$ transporter	Organic P: phospholipids, phosphate esters, phosphoproteins, phosphonucleotides		phosphate binders (CaCO$_3$, Ca-acetate, MgCO$_3$, chlorhydrate, lantane, Al) ↓drug Cl$_R$: salicylates ↓absorption of other minerals: Mn
K	A: fast and complete in jejunum, ileum passive diffusion – solvent drag and electrochemical gradient through lateral spaces and tight junctions	Hormonal regulation (glucagon, insulin, aldosteron, catecholamines), osmolarity, exercise, acid-base status Na-K-ATPase for cell uptake	90% of K$^+$ by GF and TR (paracellular diffusion, K-channels, Na-K-2Cl-cotransporter) in PT and ascending limb of Henley loop 10% faeces	↑K Cl$_R$: thiazide diuretics, gentamicin, penicillamin, corticosteroids ↓K Cl$_R$: ACE inhibitors, potassium sparing diuretics, aldosterone II antagonists, trimethoprim, NSAID ↓K c$_p$: heparin, digoxin, glycyrrhizin, cyclosporin A ↑K c$_p$: adrenergic α-mimetics, β-blokers, suxamethonium

A – absorption; AP – apical; BL – basolater; CLCNKB – voltage gated chloride channel Kb; c$_p$ – plasma levels; CRIPs – cysteine-rich proteins; DCT-1 – divalent cation transporter 1; DMT1 – divalent metal transporter 1; DT – distal tubule; Ent – enterocytes; Erc- erythrocyte; FGF-23 – fibroblast growth factor 23, sFRP-4 – secreted frizzled-related protein 4; GF – glomerular filtration; MEPE – matrix extracellular phosphoglycoprotein; NCX1 – Ca^{2+}-Na$^+$ exchanger; PMCA1b – Ca-dependent ATPase; PT – proximal tubule; Rec – receptor; ROMK – renal outer medullary potassium channel; TRPV6/V5 – transient receptor potential cation channel subfamily V member 5/6; TR – tubular reabsorption; vit – vitamin; ZnT – zinc transporters; W – women; (?) – unknown.

Sources: Hamad and Al-Jamaien, 2010; Kalkwarf and Harrast, 1998; Hallberg, 1998; Straub, 2007; Fujita, 2004; Dawson-Hughes, 1991; Heaney, 2008; Patrick, 1999; Bronner, 1998; Nair and Iyengar, 2009; Whittaker, 1998; Domellöf et al., 2009; Hunt and Vanderpool, 2001; Wapnir, 1998; Olivares et al., 2002; Puig-Domingo and Vila, 2010; Yu et al., 2003; Abdel-Monem and Anderson, 2008; Riley et al., 1986; Ducros, 1992; Daniels, 1996; Leung et al., 2012; Alexander et al., 1967; Nelson et al., 1947; Zimmermann, 2007; Ebel and Günther, 1980; Swaminathan, 2003; Nakel and Miller, 1988; Merizzi, 2012; Lukaski, 2004; Tahiri et al., 2001; Intakes, 1997.

Table 6.6 Physio-chemical properties of minerals

Calcium salts
- $CaCO_3$ (coral calcium, aragonite or calcite) – precipitation in alkaline pH; F_{abs} 30% in fed and fasted state; should be taken with meals. Take before bedtime, if you take iron supplements.
- $Ca_3(PO_4)_2$, $CaSO_4$, $CaCl_2$, Ca-acetate, $Ca(HCO_3)_2$, CaO, $CaHPO_4$, $Ca(H_2PO_4)_2$, $Ca(OH)_2$, Ca-caseinate, Ca-glubionate, Ca-levulinate, Ca-oxalate (the lowest F_{abs}).
- Ca-lactate, Ca-gluconate – less concentrated Ca-salts, not practical for oral supplementation. F_{abs} values increase with increasing doses of Ca-gluconate.
- Hydroxyapatite – not enough studies to recommend its use.
- Ca-citrate, Ca-citrate maleate – better absorbed than $CaCO_3$, indicated for patient with achlorhydria, inflammatory bowel disease, absorption disorders or when takin H_2-antagonists, proton pump inhibitors (soluble in alkaline). Absorbed citrate ions affect urinary pH (which may affect renal clearance of ionizable drugs).
- Aminoacid chelates (bisglycinocalcium, yeast) – higher bioavailability than anorganic salts.
- Bone meal – second generation calcium supplements contaminated with growth factors, proteins and Pb (obtained from bovine bones).
- Active absorbable algal calcium (CaO) – less irritable for gastric mucosa.

Iron salts
- Immediate release of high iron doses – GIT distress due to poor solubility and slow dissolution rates (i.e. slow absorption rate)
- Ferrous salts: $FeSO_4$, $FeCO_3$, $FeCl_2$, FeI_2, $Fe(NO_3)_2$, $Fe_3(PO_4)_2$, ferrous (folate, succinate, lactate, fumarate, glutamate, gluconate, citrate, tartrate, pyrophosphate, glycerophosphate, ascorbate, glycinosulphate, bis glycinate, dextran, fructate maleate, glucate maleate, sucrate maleate, sucrate citrate, sucrate tartrate, sucrate ascorbate).
- Ferric salts: $Fe_2(SO_4)_3$, $FeCl_3$, $FePO_4$, $Fe(OH)_3$, ferric- (pyrophosphate, orthophosphate, albuminate, cacodylate, valerate, ammonium citrate, ammonium tartrate, citrate, potassium tartrate, cholinisocitrate).
- Elemental iron
- Combine slow and fast dissolving salts to modify GIT release and absorption; micronization and emulsification modifies dissolution profiles, film coated sustained release systems prevent unwanted complexation with other minerals in DS or in the diet (higher compliance, no pill burden).
- Add absorption enhancers (i.e. chondroitin sulphate) and antioxidants (mixture of hydrophilic and hydrophobic – vit C and E, bioflavonoids) to prevent oxidation into Fe^{3+} with lower F_{abs} values.
- $FeSO_4$: highly bioavailable but expensive and may oxidize other present substances (organoleptic/stability issues).

Magnesium salts
- Anorganic: $MgCl_2$ and hydrates, MgO, $Mg(OH)_2$, $MgCO_3$, $Mg_3(PO_4)_2$, $MgHPO_4$,
- Organic: K-Mg-citrate, Mg-citrate, -gluconate, -lactate, -asparate, -taurin, -picolinate, -pidolate, -maleate, -orotate, -glycinate, -levulinate
- Organic salts tend to exhibit higher bioavailability than anorganic.

Continued

Table 6.6 Continued

Zinc salts
- $ZnSO_4$, ZnO, $ZnCl_2$, $ZnCO_3$, Zn-gluconate, Zn-stearate, Zn-acetate, Zn-picolinate, Zn-amino acid complexes.
- $ZnSO_4$ and Zn-acetate exhibit good absorbability; ZnO and $ZnCO_3$ are insoluble and poorly absorbed.

Copper salts
- Anorganic: $CuCl_2$, $CuSO_4$, $CuCO_3$, CuO (bioavailability: $CuSO_4 > CuCO_3 > CuO$)
- Organic: Cu-acetate, Cu-picolinate, Cu-gluconate, Cu-citrate, aminoacid complexes with cysteine, methionine, lysine, glycine
- Amino acid complexes exert higher bioavailability than anorganic salt; exception Cu-cysteine; cysteine reduces Cu^{2+} to Cu^+, which lowers F_{abs} values (solubility issues); competition between amino acids and Cu for uptake transporters.

Iodine salts
- NaI, KI, kelp (brown algae), iodized oil, salt fortification

Selenium salts
- Organic: seleno analogues of aminoacids (seleno methionine/cysteine), selenosulfides
- Anorganic: selenite (SeO_3^{2-}), selenate (SeO_4^{2-})

Chromium salts
- Anorganic: $CrCl_3$
- Organic: Cr(III)-picolinate, nicotinate, glutathione, acetate, tris-acetylacetonate, proprionate, creatine, aminoacid complexes, tris-nuclear Cr complex $(Cr_3O(O_2CCH_2CH_3)_6(H_2O)3)^+$, chromate L-threonate
- Cr^{3+}:amino acid = 1:3 complexes (methionine); higher bioavailability because complexation to amino acids prevents Cr precipitation in alkaline intestinal pH.
- Cr-picolinate: questionable safety (DNA damage in animal studies), poor aqueous solubility, popular salt, the most widely used in supplements.

Manganese salts
- Mn-gluconate, Mn-ascorbate, $MnSO_4$, $MnCl_2$, Mn-amino acid complexes, chondroitin sulphate, glucosamine hydrochloride

Molybdenum salts
- Na-molybdate, ammonium molybdate

Cobalt salts
- $CoSO_4$, $CoCl_2$, Co-complexes with α-hydroxy organic acids (glyceric, glucoheptonic, erythronic, threonic, arabinonic, ribonic, xylonic, gluconic acids).

Phosphor salts
- Monovalent (preferentially Na^+), divalent (Ca^{2+}, Mg^{2+}), trivalent ($Fe3^+$) salts, pyrophosphates (Fe^{3+} or Ca^{2+}); other monovalent inorganic phosphorous salts allowed as food additives.
- K-, Mn-, Ca-glycerophosphates, Mn-hypophosphite

Sources: Saris et al., 2000; Intakes, 1997; Moe, 2008; Guéguen and Pointillart, 2000; Cavalier et al., 2009; Romani, 2008; Heaney et al., 2003; Hansen et al., 2008; Ziegler and Filer Jr, 1996; Lynch, 1997; Brody, 1999; Anderson, 1997; Kobla and Volpe, 2000; Rubin et al., 1998; Shils et al., 2005; Krupanidhi et al., 2008; Rosado, 2003; Cousins et al., 2006; McKenna et al., 1997; Santamaria, 2008; Turnlund et al., 1995; Cerklewski, 1997; Herbert, 1999; Finley, 2008.

than specified on the packaging. Therefore, the degree of mineral–drug PK interactions may be less pronounced than was identified in the literature review.

The most pronounced and clinically relevant PK interactions were identified between divalent and polyvalent minerals and bisphosphonates, quinolones, tetracyclines, levothyroxine, and penicillamine, which form unabsorbable complexes. Minerals also compete among themselves for active uptake in the intestine and kidneys. Additionally, drugs frequently change renal elimination of minerals and vice versa. No interactions pertaining to drug metabolizing enzymes were identified.

6.11 Minerals: summary

Key points to note are:

- Gut lumen and kidneys are the predominant sites for PK mineral–drug interactions.
- Minerals should thus be taken 2 h before, or 2–4 h after, drug intake to avoid changing luminal pH and drug complexation to insoluble complexes in the gut.
- Populations at risk for deficiency should administer minerals as mono-mineral products to avoid interactions between consumed minerals in the gut or in the kidneys.

References

Abdel-Monem, M. M. and Anderson, M. D. (2008). Chromium (III) alpha amino acid complexes. Google Patents.

Abrahamsson, K., Holme, E., Jodal, U., Lindstedt, S. and Nordin, I. (1995). Effect of short-term treatment with pivalic acid containing antibiotics on serum carnitine concentration – a risk irrespective of age. *Biochem Mol Med*, 55, 77–79.

Alexander, W., Harden, R. M., Harrison, M. and Shimmins, J. (1967). Some aspects of the absorption and concentration of iodide by the alimentary tract in man. *Proc Nutr Soc*, 26, 62–67.

Alvarez, L. I., Saumell, C. A., Sanchez, S. F. and Lanusse, C. E. (1996). Plasma disposition kinetics of albendazole metabolites in pigs fed different diets. *Res Vet Sci*, 60, 152–156.

Amidon, G. L. and Lee, H. J. (1994). Absorption of peptide and peptidomimetic drugs. *Annu Rev Pharmacol Toxicol*, 34, 321–341.

Atkinson, H. C. and Begg, E. J. (1988). The binding of drugs to major human milk whey proteins. *Br J Clin Pharmacol*, 26, 107–109.

Augustin, K., Frank, J., Augustin, S., Langguth, P., Ohrvik, V., Witthoft, C., Rimbach, G. and Wolffram, S. (2009). Green tea extracts lower serum folates in rats at very high dietary concentrations only and do not affect plasma folates in a human pilot study. *Acta Physiol Polonica*, 12, 103.

Barditch-Crovo, P., Toole, J., Hendrix, C. W., Cundy, K. C., Ebeling, D., Jaffe, H. S. and Lietman, P. S. (1997). Anti-human immunodeficiency virus (HIV) Activity, Safety, and pharmacokinetics of adefovir dipivoxil (9-[2-(bis-pivaloyloxymethyl)-phosphonylmethoxyethyl]adenine) in HIV-infected patients. *J Infect Dis*, 176, 406–413.

Barrowma, J., Dmello, A. and Herxheim, A. (1973). Single dose of neomycin impairs absorption of vitamin-a (retinol) in man. *Eur J Clin Pharmacol*, 5, 199–201.

Belli, D. C., Levy, E., Darling, P., Leroy, C., Lepage, G., Giguere, R. and Roy, C. C. (1987). Taurine improves the absorption of a fat meal in patients with cystic fibrosis. *Pediatrics,* 80, 517–523.

Beneke, C. E., Viljoen, A. M. and Hamman, J. H. (2009). Polymeric plant-derived excipients in drug delivery. *Molecules,* 14, 2602–2620.

Blanchard, J., Tozer, T. N. and Rowland, M. (1997). Pharmacokinetic perspectives on megadoses of ascorbic acid. *Am J Clin Nutr,* 66, 1165–1171.

Booth, S. L., Lichtenstein, A. H. and Dallal, G. E. (2002). Phylloquinone absorption from phylloquinone-fortified oil is greater than from a vegetable in younger and older men and women. *J Nutr,* 132, 2609–2612.

Borel, P., Pasquier, B., Armand, M., Tyssandier, V., Grolier, P., Alexandre-Gouabau, M. C., Andre, M., Senft, M., Peyrot, J., Jaussan, V., Lairon, D. and Azais-Braesco, V. (2001). Processing of vitamin A and E in the human gastrointestinal tract. *Am J Physiol Gastrointest Liver Physiol,* 280, G95-G103.

Botez, M. I. and Young, S. N. (1991). Effects of anticonvulsant treatment and low levels of folate and thiamine on amine metabolites in cerebrospinal fluid. *Brain,* 114 (Pt 1A), 333–348.

Boudry, G., David, E. S., Douard, V., Monteiro, I. M., Le Huërou-Luron, I. and Ferraris, R. P. (2010). Role of intestinal transporters in neonatal nutrition: carbohydrates, proteins, lipids, minerals, and vitamins. *J Pediatr gastroenterol Nutr,* 51, 380–401.

Boullata, J. I. and Armenti, V. T. (2009). *Handbook of Drug-Nutrient Interactions,* Humana Press, New Jersey NJ.

Brodin, B., Nielsen, C. U., Steffansen, B. and Frokjaer, S. (2002). Transport of peptidomimetic drugs by the intestinal Di/tri-peptide Transporter, PepT1. *Pharmacol Toxicol,* 90, 285–296.

Brody, T. (1999). *Nutritional Biochemistry,* Academic Press, California USA.

Bronner, F. (1998). Calcium absorption – a paradigm for mineral absorption. *J Nutr,* 128, 917–920.

Cannell, J. J. and Hollis, B. W. (2008). Use of vitamin D in clinical practice. *Altern Med Rev,* 13, 6–20.

Cao, F., Gao, Y. and Ping, Q. (2012). Advances in research of PepT1-targeted prodrug. *Asian J Pharm Sci,* 7, 110–122.

Carmel, R. (2008). Efficacy and safety of fortification and supplementation with vitamin B12: biochemical and physiological effects. *Food Nutr Bulletin,* 29, 177–187.

Cavalier, E., Delanaye, P., Chapelle, J.-P. and Souberbielle, J.-C. (2009). Vitamin D: current status and perspectives. *Clin Chem Lab Med,* 47, 120–127.

Cerklewski, F. L. (1997). Fluoride bioavailability – nutritional and clinical aspects. *Nutr Res,* 17, 907–929.

Christian, P. and West, K. P. (1998). Interactions between zinc and vitamin A: an update. *American J Clin Nutr,* 68, 435s-441s.

Civitelli, R. (1993). The 1992 John M. Kinney International Award for Nutrition and Metabolism. Dietary L-lysine and calcium metabolism in humans: background. *Nutrition,* 9, 299–300.

Cousins, R. J., Liuzzi, J. P. and Lichten, L. A. (2006). Mammalian zinc transport, trafficking, and signals. *J Biol Chem,* 281, 24085–24089.

Daniels, L. A. (1996). Selenium metabolism and bioavailability. *Biol Trace Element Res,* 54, 185–199.

Dawson-Hughes, B. (1991). Calcium supplementation and bone loss: a review of controlled clinical trials. *Am J Clin Nutr,* 54, 274S–280S.

Debier, C. and Larondelle, Y. (2005). Vitamins A and E: metabolism, roles and transfer to offspring. *Br J Nutr,* 93, 153–174.

DI Salvo, M. L., Contestabile, R. and Safo, M. K. (2011). Vitamin B(6) salvage enzymes: Mechanism, structure and regulation. *Biochim Biophys Acta (BBA)-Proteins Proteom,* 1814, 1597–1608.

Diao, L. and Polli, J. E. (2011). Synthesis and in vitro characterization of drug conjugates of l-carnitine as potential prodrugs that target human Octn2. *J Pharm Sci,* 100, 3802–3816.

Domellöf, M., Hernell, O., Abrams, S. A., Chen, Z. and LÖnnerdal, B. (2009). Iron supplementation does not affect copper and zinc absorption in breastfed infants. *Am J Clin Nutr,* 89, 185–190.

Ducros, V. (1992). Chromium metabolism. *Biolo Trace Element Res,* 32, 65–77.

Ebel, H. and GÜnther, T. (1980). Magnesium metabolism: a review. *Clin Chem Lab Med,* 18, 257–270.

Ekins, S., Diao, L. and Polli, J. E. (2012). A substrate pharmacophore for the human organic cation/carnitine transporter identifies compounds associated with rhabdomyolysis. *Mol Pharm,* 9, 905–913.

El-Kattan, A. and Varma, M. (2012). Oral absorption, intestinal metabolism and human oral bioavailability. http://www.intechopen.com/books/topics-on-drug-metabolism/oral-absorption-intestinal-metabolism-and-human-oral-bioavailability-

Finley, J. W. (2008). Bioavailability of selenium from foods. *Nutr Rev,* 64, 146–151.

Fleisher, D., Li, C., Zhou, Y., Pao, L. H. and Karim, A. (1999). Drug, meal and formulation interactions influencing drug absorption after oral administration. Clinical implications. *Clin Pharmacokinet,* 36, 233–254.

Fujita, T. (2004). Active Absorbable Algal Calcium (AAA Ca): new Japanese technology for osteoporosis and calcium paradox disease. *Japi,* 52, 563–567. http://japi.org/july2004/U-564.pdf?origin=publication_detail.

Fujita, T., Nakamura, K., Yamazaki, A., Ozaki, M., Sahashi, K., Shichijo, K., Nomura, K., Maeda, M., Nakamura, T., Yokota, S., Kuroyama, S., Kumagai, Y., Majima, M. and Ohtani, Y. (2007). Effect of L-phenylalanine supplementation and a high-protein diet on pharmacokinetics of cefdinir in healthy volunteers: an exploratory study. *J Clin Pharm Ther,* 32, 277–285.

Fukumori, S., Murata, T., Takaai, M., Tahara, K., Taguchi, M. and Hashimoto, Y. (2008). The apical uptake transporter of levofloxacin is distinct from the peptide transporter in human intestinal epithelial Caco-2 cells. *Drug Metab Pharmacokinet,* 23, 373–378.

Gibney, M. J., Lanham-New, S. A., Cassidy, A. and Vorster, H. H. (2009). *Introduction to Human Nutrition,* John Wiley & Sons Ltd, The Atrium, Southern Gate, Chichester, West Sussex, UK.

Gidal, B. E., Maly, M. M., Budde, J., Lensmeyer, G. L., Pitterle, M. E. and Jones, J. C. (1996). Effect of a high-protein meal on gabapentin pharmacokinetics. *Epilepsy Res,* 23, 71–76.

Gijsbers, B. L., Jie, K. S. and Vermeer, C. (1996). Effect of food composition on vitamin K absorption in human volunteers. *Br J Nutr,* 76, 223–229.

Goldman, R. D., Rogovik, A. L., Lai, D. and Vohra, S. (2008). Potential interactions of drug–natural health products and natural health products–natural health products among children. *J Pediatr,* 152, 521–526. e4.

Goodman, B. E. (2010). Insights into digestion and absorption of major nutrients in humans. *Adv Physiol Educ,* 34, 44–453.

Goole, J., Lindley, D. J., Roth, W., Carl, S. M., Amighi, K., Kauffmann, J.-M. and Knipp, G. T. (2010). The effects of excipients on transporter mediated absorption. *Int J Pharm,* 393, 17–31.

Gropper, S. S. and Smith, J. L. (2012). *Advanced Nutrition and Human Metabolism*, Wadsworth Publishing Company, Belmont USA.
Guéguen, L. and Pointillart, A. (2000). The bioavailability of dietary calcium. *J Am Coll Nutr,* 19, 119S–136S.
Halestrap, A. P. and Meredith, D. (2004). The SLC16 gene family-from monocarboxylate transporters (MCTs) to aromatic amino acid transporters and beyond. *Pflugers Arch,* 447, 619–628.
Hallberg, L. (1998). Does calcium interfere with iron absorption? *Am J Clin Nutr,* 68, 3–4.
Hamad, A.-W. R. and AL-Jamaien, H. H. (2010). Study of the bioavailability and clinical studies of calcium-magnesium tablets. *Pak J Nutr,* 9, 1162–1165.
Hanhineva, K., Torronen, R., Bondia-Pons, I., Pekkinen, J., Kolehmainen, M., Mykkanen, H. and Poutanen, K. (2010). Impact of dietary polyphenols on carbohydrate metabolism. *Int J Mol Sci,* 11, 1365–1402.
Hansen, K. E., Jones, A. N., Lindstrom, M. J., Davis, L. A., Engelke, J. A. and Shafer, M. M. (2008). Vitamin D insufficiency: disease or no disease? *J Bone Miner Res,* 23, 1052–1060.
Harrison, E. H. and Hussain, M. M. (2001). Mechanisms involved in the intestinal digestion and absorption of dietary vitamin A. *J Nutr,* 131, 1405–1408.
Heaney, R. P. (2008). Vitamin D and calcium interactions: functional outcomes. *Am J Clin Nutr,* 88, 541S-544S.
Heaney, R. P., Dowell, M. S., Hale, C. A. and Bendich, A. (2003). Calcium absorption varies within the reference range for serum 25-hydroxyvitamin D. *J Am Coll Nutr,* 22, 142–146.
Herbert, V. (1999). Advanced nutrition micronutrients. *Am J Clin Nutr,* 69, 161–161.
Heuberger, W., Berardi, S., Jacky, E., Pey, P. and Krahenbuhl, S. (1998). Increased urinary excretion of carnitine in patients treated with cisplatin. *Eur J Clin Pharmacol,* 54, 503–508.
Hirano, T., Yasuda, S., Osaka, Y., Asari, M., Kobayashi, M., Itagaki, S. and Iseki, K. (2008). The inhibitory effects of fluoroquinolones on L-carnitine transport in placental cell line BeWo. *Int J Pharm,* 351, 113–118.
Hite, A. H., Feinman, R. D., Guzman, G. E., Satin, M., Schoenfeld, P. A. and Wood, R. J. (2010). In the face of contradictory evidence: Report of the Dietary Guidelines for Americans Committee. *Nutrition,* 26, 915–924.
Holme, E., Greter, J., Jacobson, C. E., Lindstedt, S., Nordin, I., Kristiansson, B. and Jodal, U. (1989). Carnitine deficiency induced by pivampicillin and pivmecillinam therapy. *Lancet,* 2, 469–473.
Howarth, N. C., Saltzman, E. and Roberts, S. B. (2001). Dietary fiber and weight regulation. *Nutr Rev,* 59, 129–139.
Hug, G., Mcgraw, C. A., Bates, S. R. and Landrigan, E. A. (1991). Reduction of serum carnitine concentrations during anticonvulsant therapy with Phenobarbital, valproic Acid, Phenytoin, and carbamazepine in children. *J Pediatr,* 119, 799–802.
Hulmi, J. J., Volek, J. S., Selanne, H. and Mero, A. A. (2005). Protein ingestion prior to strength exercise affects blood hormones and metabolism. *Med Sci Sports Exerc,* 37, 1990–1997.
Hunt, J. R. and Vanderpool, R. A. (2001). Apparent copper absorption from a vegetarian diet. *Am J Clin Nutr,* 74, 803–807.
Indiveri, C., Pochini, L., Oppedisano, F. and Tonazzi, A. (2010). The carnitine transporter network: interactions with drugs. *Curr Chem Biol,* 4, 108–123.
Intakes, Institute of Medicine Dietary Reference Intakes for Calcium, Phosphorus, Magnesium, Vitamin D, and Fluoride (1997). *Dietary Reference Intakes: For Calcium, Phosphorus, Magnesium, Vitamin D, and Fluoride,* National Academies Press, Washington, DC.

Isaji, M. (2011). SGLT2 inhibitors: molecular design and potential differences in effect. *Kidney Int Suppl*, S14-9.
Ismail, M. Y. M. (2009). Drug-food interactions and role of pharmacist. *Asian J Pharmaceu Clin Res*, 2(4), http://www.ajpcr.com/Vol2Issue4/226.pdf.
Jabbour, S. A. and Goldstein, B. J. (2008). Sodium glucose co-transporter 2 inhibitors: blocking renal tubular reabsorption of glucose to improve glycaemic control in patients with diabetes. *Int J Clin Pract*, 62, 1279–1284.
Jeffries, G., Todd, J. and Sleisenger, M. (1966). The effect of prednisolone on gastric mucosal Histology, gastric Secretion, and vitamin B 12 absorption in patients with pernicious anemia. *J Clin Invest*, 45, 803.
Jones, G. (2008). Pharmacokinetics of vitamin D toxicity. *Am J Clin Nutr*, 88, 582S-586S.
Juan, D., Worwag, E. M., Schoeller, D. A., Kotake, A. N., Hughes, R. L. and Frederiksen, M. C. (1986). Effects of dietary protein on theophylline pharmacokinetics and caffeine and aminopyrine breath tests. *Clin Pharmacol Ther*, 40, 187–194.
Kagan, L., Lapidot, N., Afargan, M., Kirmayer, D., Moor, E., Mardor, Y., Friedman, M. and Hoffman, A. (2006). Gastroretentive accordion pill: enhancement of riboflavin bioavailability in humans. *J Control Release*, 113, 208–215.
Kalkwarf, H. J. and Harrast, S. D. (1998). Effects of calcium supplementation and lactation on iron status. *Am J Clin Nutr*, 67, 1244–1249.
Kappas, A., Anderson, K. E., Conney, A. H., Pantuck, E. J., Fishman, J. and Bradlow, H. L. (1983). Nutrition-endocrine interactions: induction of reciprocal changes in the delta 4–5 alpha-reduction of testosterone and the cytochrome P-450-dependent oxidation of estradiol by dietary macronutrients in man. *Proc Natl Acad Sci*, 80, 7646–7649.
Katz, H. I., Waalen, J. and Leach, E. E. (1999). Acitretin in psoriasis: an overview of adverse effects. *J Am Acad Dermatol*, 41, S7-S12.
Kobla, H. V. and Volpe, S. L. (2000). Chromium, exercise, and body composition. *Crit Rev Food Sci and Nutr*, 40, 291–308.
Kreider, R. B., Almada, A. L., Antonio, J., Broeder, C., Earnest, C., Greenwood, M., Incledon, T., Kalman, D. S., Kleiner, S. M. and Leutholtz, B. (2004). ISSN exercise and sport nutrition review: research and recommendations. *Sports Nutr Rev J*, 1, 1–44.
Krupanidhi, S., Sreekumar, A. and Sanjeevi, C. (2008). Copper and biological health. *Indian J Med Res*, 128, 448.
Lamon-Fava, S., Sadowski, J. A., Davidson, K. W., O'Brien, M. E., Mcnamara, J. R. and Schaefer, E. J. (1998). Plasma lipoproteins as carriers of phylloquinone (vitamin K1) in humans. *Am J Clin Nutr*, 67, 1226–1231.
Lenz, T. L., Lenz, N. J. and Faulkner, M. A. (2004). Potential interactions between exercise and drug therapy. *Sports Med*, 34, 293–306.
Leung, A. M., Braverman, L. E. and Pearce, E. N. (2012). History of US Iodine Fortification and Supplementation. *Nutrients*, 4, 1740–1746.
Lo, C., Paris, P., Clemens, T., Nolan, J. and Holick, M. (1985). Vitamin D absorption in healthy subjects and in patients with intestinal malabsorption syndromes. *Am J Clin Nut*, 42, 644–649.
Löbenberg, R. and Steinke, W. (2006). Investigation of vitamin and mineral tablets and capsules on the Canadian market. *J Pharm Pharm Sci*, 9, 40–49.
Lukaski, H. C. (2004). Vitamin and mineral status: effects on physical performance, *Nutrition*, 20(7), 632–644.
Lynch, S. R. (1997). Interaction of iron with other nutrients. *Nutr Rev*, 55, 102–110.
Ma, K. (2010). *Role, Relevance and Regulation of Pept1 in Peptide Intestinal Absorption.* The University of Michigan.

Marcuard, S. P., Albernaz, L. and Khazanie, P. G. (1994). Omeprazole therapy causes malabsorption of cyanocobalamin (vitamin B12). *Ann Intern Med,* 120, 211.
Marthaler, N. P., Visarius, T., Kupfer, A. and Lauterburg, B. H. (1999). Increased urinary losses of carnitine during ifosfamide chemotherapy. *Cancer Chemother Pharmacol,* 44, 170–172.
Maswadeh, H. and AL-Jarbou, A. (2011). An investigation on physical quality control parameters of dietary supplements tablets commercially available on the Kingdom of Saudi Arabia. *Int J Appl Res Nat Prod,* 4, 22–26.
Mckenna, A. A., Ilich, J. Z., Andon, M. B., Wang, C. and Matkovic, V. (1997). Zinc balance in adolescent females consuming a low-or high-calcium diet. *Am J Clin Nutr,* 65, 1460–1464.
Meletis, C. D. and Zabriskie, N. (2007). Common nutrient depletions caused by pharmaceuticals. *Altern Complement Ther,* 13, 10–17.
Menon, R. M., González, M. A., Adams, M. H., Tolbert, D. S., Leu, J. H. and Cefali, E. A. (2007). Effect of the rate of niacin administration on the plasma and urine pharmacokinetics of niacin and its metabolites. *J Clin Pharmacol,* 47, 681–688.
Merizzi, G. (2012). Food supplement composition suitable for promoting iron absorption. Google Patents.
Moe, S. M. (2008). Disorders involving calcium, phosphorus, and magnesium. *Primary Care: Clin Office Practice,* 35, 215–237.
Nabokina, S. M., Kashyap, M. L. and Said, H. M. (2005). Mechanism and regulation of human intestinal niacin uptake. *Am J Physiol Cell Physiol,* 289, C97-103.
Nagaoka, K., Aoki, F., Hayashi, M., Muroi, Y., Sakurai, T., Itoh, K., Ikawa, M., Okabe, M., Imakawa, K. and Sakai, S. (2009). L-amino acid oxidase plays a crucial role in host defense in the mammary glands. *FASEB J,* 23, 2514–2520.
Nair, K. M. and Iyengar, V. (2009). Iron content, bioavailability and factors affecting iron status of Indians. *Indian J Med Res,* 130, 634.
Nakel, G. M. and Miller, S. M. (1988). Iron mineral supplements. Google Patents.
Nelson, N., Palmes, E. D., Park, C. R., Weymouth, P. P. and Bean, W. B. (1947). The Absorption, Excretion, and physiological effect of iodine in normal human subjects. *J Clin Invest,* 26, 301.
Nutescu, E. A., Shapiro, N. L., Ibrahim, S. and West, P. (2006). Warfarin and its interactions with foods, herbs and other dietary supplements. *Expert Opin Drug Saf,* 5, 433–451.
Ohnishi, N. and Yokoyama, T. (2004). Interactions between medicines and functional foods or dietary supplements. *Keio J Med,* 53, 137–150.
Olivares, M., Lönnerdal, B., Abrams, S. A., Pizarro, F. and Uauy, R. (2002). Age and copper intake do not affect copper absorption, measured with the use of 65Cu as a tracer, in young infants. *Am J Clin Nutr,* 76, 641–645.
Panakanti, R. and Narang, A. S. (2012). Impact of Excipient Interactions on Drug Bioavailability from Solid Dosage Forms. *Pharm Res,* 1–21.
Patrick, L. (1999). Comparative absorption of calcium sources and calcium citrate malate for the prevention of osteoporosis. *Alter Med Rev: J Clin Ther,* 4, 74.
Persky, A. M. and Brazeau, G. A. (2001). Clinical pharmacology of the dietary supplement creatine monohydrate. *Pharmacol Rev,* 53, 161–176.
Persky, A. M., Brazeau, G. A. and Hochhaus, G. (2003). Pharmacokinetics of the dietary supplement creatine. *Clin Pharmacokinet,* 42, 557–574.
Phillips, G. O. (1998). Acacia gum (Gum Arabic): a nutritional fibre; metabolism and calorific value. *Food Addit Contam,* 15, 251–264.
Pinto, J. T. and Rivlin, R. S. (1987). Drugs That Promote Renal Excretion of Riboflavin. *Drug-Nutrient Interactions,* 5, 143–151.

Preedy, V. R. and Watson, R. (2007). *The Encyclopedia of Vitamin E*, CABI.
Prosser, D. E. and Jones, G. (2004). Enzymes involved in the activation and inactivation of vitamin D. *Trends Biochem Sci*, 29, 664–673.
Puig-Domingo, M. and Vila, L. (2010). Iodine status, thyroid and pregnancy. *Hot Thyroidol Eta*, 1.
Puntheeranurak, T., Wimmer, B., Castaneda, F., Gruber, H. J., Hinterdorfer, P. and Kinne, R. K. (2007). Substrate specificity of sugar transport by rabbit SGLT1: single-molecule atomic force microscopy versus transport studies. *Biochemistry*, 46, 2797–2804.
Quan, Z. F., Yang, C., Li, N. and Li, J. S. (2004). Effect of glutamine on change in early post-operative intestinal permeability and its relation to systemic inflammatory response. *World J Gastroenterol*, 10, 1992–1994.
Ravi Kumar, M. N. (2000). A review of chitin and chitosan applications. *Reactive Funct Polym*, 46, 1–27.
Riley, D. P., Anderson, M. M. and Rotruck, J. T. (1986). Chromium acetylacetonate as a dietary supplement and pharmaceutical agent. Google Patents.
Robert, B. S., David, M. E. and Russell, S. P. (2004). Common dietary supplements for weight loss. *Am Fam Physician*, 70, 1731–1738.
Robertson, D. R., Higginson, I., Macklin, B. S., Renwick, A. G., Waller, D. G. and George, C. F. (1991). The influence of protein containing meals on the pharmacokinetics of levodopa in healthy volunteers. *Br J Clin Pharmacol*, 31, 413–417.
Rogovik, A. L., Vohra, S. and Goldman, R. D. (2010). Safety considerations and potential interactions of vitamins: should vitamins be considered drugs? *Ann Pharmacother*, 44, 311–324.
Romani, A. (2008). Magnesium homeostasis and alcohol consumption. *Magnes Res*, 21, 197–204.
Rosado, J. L. (2003). Zinc and copper: proposed fortification levels and recommended zinc compounds. *J Nutr*, 133, 2985S-2989S.
Ross, A. H., Eastwood, M. A., Brydon, W. G., Anderson, J. R. and Anderson, D. M. 1983. A study of the effects of dietary gum arabic in humans. *Am J Clin Nutr*, 37, 368–375.
Rowe, D. J. and Baker, A. C. (2009). Perioperative risks and benefits of herbal supplements in aesthetic surgery. *Aesthet Surg J*, 29, 150–157.
Rubin, M. A., Miller, J. P., Ryan, A. S., Treuth, M. S., Patterson, K. Y., Pratley, R. E., Hurley, B. F., Veillon, C., MOSER-Veillon, P. B. and Anderson, R. A. (1998). Acute and chronic resistive exercise increase urinary chromium excretion in men as measured with an enriched chromium stable isotope. *J Nutr*, 128, 73–78.
Rumsey, S. C. and Levine, M. (1998). Absorption, Transport, and disposition of ascorbic acid in humans. *J Nutr Biochem*, 9, 116–130.
Russell, R. M., Golner, B. B., Krasinski, S. D., Sadowski, J. A., Suter, P. M. and Braun, C. L. (1988). Effect of antacid and H2 receptor antagonists on the intestinal absorption of folic acid. *J Lab Clin Med*, 112, 458–463.
Rustom, R., Maltby, P., Grime, J. S., Stockdale, H. R., Critchley, M. and Bone, J. M. (1992). Effects of lysine infusion on the renal metabolism of aprotinin (Trasylol) in man. *Clin Sci (Lond)*, 83, 295–299.
Sachan, D. S. (1975). Effects of low and high protein diets on the induction of microsomal drug-metabolizing enzymes in rat liver. *J Nutr*, 105, 1631–1639.
Sahai, J., Gallicano, K., Garber, G., Mcgilveray, I., Hawley-Foss, N., Turgeon, N. and Cameron, D. W. (1992). The effect of a protein meal on zidovudine pharmacokinetics in HIV-infected patients. *Br J Clin Pharmacol*, 33, 657–660.
Said, H. M. (2004). Recent advances in carrier-mediated intestinal absorption of water-soluble vitamins. *Annu Rev Physiol*, 66, 419–446.

Said, H. M. (2009). Cell and molecular aspects of human intestinal biotin absorption. *J Nutr,* 139, 158–162.

Said, H. M. (2011). Intestinal absorption of water-soluble vitamins in health and disease. *Biochem J,* 437, 357–372.

Santamaria, A. (2008). Manganese Exposure, essentiality and toxicity. *Indian J Med Res,* 128, 484.

Sayed-Ahmed, M. M. (2010). Progression of cyclophosphamide-induced acute renal metabolic damage in carnitine-depleted rat model. *Clin Exp Nephrol,* 14, 418–426.

Schaafsma, G. (2009). Safety of protein hydrolysates, fractions thereof and bioactive peptides in human nutrition. *Eur J Clin Nutr,* 63, 1161–1168.

Schmidt, L. E. and Dalhoff, K. 2002. Food-drug interactions. *Drugs,* 62, 1481–1502.

Selhub, J., Dhar, G. J. and Rosenberg, I. H. (1978). Inhibition of folate enzymes by sulfasalazine. *J Clin Invest,* 61, 221–224.

Semino-Mora, M. C., Leon-Monzon, M. E. and Dalakas, M. C. (1994). Effect of L-carnitine on the zidovudine-induced destruction of human myotubes. Part I: L-carnitine prevents the myotoxicity of AZT in vitro. *Lab Invest,* 71, 102–112.

Shils, M. E., Shike, M., Ross, A. C., Caballero, B. and Cousins, R. J. (2005). *Modern nutrition in Health and Disease,* Lippincott Williams and Wilkins, http://books.google.com/books?hl=en&lr=&id=S5oCjZZZ1ggC&oi=fnd&pg=PA3&ots=2xHCt0iMvC&sig=0znPqZkdMd2iZUrmpgFqDjvjU40#v=onepage&q&f=false.

Shimizu, K., Saito, A., Shimada, J., Ohmichi, M., Hiraga, Y., Inamatsu, T., Shimada, K., Tanimura, M., Fujita, Y., Nishikawa, T. and ET AL. (1993). Carnitine status and safety after administration of S-1108, a new oral Cephem, to patients. *Antimicrob Agents Chemother,* 37, 1043–1049.

Sirdah, M. M., EL-Agouza, I. M. and ABU Shahla, A. N. (2002). Possible ameliorative effect of taurine in the treatment of iron-deficiency anaemia in female university students of Gaza, Palestine. *Eur J Haematol,* 69, 236–242.

Steffansen, B., Nielsen, C. U., Brodin, B., Eriksson, A. H., Andersen, R. and Frokjaer, S. (2004a). Intestinal solute carriers: an overview of trends and strategies for improving oral drug absorption. *Eur J Pharm Sci,* 21, 3–16.

Steffansen, B., Nielsen, C. U., Brodin, B., Eriksson, A. H., Andersen, R. and Frokjaer, S. (2004b). Intestinal solute carriers: an overview of trends and strategies for improving oral drug absorption. *Eur J Pharm Sci,* 21, 3–16.

Stoimenova, A. (2010). Food supplements in Central and Eastern European countries. *Acta Med Bulg,* 1, 71–77.

Straub, D. A. (2007). Calcium supplementation in clinical practice: a review of forms, doses, and indications. *Nutr Clin Practice,* 22, 286–296.

Sundlof, S. F. and Kellermann, P. (2009). Multivitamins: Supplements or Substitutes? http://www.personal.psu.edu/users/p/m/pmk8/202C/RecReport-sample-09a.pdf.

Swaminathan, R. (2003). Magnesium metabolism and its disorders. *Clin Biochem Rev,* 24, 47.

Tahiri, M., Tressol, J. C., Arnaud, J., Bornet, F., Bouteloup – Demange, C., Feillet – Coudray, C., Ducros, V., PÉpin, D., Brouns, F. and Roussel, A. M. (2001). Five – week intake of short – chain fructo – oligosaccharides increases intestinal absorption and status of magnesium in postmenopausal women. *J Bone Miner Res,* 16, 2152–2160.

Ten Dam, M. A., Zwiers, A., Crusius, J. B., Pals, G., Van Kamp, G. J., Meuwissen, S. G., Donker, A. J. and TEN Kate, R. W. (1991). Tubular reabsorption of pepsinogen isozymogens in man studied by the inhibition of tubular protein reabsorption with dibasic amino acids. *Clin Sci (Lond),* 80, 161–166.

Thomas, J. A. and Burns, R. A. (1998). Important drug-nutrient interactions in the elderly. *Drugs Aging*, 13, 199–209.
Thorp, V. J. (1980). Effect of oral contraceptive agents on vitamin and mineral requirements. *J Am Diet Assoc*, 76, 581–584.
Thurnham, D. I. (2004). An overview of interactions between micronutrients and of micronutrients with drugs, genes and immune mechanisms. *Nutr Res Rev*, 17, 211–240.
Trovato, A., Nuhlicek, D. N. and Midtling, J. E. (1991). Drug-nutrient interactions. *Am Fam Phys*, 44, 1651–1658.
Turnlund, J., Keyes, W. R. and Peiffer, G. L. (1995). Molybdenum absorption, excretion, and retention studied with stable isotopes in young men at five intakes of dietary molybdenum. *Am J Clin Nutr*, 62, 790–796.
Tyson, J. E., Lasky, R., Flood, D., Mize, C., Picone, T. and Paule, C. L. (1989). Randomized trial of taurine supplementation for infants less-than-or-equal-to 1,300-gram birthweight – effect on auditory Brainstem-Evoked responses. *Pediatrics*, 83, 406–415.
Uchino, H., Kanai, Y., Kim, D. K., Wempe, M. F., Chairoungdua, A., Morimoto, E., Anders, M. W. and Endou, H. (2002). Transport of amino acid-related compounds mediated by L-type amino acid transporter 1 (LAT1): Insights into the mechanisms of substrate recognition. *Mole Pharmacol*, 61, 729–737.
Van den Berg, H. (1997). Bioavailability of pantothenic acid. *Eur J Clin Nutr*, 51, S62.
Vitaglione, P., Napolitano, A. and Fogliano, V. (2008). Cereal dietary fibre: a natural functional ingredient to deliver phenolic compounds into the gut. *Trends Food Sci Technol*, 19, 451–463.
Voss, A. A., Diez-Sampedro, A., Hirayama, B. A., Loo, D. D. and Wright, E. M. (2007). Imino sugars are potent agonists of the human glucose sensor SGLT3. *Mole Pharmacol*, 71, 628–634.
Walgren, R. A., Lin, J. T., Kinne, R. K. and Walle, T. (2000). Cellular uptake of dietary flavonoid quercetin 4′-beta-glucoside by sodium-dependent glucose transporter SGLT1. *J Pharmacol Exp Ther*, 294, 837–843.
Walter, E., Kissel, T. and Amidon, G. L. (1996). The intestinal peptide carrier: A potential transport system for small peptide derived drugs. *Adv Drug Deliv Rev*, 20, 33–58.
Wang, W. Y. and Liaw, K. Y. (1991). Effect of a taurine-supplemented diet on conjugated bile acids in biliary surgical patients. *JPEN J Parenter Enteral Nutr*, 15, 294–297.
Wapnir, R. A. (1998). Copper absorption and bioavailability. *Am J Clin Nutr*, 67, 1054S–1060S.
Welsh, J. A., Sharma, A., Abramson, J. L., Vaccarino, V., Gillespie, C. and Vos, M. B. (2010). Caloric sweetener consumption and dyslipidemia among US adults. *JAMA: J Am Med Assoc*, 303, 1490–1497.
White, R. (2010). Drugs and nutrition: how side-effects can influence nutritional intake. *Proc Nutr Soc*, 69, 558–564.
Whittaker, P. (1998). Iron and zinc interactions in humans. *Am J Clin Nutr*, 68, 442S–446S.
Williams, M. (2005). Dietary supplements and sports performance: amino acids. *J Int Soc Sports Nutr*, 2, 63–67.
Wood, I. S. and Trayhurn, P. (2003). Glucose transporters (GLUT and SGLT): expanded families of sugar transport proteins. *Br J Nutr*, 89, 3–9.
Wortsman, J., Matsuoka, L. Y., Chen, T. C., Lu, Z. and Holick, M. F. (2000). Decreased bioavailability of vitamin D in obesity. *Am J Clin Nutr*, 72, 690–693.
Yamamoto, S., Inoue, K., Ohta, K. Y., Fukatsu, R., Maeda, J. Y., Yoshida, Y. and Yuasa, H. (2009). Identification and functional characterization of rat riboflavin transporter 2. *J Biochem*, 145, 437–443.

Yanagida, O., Kanai, Y., Chairoungdua, A., Kim, D. K., Segawa, H., Nii, T., Cha, S. H., Matsuo, H., Fukushima, J., Fukasawa, Y., Tani, Y., Taketani, Y., Uchino, H., Kim, J. Y., Inatomi, J., Okayasu, I., Miyamoto, K., Takeda, E., Goya, T. and Endou, H. (2001). Human L-type amino acid transporter 1 (LAT1): characterization of function and expression in tumor cell lines. *Biochim Biophys Acta*, 1514, 291–302.

Yetley, E. A. (2007). Multivitamin and multimineral dietary supplements: Definitions, Characterization, Bioavailability, and drug interactions. *Am J Clin Nutr*, 85, 269S-276S.

Yoshida, S., Kaibara, A., Ishibashi, N. and Shirouzu, K. (2001). Glutamine supplementation in cancer patients. *Nutrition*, 17, 766–768.

Younis, I. R. (2003). *Pharmaceutical Quality Performance of Folic Acid Supplements*. West Virginia University.

Yu, K., Kou, F. and Wang, Z. (2003). Chromium L-Threonate, process for preparation of the same and their use. Google Patents.

Zangen, A., Botzer, D., Zangen, R. and Shainberg, A. (1998). Furosemide and digoxin inhibit thiamine uptake in cardiac cells. *Eur J Pharmacol*, 361, 151–155.

Zempleni, J. (2005). Uptake, localization, and noncarboxylase roles of biotin*. *Annu Rev Nutr*, 25, 175–196.

Zhao, R., Matherly, L. H. and Goldman, I. D. (2009). Membrane transporters and folate homeostasis: intestinal absorption and transport into systemic compartments and tissues. *Expert Rev Mol Med*, 11, S1462399409000969.

Ziegler, E. E. and Filer Jr, L. (1996). *Present Knowledge of NUTRITION*, International Life Sciences Institute (ILSI Press).

Zimmermann, M. B. (2007). The impact of iodised salt or iodine supplements on iodine status during Pregnancy, lactation and infancy. *Public Health Nutr*, 10, 1584–1595.

Zlotkin, S. H. and Buchanan, B. E. (1988). Amino acid intake and urinary zinc excretion in newborn infants receiving total parenteral nutrition. *Am J Clin Nutr*, 48, 330–334.

Pharmacodynamic interactions between drugs and dietary supplements

S. Kreft
University of Ljubljana, Ljubljana, Slovenia

7.1 Introduction

Interaction between a food supplement and drug is a situation in which an ingredient of the food supplement affects the activity of some drug when they are administered simultaneously, or within a short time period (e.g. in the same day). In some cases, the interaction can also be reversed: an ingredient of a drug can affect the (nutritional) activity/availability of a food supplement. The interaction can be synergistic (the effect is increased) or antagonistic (the effect is decreased). Interaction can change (increase or decrease) the therapeutic effect, but it can also change an adverse effect. In some cases, a new effect can be induced.

According to the mechanism involved, there are two types of interaction: pharmacokinetic and pharmacodynamic. In pharmacokinetic interactions, changes in the effect of a drug are caused by changes in the absorption, distribution, metabolism or excretion (ADME) of the drug, which result in changed concentration of the drug in the blood and at its action site. Pharmacokinetic interactions have been described in the previous three chapters of this book.

In pharmacodynamic interactions, which are the scope of this chapter, the response of the organism to the drug (the drug's efficacy) is changed without changes in drug concentration.

Interactions vary largely in severity and significance. Patients often do not share information about the supplements they take with their pharmacist and physicians. They assume that supplements are harmless and irrelevant to their medication therapy.

Investigation of interaction is not an easy task. It is often done only after a suspicion of interaction has been raised by observing side effects of concomitant use of food supplements and the medicinal product in practice and/or by theoretical consideration of pharmacological activity of the two products. There are many possible combinations of nutrients and drugs, preventing systematic research of them all. On many occasions, the case reports of interactions are inspired by known pharmacological activities (e.g. valerian and synthetic sedatives), but later systematic research finds no clinical importance of interaction. In this chapter we review only the most important pharmacodynamic interactions, with higher levels of evidence, not based just on suspicion.

7.2 Vitamins

Several minerals are involved in pharmacokinetic interactions with medicinal products, but in most cases the interactions appear only at doses much above the RDA. In this chapter, we report on six vitamins with most clinically relevant interactions.

7.2.1 Vitamin A

Vitamin A can interact with retinoid drugs. Retinoid drugs are compounds similar to vitamin A, such as isotretinoin and acitretin. They are indicated for the treatment of acne and psoriasis. With concomitant use of retinoids and vitamin A, there is concern over vitamin A toxicity.

Owing to ethical concerns, there is not much clinical research available on these topics. In a study from 1986, the disposition of oral isotretinoin to the skin and its effects on the vitamin A levels in serum and skin were studied in 17 patients with nodulocystic acne.[1] All patients received 0.5 mg/kg/day for 3 months and eight patients continued treatment with 0.75 mg/kg/day for another 3 months. The parent drug, the major metabolite (4-oxo-isotretinoin), and two natural retinoids (retinol and dehydroretinol) were monitored in serum and biopsies of uninvolved skin. During the initial 3 months of treatment the mean isotretinoin level in the serum was 145 ng/mL and in the epidermis 73 ng/g. The corresponding values for 4-oxo-isotretinoin were 615 and 113 ng/g, respectively. Even at the highest dosage there was no progressive accumulation of isotretinoin in serum, epidermis or subcutis. After discontinuation of therapy the drug disappeared from both serum and skin within 2–4 weeks. The serum transport of vitamin A, monitored by the concentrations of retinol, retinol-binding protein, and prealbumin (transthyretin), was not affected by the treatment. By contrast, the retinol level in the epidermis increased by an average of 53% and the dehydroretinol level decreased by 79% during 3 months of treatment. Both changes were reversible. The results suggest that isotretinoin therapy interferes with the endogenous vitamin A metabolism in the skin.

Using food supplements with vitamin A is therefore not recommended for patients using retinoid drugs.

7.2.2 Folic acid

Folic acid supplementation is commonly recommended before and during pregnancy, but also during methotrexate therapy as a prophylaxis against toxicities in patients with rheumatoid arthritis and psoriasis. Folic acid deficiency is common in these patients, since methotrexate inhibits dihydrofolate reductase. Folic acid supplementation reduces toxicities of methotrexate without affecting efficacy in long-term, low-dose methotrexate therapy for rheumatoid arthritis or psoriasis, but it might reduce the efficacy of methotrexate in cancer therapy.[2]

7.2.3 Vitamin B3

Vitamin B3 (niacin) is used for the treatment of hyperlipidaemia and pellagra. The combination of niacin and statins increases the risk of myopathies or rhabdomyolysis. The interaction occurs at doses of niacin over 1 g/day,[3,4] which is more than 60 × above the recommended daily allowance and is generally not available in niacin supplements.

7.2.4 Vitamin K

Vitamin K is indicated to reverse insufficient blood coagulation (high prothrombin time) caused by warfarin.[5] If vitamin K supplementation is taken together with warfarin, the activity of warfarin is decreased and can result in dangerously elevated blood coagulation (decreased prothrombin time) and can lead to thromboembolic events such as thrombosis. It is important to avoid inconsistent use of vitamin K supplements or foods with high content of vitamin K (spinach, broccoli).

7.2.5 Vitamin B6

Vitamin B6 (pyridoxine, pyridoxal and pyridoxamine) was found to decrease the effects of phenytoin and levodopa at small doses, such as 10–25 mg, which are only 5–10-fold above the RDA.[6] If levodopa is used in combination with carbidopa, the interaction does not occur.

7.2.6 Vitamin E

Vitamin E (tocopherols and tocotrienols) is a fat-soluble vitamin used in vitamin E deficiency, atherosclerosis, Alzheimer's disease, cancer and cardiovascular disease. Case reports have shown a possible interaction in patients taking vitamin E and warfarin concomitantly, which leads to increased risk of bleeding.[7,8] The interaction occurs at larger doses of vitamin E (>800 IU) which is cca 30 × above the RDI and such doses are usually not found in food supplements.

7.3 Minerals

Minerals are involved in many pharmacokinetic interactions with medicinal products, but there are only two pharmacodynamic interactions with clinical significance.

7.3.1 Calcium

Long-term use of high doses of calcium supplementation can lead to hypercalcaemia. Hypercalcaemia by itself is infrequently associated with a clinical manifestation of arrhythmia; however, concomitant therapy with cardiac glycosides (e.g. digoxin) can lead to a symptomatic rhythm disorder.[9] Patients using calcium supplementation with cardiac glycosides should be monitored by electrocardiogram (ECG) and serum calcium levels.

7.3.2 Iodine

Extensive supplementation with iodine reduces the effect of antithyroid treatment (e.g. carbimazole) in hyperthyroidism.[10] Iodine may decrease the response to the therapy, requiring an increase in dosage or longer duration of therapy with antithyroid drug.

7.4 Herbal supplements

Plants are a rich source of many different substances. These phytochemicals can have nutritional value, but also have other biological effects, physiological, pharmacological and toxicological. Owing to these effects, plants can be used as food, as food supplements and as medicinal products. There is no clear borderline between these types of products, and the same product can be marketed as a food supplement in one country and as a medicinal product in another. Very similar products can be marketed side by side in the same market as food supplements and as medicinal products. The labelling of medicinal products is strictly regulated and contains all required warnings and contraindications, including warnings about interactions with other medicinal products. Labelling of food supplements is not strictly regulated and often contains no warning. It is important that consumers and health care professionals are aware of their possible interactions.

The use of herbal medicinal products and/or herbal food supplements is very popular and the proportion of the population taking them ranges from 10% to 70% depending on the population, the country and research methodology.[11-15]

The vast majority of people do not inform their doctors about the use of herbal products. A questionnaire research on the parents of 601 children attending ambulatory surgery showed that 89.8% of them did not inform the surgical team about their use of herbal products.[11] Many of them were using products with potential interaction with anaesthesia or surgical procedures (garlic, ginkgo, ginseng, valerian and St John's Wort).

A cross-sectional, point-of-care survey was conducted and combined with a review of patient medical records to assess the frequency of clinically significant interactions caused by concurrent use of herbal supplements and prescription medication.[16] One thousand one hundred and eighteen patients treated at Mayo Clinic were surveyed (1795 responded) on their use of herbal supplements, and concurrent use of prescription medications was obtained from patients' medical records. The potential clinical significance of each interaction was assessed from the database. Seven hundred and ten patients (39.6%) reported use of dietary supplements. In total, 107 interactions with potential clinical significance were identified. The five most common natural products with a potential for interaction (garlic, valerian, kava, ginkgo, and St John's Wort) accounted for 68% of the potential clinically significant interactions. The four most common classes of prescription medications with a potential for interaction (antithrombotic medications, sedatives, antidepressant agents, and antidiabetic agents) accounted for 94% of the potential clinically significant interactions. No patient was harmed seriously from any interaction.

7.4.1 Garlic

Garlic (*Allium sativum* L., fam.: Liliaceae) is a close relative of onion and leek. Its underground parts (bulb) are used in human nutrition (as food or spice) but also in herbal medicinal products and in food supplements. It is the top-selling herbal supplement in the USA, with sales estimated at 26 million dollars.[17]

Pharmacological tests of garlic showed antimicrobial (antibacterial, antiviral, antifungal), antihypertensive, blood glucose lowering, antithrombotic, antiplatelet and antimutagenic actions. Activities are attributed to the pungent tasting volatile sulphur compounds such as alliin, allicin, diallyl disulfide and ajoene.[18]

The regulatory status of products containing garlic in pharmaceutical form (capsules) has been subject of court trials. European Court of Justice decided in 2007 that such products can be marketed as food supplements if they are not presented for treating or preventing disease.[19] On the other hand, garlic capsules are also marketed as medicinal products for the treatment of hypercholesterolaemia. Interactions of garlic products with drugs ("suppression of the effects of certain anti-retroviral drugs and an interaction with some anticoagulants") were stated as the arguments in favour of the view that garlic products in pharmaceutical form should be sold only as medicinal products where appropriately regulated labelling would prevent risk to public health.

Garlic products can have pharmacokinetic or pharmacodynamic interactions with medicinal products. Pharmacokinetic interactions are described in Chapter 4 of this book, and here we describe pharmacodynamic interactions.

7.4.1.1 Interaction with anticoagulants

Garlic can on its own (without concomitant use of other drugs) alter the platelet function and coagulation with a possible risk of bleeding.[18] Several case reports showed increased risk of bleeding in patients undergoing surgery.[20–23] The effect is even more pronounced with concomitant use of garlic with other oral anticoagulants drugs. Oral anticoagulant drugs have narrow therapeutic index and are consequently more susceptible to interactions.

In an article from 1991 it was reported that in two patients extrinsic pathway of blood coagulation has decreased (International normalized ratio (INR) increased) on warfarin after garlic intake.[24] On the other hand, two recent trials have reported that garlic did not alter the pharmacokinetics or pharmacodynamics of warfarin.[25,26] The first was a double-blind, randomized, placebo-controlled trial with 48 patients (30 men and 18 women, with a mean age of 56 ± 10 years) completing the study,

22 receiving aged garlic extract 5 mL twice a day for 12 weeks and 26 receiving a placebo.[25] No difference was found in blood coagulation, dose of warfarin or any adverse event.

The second was an open-label, randomized crossover clinical trial on 12 healthy men.[26] A single dose of 25 mg warfarin was administered alone or after 2 weeks of pre-treatment with garlic (Garliplex 2000 enteric-coated garlic tablets, containing 2000 mg of fresh garlic bulb equivalent to 3.71 mg of allicin per tablet, one tablet twice daily). Garlic did not alter warfarin enantiomer concentrations, INR, platelet aggregation or clotting factor activity.

There is also one case report on antagonistic interaction of oral anticoagulant and garlic.[27] An 82-year-old man was on a well-balanced (INR = 2–3) therapy with fluindione (5 mg) for more than 1 year. After the man started to take garlic supplement (600 mg/day, herbal preparation not reported), INR dropped to below 2 and even with duplicated dose (10 mg) of fluindione INR stayed below 2 for 12 days. When garlic supplementation was stopped, INR normalized in 4 days and stayed normal with the original dose (5 mg) of fluindione.

7.4.1.2 Other interactions

Since garlic possesses hypoglycaemic[28,29] and hypolipaemic effects, the interaction with antidiabetic drugs and cholesterol/triglyceride lowering drugs is possible. In an unreliable report from 1979, a fall in glucose levels in a 40-year-old diabetic woman taking chlorpropamide and a curry containing garlic and karela has been reported.[30,31]

7.4.2 Cranberry

Cranberry (*Vaccinium macrocarpon* fruit juice or dried juice) supplements are among the top herbal supplements sold in the United States.[17] They are used for prevention of urinary tract infections.[32] Case reports showed possible interactions between cranberry and warfarin,[33] including one fatal case.[34]

An open-label, randomized crossover clinical trial was conducted on 12 healthy men.[26] A single dose of 25 mg warfarin was administered alone or after 2 weeks of pre-treatment with cranberry (GNC cranberry juice concentrate, 500 mg, two capsules three times daily, equivalent to 57 g of fruit per day). Cranberry significantly increased the area under the INR–time curve by 30% when administered with warfarin compared with treatment with warfarin alone. Cranberry did not alter S- or R-warfarin pharmacokinetics or plasma protein binding.

7.4.3 Echinacea

No cases of interactions were found for Echinacea,[31] but due to its immunostimulatory activity, its concomitant use with immunosuppressants is not recommended, as a general precaution.[35,36]

7.4.4 Red yeast rice

Red yeast rice (*Monascus purpureus*) is rice fermented with red yeast. It contains several derivatives of mevinic acids, including lovastatin. Lovastatin is an active ingredient in cholesterol-lowering medicinal products, but when found in red yeast rice it is more often referred to by its synonymous name monacolin K. Rhabdomyolysis is a known complication of statin therapy. There is a case report of rhabdomyolysis in a stable renal-transplant recipient, induced by the use of a food supplement containing red yeast rice.[37] The authors postulated that the interaction of cyclosporine and these statins through the cytochrome P450 system resulted in the adverse effect seen in this patient.

7.5 Antioxidants

There is an on-going controversy over the interaction of antioxidants with chemotherapy and radiotherapy in cancer patients.[38] Interaction has been theoretically based on the possibility of antioxidants interfering with the oxidative mechanism of the therapeutic agents, thereby reducing their efficacy.

On the other hand, antioxidants were shown to prevent or lessen the toxic effects of chemotherapy. Administration of antineoplastic agents results in oxidative stress, which contributes to certain side effects that are common to many anticancer drugs (e.g. gastrointestinal toxicity and mutagenesis) or they occur only with individual agents (e.g. doxorubicin-induced cardiotoxicity, cisplatin-induced nephrotoxicity, and bleomycin-induced pulmonary fibrosis). Antioxidants can reduce or prevent many of these side effects.[39]

7.6 Conclusion

The list of known interactions between food supplements and medicinal products is not final. Since they are not easy to observe, many more may be found in the future. On the other hand, the interactions that used to be considered clinically very important (e.g. garlic and anticoagulants), are now shown to be less critical.

References

1. Rollman O and Vahlquist A. (1986) Oral isotretinoin (13-cis-retinoic acid) therapy in severe acne: drug and vitamin A concentrations in serum and skin. *J Invest Dermatol*, 86(4): 384–389.
2. Endresen GK and Husby G. (2001) Folate supplementation during methotrexate treatment of patients with rheumatoid arthritis. An update and proposals for guidelines. *Scand J Rheumatol*, 30: 129–134.

3. Cooke HM. (1994) Lovastatin- and niacin-induced rhabdomyolysis. *Hosp Pharm,* 29: 33–34.
4. Malloy MJ, Kane JP, Kunitake ST and Tun P. (1987) Complementarity of colestipol, niacin, and lovastatin in treatment of severe familial hyper cholesterolemia. *Ann Intern Med,* 107: 616–623.
5. Greenblatt DJ and von Moltke LL. (2005) Interaction of warfarin with drugs, natural substances, and foods. *J Clin Pharmacol,* 45: 127–132.
6. Leon AS, Spiegel HE, Thomas G and Abrams WB. (1971) Pyridoxine antagonism of levodopa in parkinsonism. *JAMA,* 218:1924–1927.7. Corrigan JJ and Marcus FI. (1974) Coagulopathy associated with vitamin E ingestion. *JAMA,* 230: 1300–1301.
7. Corrigan JJ, Marcus FI. (1974) Coagulopathy associated with vitamin E ingestion. *JAMA,* 230: 1300–1301.
8. Schrogie JJ. (1975) Coagulopathy and fat-soluble vitamins. *JAMA,* 232: 19.
9. Vella A, Gerber TC, Hayes DL and Reeder GS (1999) Digoxin, hypercalcaemia, and cardiac conduction. *Postgrad Med J,* 75: 554–556.
10. Roy G, Nethaji M and Mugesh G. (2006) Interaction of anti-thyroid drugs with iodine: the isolation of two unusual ionic compounds derived from Se-methimazole. *Org Biomol Chem,* 7 August, 4(15): 2883–2887.
11. Crowe S and Lyons B. (2004) Herbal medicine use by children presenting for ambulatory anaesthesia and surgery. *Paediatr Anaesth,* 14(11): 916–919.
12. Ayranci U, Son N and Son O. (2005) Prevalence of nonvitamin, nonmineral supplement usage among students in a Turkish University. *BMC Public Health,* 16 May, 5(1): 47.
13. Newberry H, Beerman K, Duncan S, McGuire M and Hillers V. (2001) Use of nonvitamin, nonmineral dietary supplements among college students. *J Am Coll Health,* November, 50(3): 123–129.
14. Knudtson MD, Klein R, Lee KE, Reinke JO, Danforth LG, Wealti AM, Moore E and Klein BE. (2007) A longitudinal study of nonvitamin, nonmineral supplement use: prevalence, associations, and survival in an aging population. *Ann Epidemiol,* 17(12): 933–939.
15. Hümer M, Scheller G, Kapellen T, Gebauer C, Schmidt H and Kiess W. (2010) Use of herbal medicine in German children – prevalence, indications and motivation. *Dtsch Med Wochenschr,* 135(19): 959–964.
16. Sood A, Sood R, Brinker FJ, Mann R, Loehrer LL and Wahner-Roedler DL. (2008) Potential for interactions between dietary supplements and prescription medications. *Am J Med,* March, 121(3): 207–211.
17. Blumenthal M, Ferrier, GKL and Cavaliere C. (2006) Total sales of herbal supplements in United States show steady growth. *HerbalGram,* 71, 64–66.
18. Borrelli F, Capasso R and Izzo AA. (2007) Garlic (Allium sativum L.): adverse effects and drug interactions in humans. *Mol Nutr Food Res,* November, 51(11): 1386–1397.
19. European Court of Justice, Case C-319/05 Judgment of the Court 15 November 2007 http://eur-lex.europa.eu/LexUriServ/LexUriServ.do?uri=CELEX:62005J0319:EN:HTML.
20. Rose KD, Croissant PD, Parliament CF and Levin MB. (1990) Spontaneous spinal epidural hematoma with associated platelet dysfunction from excessive garlic ingestion: a case report. *Neurosurgery,* 26, 880–882.
21. Burnham BE. (1995) Garlic as a possible risk for postoperative bleeding. *Plast Reconstr Surg,* 95: 213.
22. German K, Kumar U and Blackford HN. (1995) Garlic and the risk of TURP bleeding. *Br J Urol,* 76: 518.
23. Carden SM, Good WV, Carden PA and Good RM. (2002)Garlic and the strabismus surgeon. *Clin Exp Ophthalmol,* 30: 303–304.

24. Sunter WH. (1991) Warfarin and garlic. *Pharm J*, 246: 722.
25. Macan H, Uykimpang R, Alconcel M et al. (2006) Aged garlic extract may be safe for patients on warfarin therapy. *J Nutr*, 136: 793S–795S.
26. Mohammed Abdul MI, Jiang X, Williams KM et al. (2008) Pharmacodynamic interaction of warfarin with cranberry but not with garlic in healthy subjects. *Br J Pharmacol*, 154: 1691–700.
27. Pathak A, Leger P, Bagheri H, Senard JM. et al. (2003) Garlic interaction with fluindione: a case report. *Therapie*, 58: 380–381.
28. Jalal R, Bagheri SM, Moghimi A and Rasuli MB. (2007) Hypoglycemic effect of aqueous shallot and garlic extracts in rats with fructose-induced insulin resistance. *J Clin Biochem Nutr*, November, 41(3): 218–223.
29. Sher A, Fakhar-ul-Mahmood M, Shah SN, Bukhsh S and Murtaza G. (2012) Effect of garlic extract on blood glucose level and lipid profile in normal and alloxan diabetic rabbits. *Adv Clin Exp Med*, November–December, 21(6): 705–711.
30. Aslam M and Stockley IH. (1979) Interaction between curry ingredient (karela) and drug (chlorpropamide). *Lancet*, 313: 607.
31. Izzo AA and Ernst E. (2009) Interactions between herbal medicines and prescribed drugs: an updated systematic review. *Drugs*, 69(13): 1777–1798.
32. Jepson RG and Craig JC. (2008) Cranberries for preventing urinary tract infections. *Cochrane Database Syst Rev1*:Art. No.: CD001321. DOI.10.1002/14651858.CD001321.pub4.
33. Medicines and Healthcare Products Regulatory Agency (MHRA) and Committee on Safety of Medicines (CSM) (2004) Possible interaction between warfarin and cranberry juice. *Cur Probl Pharmacovigilance*, 30: 9.
34. Suvarna R, Pirmohamed M and Henderson L. (2003) Possible interaction between warfarin and cranberry juice. *BMJ*, 327: 1454.
35. Kreft S (2008) Assessment report on Echinacea purpurea (L.) Moench., herba recens. *European Medicines Agency*. Doc. Ref: EMEA/HMPC/104918/2006. http://www.ema.europa.eu/docs/en_GB/document_library/Herbal_-_HMPC_assessment_report/2009/12/WC500018261.pdf.
36. HMPC (2008) Community herbal monograph on Echinacea purpurea (L.) Moench, herba recens. European Medicines Agency. Doc. Ref. EMEA/HMPC/104945/2006Corr.1. http://www.ema.europa.eu/docs/en_GB/document_library/Herbal_-_Community_herbal_monograph/2009/12/WC500018263.pdf.
37. Prasad GV, Wong T, Meliton G and Bhaloo S. (2002) Rhabdomyolysis due to red yeast rice (Monascus purpureus) in a renal transplant recipient. *Transplantation*, 27 October, 74(8): 1200–1201.
38. Fuchs-Tarlovsky V. (2013) Role of antioxidants in cancer therapy. *Nutrition*, January, 29(1): 15–21.
39. Conklin KA. (2000) Dietary antioxidants during cancer chemotherapy: impact on chemotherapeutic effectiveness and development of side-effects. *Nutr Cancer*, 37(1): 1–18.

Part Three

Vitamins, minerals and probiotics as dietary supplements

Vitamins/minerals as dietary supplements: a review of clinical studies

G. P. Webb
University of East London, London, UK

8.1 Introduction: efficacy in clinical trials does not guarantee practical impact

Vitamin and mineral supplements make up over a third of the value of dietary supplements sold in the UK (Mintel, 2009). These substances are proven to be essential components of the diet, and firm quantitative estimates of requirements are published. Well-defined deficiency syndromes are caused by inadequacies of these substances and some of these are or have been major causes of human morbidity and mortality e.g. scurvy, rickets, pellagra, cretinism and beriberi. Supplements can undoubtedly provide a cheap and effective means of preventing or curing these deficiency diseases, and could also eradicate any subclinical consequences of deficiency.

Early in the twentieth century it was established that supplemental iodine (as iodised salt) could eradicate endemic goitre and cretinism. In 1915, David Marine, who is credited with this discovery, said that "endemic goitre is the easiest known disease to prevent" (see Kimball, 1953). Despite this, iodine deficiency is still the leading cause of preventable mental retardation in children, with around 2 billion people and 266 million school-aged children in the world still classified as iodine deficient (de Benoist et al., 2008). Likewise, millions of children in some Asian, African and South American countries are affected by xerophthalmia due to vitamin A deficiency. It causes child blindness, depresses immune function and results in high child mortality due to infections. Mayo-Wilson et al. (2011) estimated that worldwide, 190 million pre-school children may be vitamin A deficient and supplements could reduce mortality rates by a quarter in some areas and thus would have the potential to annually save 600 000 child deaths and reduce blindness and other morbidities.

Inadequate micronutrient intakes are not confined to developing countries. Data from the UK National Dietary and Nutritional Survey (NDNS) programme have been used to show (e.g. Fletcher et al., 2004; Webb, 2007, 2012) that many individuals in all age groups have poor biochemical status or have measured micronutrient intakes that are classified as inadequate, i.e. more than two standard deviations below the Estimated Average Requirement (termed the Lower Reference Nutrient Intake (LRNI) in the UK). Poor biochemical status for micronutrients is the result of inadequate total intake from both food and supplements, and the percentage of people with intakes below the LRNI is essentially unaffected by the inclusion of supplemental intakes (Hoare *et al.*, 2004). Supplements are taken by those people who already have the highest intakes from food and who need them least; they are rarely taken by those with poor dietary intake.

Supplements may also be taken to compensate for some (perceived) increase in requirement as a result of physiological status, disease or drug use, e.g. the perceived increased need for iron in pregnancy or when there is chronic blood loss. Vitamins and minerals may also be taken in the belief that they may help in treating or preventing disease, e.g. the belief that mega-doses of vitamin C may help prevent or alleviate colds. Where micronutrients are taken to ensure adequacy, then maximum doses are likely to be around the RDA/RNI and so unlikely to be hazardous. However, when they are taken to treat or prevent disease then doses may be orders of magnitude greater, and so the potential for toxicity is higher, e.g. several grams per day of vitamin C may be taken to prevent or alleviate colds, and high doses of β-carotene taken as an antioxidant to prevent cancer and heart disease.

Clinical trials confirm that folic acid supplements taken peri-conceptually substantially reduce the risk of babies developing with a neural tube defect (NTD) such as spina bifida or anencephaly (De-Regil *et al.*, 2010). Recommendations that European women should take folic acid supplements when planning a pregnancy were made as early as 1992. Despite such recommendations, Botto *et al.* (2005) found that the incidence of NTD-affected pregnancies did not change in Europe between 1988 and 1998. Most pregnancies are not specifically planned, few women routinely take folic acid supplements, and it is likely that those who take supplements are those with the highest intakes from food sources. To be effective, these supplements need to be taken soon after conception and ideally should start before conception. Supplements taken only after pregnancy is confirmed are likely to be ineffective.

Thus, even clear evidence of the efficacy of a supplement does not guarantee that it will have significant practical impact, because it may not be taken by those who would benefit from taking it. In theory, supplements allow targeting of extra micronutrients to those who need them most, and high doses can be used without exposing the whole population to them. In practice, they have not prevented widespread deficiency in developing countries, have not significantly reduced the prevalence of inadequate intakes in the UK, and folic acid supplement recommendations have had little impact on the prevalence of NTD.

Increased intake of *natural* vitamins and minerals from food sources is an alternative strategy, but it is difficult to achieve and may sometimes be impractical, as in the examples listed below:

- It is probably not currently feasible to ensure that all children in developing countries receive a diet that contains adequate amounts of natural vitamin A.
- Most Northern Europeans cannot obtain enough vitamin D from natural foods to meet their needs without exposure to summer sunlight; in the UK average dietary intake is less than a quarter of estimated needs.
- Average folate intake by UK women is about 250 µg/day, and very few women of childbearing age take in the recommended supplemental intake of 400 µg/day from food and supplements.

This problem may be compounded by food preparation practices that may deplete foods of vitamins.

Another alternative to supplements is to fortify a universally consumed food with micronutrients. Everyone then gets the extra vitamin or mineral whether they benefit from it or not, and some people may be harmed by excessive intakes. Levels of fortification must be set cautiously, to avoid excessive consumption by some people. Since the 1940s it has been mandatory to fortify most bread and flour in the UK with niacin, thiamin, calcium and iron and to fortify margarine with vitamins A and D. In the USA, in 1989, folic acid was added to the existing list of vitamins that should be added to most bread and flour, and this resulted in an immediate fall in the incidence of NTD of 25–30%, and an increased fortification level has been advocated to achieve optimal NTD prevention (Pitkin, 2007). Many other countries have since introduced folic acid fortification and whilst this has undoubtedly been successful in reducing incidence of NTD, several hundred thousand people receive the extra folic acid for each NTD-affected pregnancy prevented. Is it justified to expose so many to help so few? There must be certainty that the extra folic acid is safe, and ideally there should be wider benefits from the fortification (the hazards and wider benefits of extra folic acid are discussed later in the chapter).

Depot injections are another possible means of ensuring good vitamin or mineral status that bypass the normal need for patient compliance, e.g. injections of vitamin D or iodised oil. Increased exposure of the skin to UV light (sunlight) is another way of improving vitamin D status.

8.2 Are some natural metabolites conditionally essential nutrients?

Several natural metabolites (discussed below) are sold as dietary supplements. They often fulfil similar biochemical roles to vitamins (e.g. as co-enzymes) but are not classified as vitamins because needs are thought to be met by endogenous synthesis. The underlying assumption when using these as supplements is that endogenous synthesis may not always be sufficient for optimal functioning or in disease.

The distinction between essential and non-essential nutrients is not always absolute; for example:

- Niacin (B_3) can be synthesised from the amino acid tryptophan
- Sufficient vitamin D can be synthesised if the skin is exposed to UV light.

Some nutrients are termed conditionally essential, i.e.:

> *"not ordinarily required in the diet but which must be supplied exogenously to specific groups that do not synthesise them in adequate amounts"* (Harper, 1999).

- Some normally non-essential nutrients may become essential in newborn or premature babies who have not developed the synthetic enzymes (e.g. the amino acids cysteine and tyrosine).

- The amino acid glutamine may become essential in people with serious illness because rate of utilisation exceeds synthetic capability.
- Some metabolites may become essential nutrients for people with some inborn errors of metabolism e.g. tyrosine becomes an essential amino acid in phenylketonuria (PKU).

Six *natural metabolites* used as supplements are briefly discussed below (see Webb, 2011a for fuller accounts).

L-carnitine (see Figure 8.1a) is normally synthesised from the amino acid lysine. The diets of omnivores contain substantial amounts of carnitine, but a vegan diet contains none. Fatty acids with more than 16 carbon atoms have to be converted to carnitine esters in order to pass across the mitochondrial membrane. Some rare inborn errors of fatty acid metabolism increase carnitine excretion, e.g. as propionyl carnitine in propionyl CoA carboxylase deficiency. A defect in the enzyme that transports carnitine across the plasma membrane also increases urinary carnitine excretion. These conditions may respond to pharmacological doses of carnitine. Haemodialysis may also increase urinary carnitine losses. In newborn babies and especially in premature babies, L-carnitine is regarded as a conditionally essential nutrient. It has been suggested that because of its role in fatty acid metabolism, carnitine supplements might boost athletic performance, although controlled trials have found no evidence of any beneficial effect (Broad *et al.*, 2005; Smith *et al.*, 2008). Early suggestions that carnitine supplements might slow the rate of deterioration in Alzheimer's disease have not been supported by two relatively large clinical trials (Thal *et al.*, 1996, 2000). There is generally little evidence that carnitine supplements are likely to benefit healthy adults or children.

Coenzyme Q_{10} (ubiquinone) comprises a benzoquinone component (synthesised from tyrosine) that is attached to ten isoprene units, and this is synthesised from acetyl coenzyme A via a pathway that is partly common to cholesterol biosynthesis. The benzoquinone part of the molecule can be reduced to the quinol form by addition of two hydrogen atoms (see Figure 8.1b). Coenzyme Q_{10} is a component of the electron transport system in mitochondria that generates most of the adenosine triphosphate (ATP) produced during aerobic metabolism. The reduced quinol form is present in the lipid fraction of membranes where it is believed to act in conjunction with vitamin E as an antioxidant. It has been used as a supplement largely because of its role as an antioxidant. Two major reviews found that there was no evidence at that time to support the use of coenzyme Q_{10} to prevent either cardiovascular disease (Shekelle *et al.*, 2003) or cancer (Coulter *et al.*, 2003); they noted a paucity of large extended controlled trials to support or refute its use. More recently it has been suggested that the statin type of cholesterol-lowering drugs taken by many millions of people may reduce coenzyme Q_{10} biosynthesis and so increase reliance on exogenous sources. Statins inhibit the enzyme hydroxymethyl glutaryl CoA reductase (HMG CoA reductase), which is a key rate limiting enzyme in both cholesterol and Q_{10} biosynthesis. Marcoff and Thompson (2007) found that although statin use reduced circulating levels of Q_{10} there was no evidence that they affected intramuscular levels, and so they found no case for routine use of Q_{10} supplements for those taking statins. Lowered Q_{10} concentrations in muscles had been suggested as a possible factor in the myopathy that is an occasional side-effect of statin use.

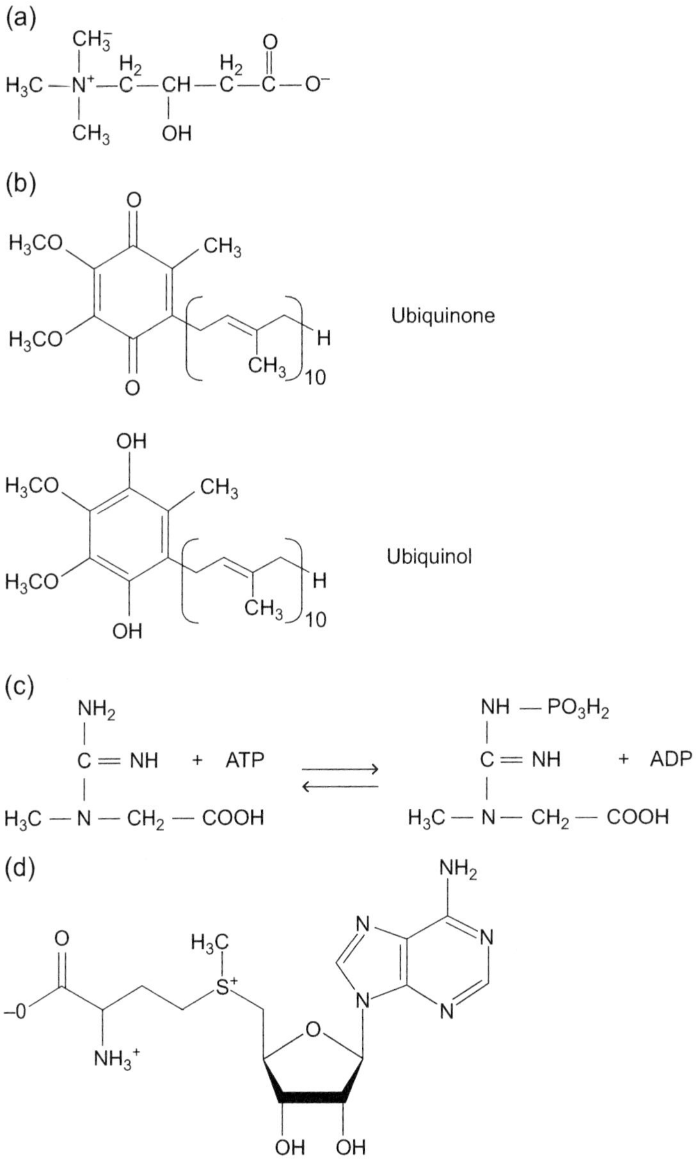

Figure 8.1 (a) The structure of L-carnitine. Acetyl-L-carnitine and propionyl-L-carnitine have acetyl of propionyl groups esterified to the OH group. (b) The structure of coenzyme Q10 (ubiquinone) and its reduced form ubiquinol (c) The structure of creatine and creatine phosphate (d) The structure of s-adenosyl methionine (SAMe) (e) The structure of α-lipoic acid and below its reduced form α-dihydrolipoic acid (DHLA) (f) The structure of phosphatidylcholine (lecithin) (g) The structure of folic acid (h) The structures of 7-dehydrocholesterol and cholecalciferol (vitamin D3).

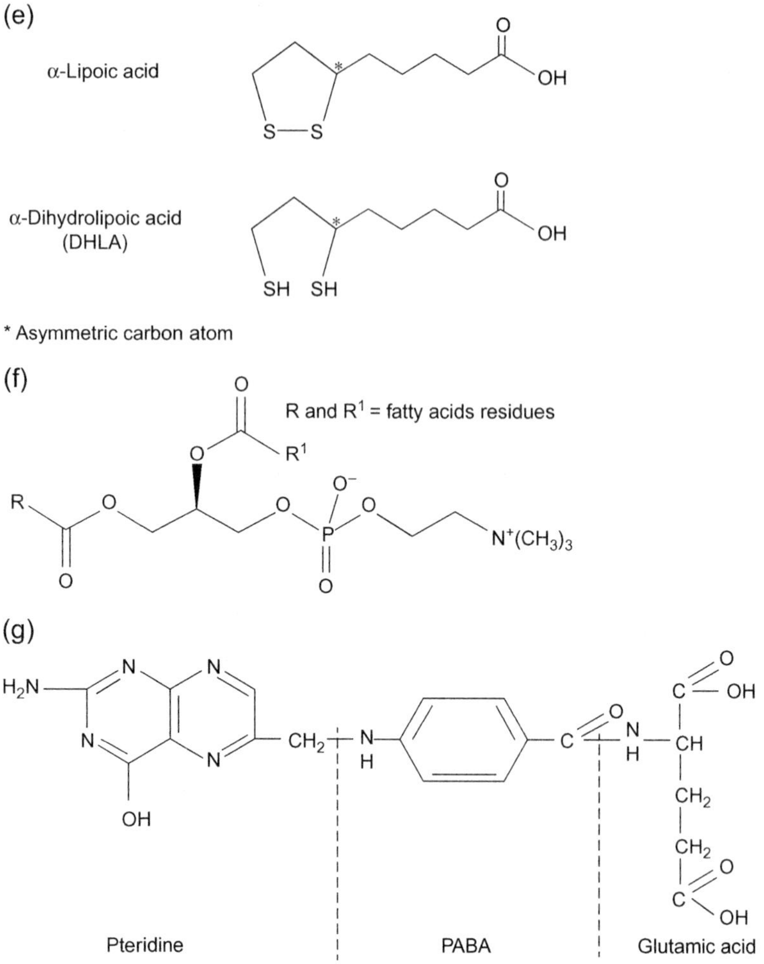

(e)

α-Lipoic acid

α-Dihydrolipoic acid
(DHLA)

* Asymmetric carbon atom

(f) R and R¹ = fatty acids residues

(g)

Pteridine | PABA | Glutamic acid

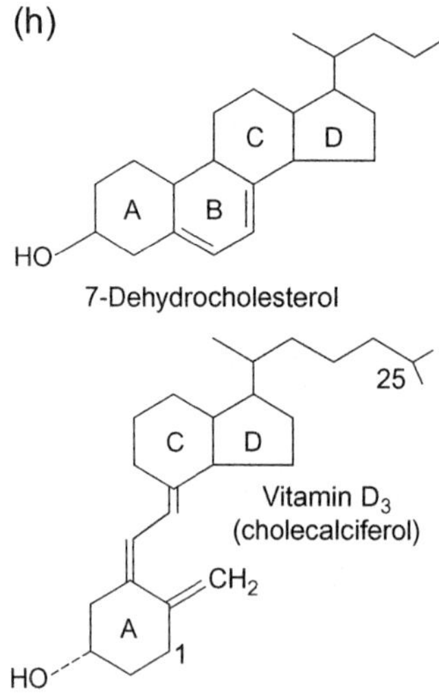

(h)

7-Dehydrocholesterol

Vitamin D₃
(cholecalciferol)

Figure 8.1 Continued

Creatine is an amino acid that is not a component of body protein and is not essential in the diet as it can be synthesised from other amino acids. Creatine in muscle can be phosphorylated to creatine phosphate (phosphocreatine) (see Figure 8.1c), and this can be used to replenish muscle ATP during short periods of intense activity. Increased muscle concentrations of creatine might thus be expected to boost performance in explosive sporting events by increasing availability of ATP. Creatine supplements at doses well beyond those in a normal diet, even a meat-rich diet, can boost phosphocreatine concentrations in muscles (Harris *et al.*, 1992). The results of trials of creatine supplements on athletic performance are variable – some controlled laboratory studies suggest that they do boost performance when it involves short periods of intense activity. Other trials, especially those using field tests, have not found any beneficial effect (see meta-analysis of Branch, 2003). It is accepted that creatine supplements will not improve performance in endurance events and, because they lead to slight increases in muscle water content and body weight, they may be more likely to hinder than enhance performance.

s-adenosylmethionine (sAME) (see Figure 8.1d) acts as an important methyl donor in several biochemical reactions involving methyl transfer, e.g. reactions in synthetic pathways for neurotransmitters and nucleic acids. sAME is synthesised endogenously from the amino acid methionine, and a typical adult synthesises several grams of it each day. It has been available only as a supplement since 1999 because of the difficulty in producing an orally active preparation. Despite the high rate of endogenous synthesis, it is suggested that supplements may be necessary because the availability of methyl groups from sAME may be rate limiting for some methyl transfer reactions in some circumstances. Supplements of sAME have been advocated as being beneficial in treating depression, osteoarthritis and liver disease. A major report on the effects of sAME supplements concluded that they might have some beneficial effect on osteoarthritic pain and some of the symptoms of severe liver disease, such as intense itching (Hardy *et al.*, 2002), but this review was published just 3 years after sAME became available as a supplement and was necessarily based on limited evidence. Subsequent meta-analyses have found no substantial evidence to support any benefits in alcoholic liver disease (Rambaldi and Gluud, 2006) or for osteoarthritis of the hip or knee (Rutjes *et al.*, 2009).

Alpha (α)-lipoic acid is a co-factor for several important enzymes including pyruvate dehydrogenase, succinyl CoA dehydrogenase and several enzymes involved in amino acid metabolism. It is covalently bound to lysine resides of these enzymes and is absorbed from food as lipolysine because human gut enzymes do not break the bonds between lipoic acid and lysine. Only when supplements are taken is free α-lipoic acid found in blood. It is synthesised by both animals and plants and not considered an essential nutrient. It can be reduced to α-dihydrolipoic acid and this has antioxidant potential (see Figure 8.1e). It has been claimed to be have beneficial effects upon memory and thus to be potentially beneficial in treating Alzheimer's disease, but Klugman *et al.* (2004) could find no clinical trials to support these claims.

Lecithin (phosphatidyl choline) and *choline* (see Figure 8.1f) were actively considered but not classified as essential nutrients in the UK (COMA, 1991), although choline was added to the US list of essential nutrients because of doubt that the synthetic pathway was capable of providing adequate amounts at all stages of the lifecycle. It is present in many foods and so dietary deficiency would be highly improbable even if there were some requirement for an exogenous supply. Lecithin can be extracted from soybean oil for use in supplements. Early suggestions of a possible beneficial effect in Alzheimer's disease (choline is a component the nerve transmitter acetylcholine) have not been supported by clinical trials (Higgins and Flicker, 2000), nor have early claims that lecithin has a cholesterol-lowering effect (Oosthuizen *et al.*, 1998).

8.3 Use of supplements to improve micronutrient adequacy

Preventing and treating deficiency disease was the original justification for using micronutrient supplements. Deficiency diseases are now uncommon in industrialised countries, except amongst those with precipitating medical conditions or those at the extremes of social and economic deprivation. Despite this, many individuals have intakes of some micronutrients that are regarded as inadequate (i.e. below the LRNI) or show biochemical evidence of unsatisfactory micronutrient status (e.g. Fletcher *et al.* 2004; Webb, 2007, 2011a, b). Table 8.1 shows a condensed synthesis of data from the last full NDNS survey of British adults (Hoare *et al.*, 2004) on the extent of vitamin and mineral inadequacy. This table shows that even apparently adequate average intakes (i.e. above the RNI) are no guarantee that substantial numbers of people will not have inadequate intakes (below the LRNI) or have unsatisfactory biochemical status. The intakes shown in Table 8.1 are from food sources only, but biochemical status is dependent upon the combined intake from food and supplements, and a third of UK adults take micronutrient supplements. Hoare *et al.* (2004) stated that supplements, make almost no difference to the number of people with intakes below the LRNI. In a survey of elderly British adults, Finch *et al.* (1999) found that supplements increased average intakes of vitamin A and folate but made almost no difference to the median intakes. This confirms that supplements are taken by those with the highest micronutrient intakes from food and thus the least likely to benefit from taking them.

Some of the estimates of poor biochemical status prevalence in Table 8.1 should to be treated with caution, e.g. an apparent zero incidence of "biochemical deficiency" for vitamin A despite low average intakes and high number of young adults with inadequate intakes. There is no sensitive and reliable biochemical test for vitamin A status, and the measure used in the table only decreases after severe depletion. The apparent high prevalence of biochemical riboflavin deficiency is probably because either the measure used is too sensitive to short-term fluctuations in riboflavin availability or the threshold for normality is set too high. Biochemical assessments of micronutrient status are usually specific, reliable and sensitive, but their interpretation depends upon the criterion for inadequacy set, and this is necessarily a matter of expert opinion. Thus, the apparent high levels of biochemical deficiency for vitamin B_6 could be inflated if the threshold of adequacy has been set too high. Conversely, the criterion used for

Vitamins/minerals as dietary supplements

Table 8.1 Vitamin and mineral adequacy of diets of adult British aged 19–64

Nutrient	Average intake as % RNI				% Subjects below LRNI				% Below biochemical threshold			
	Men (aged)		Women (aged)		Men (aged)		Women (aged)		Men (aged)		Women (aged)	
	19–64	19–24	19–64	19–24	19–64	19–24	19–64	19–24	19–64	19–24	19–64	19–24
A (retinol equivalents)	130	80	112	78	7	16	9	19	0	0	0	0
Thiamin	214	160	193	181	1	2	1	0	3	0	1	0
Riboflavin	162	129	146	126	3	8	8	15	66	82	66	77
Niacin equivalents	268	232	257	246	0	0	1	2				
B$_6$	204	189	169	165	1	0	2	5	10	4	11	12
B$_{12}$	431	296	319	266	0	1	1	1	2	0	4	5
Folate*	172	151	125	114	0	2	2	3	4	13	5	8
C	209	162	202	170	0	0	0	1	5	7	3	4
D**	3.7 (µg)	2.9 (µg)	2.8 (µg)	2.3 (µg)	–	–	–	–	14	24	15	28
Iron†	151	131	82	60	1	3	25	42	3	0	8	7
									(4)	(4)	(11)	(16)
Ca	144	123	111	99	2	5	5	8				
Iodine	154	119	114	93	2	2	4	12				
Magnesium	103	86	85	76	9	17	13	22				
Potassium	96	81	76	67	6	18	19	30				
Zinc	107	95	105	98	4	7	4	5				

* Biochemical value is red cell folate indicating marginal status
** No adult RNI or LRNI for vitamin D – absolute values given
† The two biochemical values are the value for haemoglobin indicative of anaemia and in parentheses the value for serum ferritin indicative of iron store depletion
Source: Data from Hoare et al. (2004).

vitamin D adequacy used in Table 8.1 is much lower than that set in some other countries and that suggested by some learned societies (see later in the chapter).

If the survey used to construct Table 8.1 is nationally representative, then even small percentages may translate into tens or hundreds of thousands of individuals. Those at the extremes of social and economic deprivation and those with serious medical problems will be under-represented in this survey. Many non-UK readers may be surprised at just how low the threshold for inadequate intake (LRNI) is set for some nutrients. For example, the adult LRNI for the following vitamins and minerals:

- Folate – 100 µg/day
- Vitamin C – 10 mg/day
- Vitamin B_{12} – 1 µg/day
- Calcium – 400 mg/day
- Iodine – 70 µg/day
- Vitamin A for women 250 µgRE/day
- Iron for women 8 mg/day
- Zinc for women 4 mg/day.

UK dietary standards generally tend to be conservative compared to those in other countries, as the comparisons of adult standards with those of the USA below illustrate:

- The UK RNI for vitamin C of 40 mg/day compares with US RDA of 90 mg/day for men and 75 mg/day for women
- A UK folate RNI of 200 µg/day compares with a US RDA of 400 µg/day
- An RNI of 700 mg/day for calcium compares with a US RDA of 1000 mg/day
- There is no vitamin D RNI set for most adults in the UK, but in the USA it is 15 µg/day (see later section for rationale).

The high levels of unsatisfactory intakes and status seen in Table 8.1 are almost certainly typical of many other industrialised countries, especially given the generally conservative levels of UK standards.

Several of the nutrients in Table 8.1 are discussed specifically in later sections, but iodine and iron are briefly discussed below.

Table 8.1 suggests that many women, especially those in the youngest age group, have low iron intakes. About 8% of women are classified as anaemic (low blood haemoglobin concentration) and double this proportion of younger women show evidence of depleted iron stores (low plasma ferritin concentration). There would thus seem to be a prima facie case for wider use of iron-containing supplements in women.

The high incidence of iodine deficiency in some developing countries was discussed earlier, and Table 8.1 would suggest that many people in the UK, especially young women, also have less than satisfactory intakes of iodine. Vanderpump *et al.* (2011) assessed the iodine status of a sample of 14–15 year old schoolgirls from across the UK using WHO criteria and found that 51% of those sampled had urinary iodine concentrations that were indicative of mild iodine deficiency, 18% were classified as moderately deficient and 1% severely deficient. In the UK, only 2% of the salt used is iodised compared to over 90% in some other European countries like Austria, Bulgaria, Croatia, Czech Republic and Poland (Andersson *et al.*, 2007).

Zimmerman and Delange (2004) suggested that two-thirds of Western Europeans lived in areas that were iodine deficient and that most women in Europe were iodine deficient during pregnancy. They recommended that pregnant women in Europe should take supplements of 150 μg/day of iodine. A more recent WHO survey of iodine status in 40 European countries found that 19 countries had adequate iodine status, 12 had mild iodine deficiency and 1 moderate deficiency, and there were insufficient data to classify the others (Andersson *et al.*, 2007). The authors of this report emphasise that even mild or moderate iodine deficiency affects the intellectual development of neonates. A recent UK survey by Bath *et al.* (2013) analysed the iodine content of stored urine taken during early pregnancy in over 1000 mothers of 8 year old children. They found that the children of women classified as being iodine deficient during pregnancy were more likely to be in the lowest category for verbal IQ scores and reading ability tests. These measures in the children worsened with declining iodine status of their mothers. This provides further support for measures to improve iodine status in women in the UK. Note that the UK is one of the countries where iodine status could not be classified by Andersson *et al.* (2007) because there were insufficient data.

8.4 Do folic acid supplements prevent neural tube defects (NTDs)?

Folic acid or pteroylmonoglutamic acid (Figure 8.1g) is the parent compound of a group of substances collectively termed folate (vitamin B_9). Folic acid itself is not found naturally in food, but is the form used in supplements and food fortification. It was initially specified as the only form of the vitamin that could be used in supplements within the EU, but calcium L-methylfolate has now been added to that permitted list. Folate from food has multiple units of glutamic acid (5–7 usually) rather than just one; there is also reduction of double bonds and addition of methyl units to the nitrogen atoms in the pteridine component. In people eating a natural diet, no free folic acid is detected in plasma. Natural folate is deconjugated in the intestine and absorbed as 5-methyl tetrahydrofolate. When folic acid is consumed, conversion to 5-methyl tetrahydrofolate occurs in the liver after absorption and because of the low activity of the enzyme dihyhrofolate reductase in liver, some free folic acid remains in the blood (Wright *et al.*, 2007). In the USA, where flour is fortified with folic acid, around 40% of older adults now have free folic acid in their plasma (Bailey *et al.*, 2010).

A link between poor folate status during pregnancy and increased risk of congenital NTDs was suggested in the early 1960s (see DH, 1992). Confirmation that folic acid supplements could reduce the recurrence of NTD in women with a previous affected pregnancy was provided by a large, multi-centre, randomised controlled trial (MRC, 1991). Large supplemental doses of folic acid (4 mg/day) reduced recurrence by 72% when taken before conception and in the first trimester. A meta-analysis by De-Regil *et al.* (2010) unequivocally confirms that folic acid supplements reduce both recurrence and first occurrence of NTD.

UK women planning a pregnancy were first advised to take supplements of 400 µg/day in 1992 (DH, 1992). All pre-menopausal UK women are now advised to take this supplement routinely. Similar advice has been issued in many other countries since 1992. This supplement advice had no significant impact on the incidence of NTD-affected pregnancy in Europe and Israel (Botto et al., 2005); NTD incidence did not change between 1988 and 1998 in Europe. Very few women in the UK routinely take these supplements, and those with the highest intake from food are the most likely to take them; only 13% of UK women get 400 µg/day from food and supplements combined. As many pregnancies are not specifically planned, many women do not take supplements until they know they are pregnant, which is probably too late for them to be effective; they are most effective in the month after conception.

In contrast to the lack of effect of supplement advice, fortification of flour and bread with folic acid has led to immediate and sustained falls in the incidence of NTD-affected pregnancies in the USA (Pitkin, 2007), Canada (De Wals et al., 2008) and South America (Lopez-Camelo et al., 2010). According to Solomons (2007), folic acid fortification had been introduced in 42 countries and is currently around double this value.

Folic acid supplements can undoubtedly reduce NTD incidence to a core of non-folate responsive cases, i.e. around seven to eight cases per 100, 000 pregnancies (Heseker et al., 2009). Folate deficiency per se is not a major factor in NTD occurrence, but extra folate probably compensates for some genetic variations in the functioning of folate dependent enzymes or receptors involved in folate metabolism (van der Linden et al., 2006). Folate interacts with vitamin B_{12} in methyl transfer reactions involved in DNA synthesis. Deficiency of either folate or B_{12} impairs red cell production in bone marrow, leading to macrocytic anaemia. Other rapidly dividing cells like those in the foetal neural tube are thus likely to be susceptible to deficiency of these vitamins. Increased peri-conceptual folate from supplements or fortified food may reduce the incidence of other birth defects (Czeizel, 2009) including cleft lip (Wilcox et al., 2007) and congenital heart defects (Ionescu-Ittu et al., 2009).

Concerns about the safety of synthetic folic acid have prevented introduction of mandatory fortification of flour with folic acid in the UK and some other European countries. These concerns are outlined below:

- Several hundred thousand people would receive the folic acid from fortified food for each NTD-affected pregnancy prevented (Smith et al., 2008).
- Large doses of folic acid could mask the anaemia caused by B_{12} deficiency and thus allow irreversible neurological damage to occur. At moderate levels of fortification this seems an improbable risk (Carmel, 2006).
- Folic acid might interfere with the action of various anti-folate drugs, such as methotrexate. Doses of methotrexate used to manage rheumatoid arthritis have reportedly increased in the USA since flour fortification was introduced (Arbelovic et al., 2007). However, Shea et al. (2013) reported that concurrent administration of methotrexate and folic acid supplements to treat rheumatoid arthritis reduced the gastrointestinal side-effects of methotrexate, and Prey and Paul (2009) found that folic acid supplements reduced the adverse liver effects of methotrexate used to treat inflammatory conditions (psoriasis and rheumatoid arthritis).

Pharmacokinetic and pharmacodynamic nutrient-drug interactions are discussed more fully in chapters 6 and 7.
- High dietary folate intake is associated with reduced incidence of bowel cancer (WCRF/AICR, 2007). It has paradoxically been suggested that synthetic folic acid might accelerate the growth of existing bowel tumours or stimulate the development of benign adenomas into cancers (see Mathers, 2009 for potential mechanisms). A tiny upward blip in recorded rates of bowel cancer immediately after the introduction of folic acid fortification in the USA and Canada reinforced this concern. Bowel cancer incidence in the following years continued to decline after the "blip" but remained marginally above that predicted from the pre-fortification trends (Mason et al., 2007). A large Danish cohort study found an apparent protective effect of high food folate intake against bowel cancer, but this effect was not found with supplemental folic acid (Roswall et al., 2010). A recent meta-analysis of randomised controlled trials of folic acid supplements found no significant increase in bowel cancer incidence during the first 5 years of use (Vollset et al., 2013).

Poor folate status is relatively common in the UK, Finch et al. (1998) reported that 19% of free living and 39% of institutionalised elderly people had serum folate levels below 7 nmol/L. Supplements could potentially improve folate status. Folate deficiency leads to moderate elevation of homocysteine levels in blood, as folate is required for its methylation and conversion to methionine. In the inherited condition homocystinuria, plasma levels of homocysteine are greatly elevated and there is increased risk of cardiovascular disease (Clarke et al., 1991). Extra folic acid might reduce homocysteine levels and thus reduce cardiovascular risk. However, evidence from primary and secondary intervention trials does not support any beneficial effects of folic acid, even though they do reduce plasma homocysteine levels (SEARCH Collaborative Group, 2010). Malouf and Grimley Evans (2008) found no support for suggestions that large supplements of folate and/or B_{12} might help prevent or slow progression of Alzheimer's disease.

Supplements of folic acid (400 μg/day) clearly reduce the incidence of NTD if taken prior to and immediately after conception. They may also reduce the incidence of some other developmental defects. There is no substantial evidence that these supplements would have significant risk if widely taken. There is also little clear evidence that such supplements would confer specific wider benefits although they could improve the poor folate status of many in the UK especially institutionalised elderly people. There is some evidence that folic acid supplements may reduce side-effects associated with use of the drug methotrexate.

8.5 Do supplements of the ACE vitamins and selenium reduce cancer and heart disease mortality?

Several micronutrients have inherent antioxidant activity (e.g. vitamins C and E) or act as co-factors for enzymes involved in free radical quenching (e.g. selenium and zinc). The antioxidant nutrients vitamins A (usually as β-carotene), C and E plus selenium have been the subject of a number of clinical trials to test their efficacy in reducing cancer, cardiovascular diseases and total mortality. Observational evidence is generally consistent with a protective role for antioxidants, and these micronutrients in particular, against cancer and heart disease (see examples below) and Harman (1972) went as far as to suggest that addition of an antioxidant supplement to a good natural diet might increase the average age of death by up to 7 years:

- There is an epidemiological association between high antioxidant intake (mainly from fruit and vegetables) and lowered risk of heart disease and cancer.
- Spontaneous use of vitamin E supplements has been associated with reduced rates of coronary heart disease (Rimm *et al.*, 1993; Stampfer *et al.*, 1993).
- Low blood levels of β-carotene and other carotenoids have been associated with increased cancer risk (Ziegler, 1991).
- An inverse relationship between blood levels of vitamin E and coronary heart disease (CHD) mortality has been reported (Gey *et al.*, 1991).

There are also many hundreds of studies which indicate that these and other antioxidants reduce acute measures of oxidant stress in animals and human volunteers.

Despite this weight of suggestive evidence, long-term clinical trials of these ACE vitamins and selenium have not found holistic beneficial effects of supplemental intakes. Some β-carotene trials using smokers or asbestos workers as subjects have actually reported higher total mortality and lung cancer deaths in the supplemented group (e.g. Omenn *et al.*, 1996).

In a major commissioned report, Shekelle *et al.* (2003) found no evidence from an analysis of 144 clinical trials that supplements of these vitamins had any beneficial effects upon cardiovascular or all-cause mortality, or reduced incidence of non-fatal heart attacks. Coulter *et al.* (2003) similarly found no evidence that supplements of these vitamins were useful in preventing or treating cancer. Several meta-analyses have similarly failed to find any significant beneficial effect of antioxidant micronutrient supplements in preventing cancer, cardiovascular disease or in reducing all-cause mortality (Bjelakovic *et al.*, 2008; Myung *et al.*, 2013; Vivekanathan *et al.*, 2003). The potential for net harm from large β-carotene supplements has been confirmed by such studies.

8.6 Do vitamin C supplements prevent or ameliorate the common cold?

Numerous studies have suggested that vitamin C status affects several measures of immune function (overviewed by Hemila and Chalker, 2013). Phagocytic cells (like most body tissues) have a specific transport system for the absorption of vitamin C. Evidence for a role for vitamin C in normal immune function have led to suggestions since the 1940s that large supplemental doses of vitamin C might help prevent colds or reduce their severity and duration. The double Nobel prize-winner Linus Pauling popularised this belief when he published in 1970 a book titled *Vitamin C and the Common Cold*.

In a meta-analysis of 30 trials with over 11 000 participants, Hemila and Chalker (2013) found no evidence that vitamin C supplements of at least 200 mg/day reduced the incidence of colds in the general community (RR 0.97 CI 0.94–1.00). Studies with subjects (c600) who were exposed to severe physical exercise (e.g. marathon runners and skiers) did suggest that vitamin C supplements significantly reduced colds incidence. There was no consistent evidence that vitamin C taken at the onset of a cold had any beneficial effects upon the duration or severity of the symptoms. In those routinely taking large supplements of vitamin C, it may have had a moderate effect on the duration or severity of symptoms. There is still no justification for the routine use of large vitamin C supplements by the general population despite 70 years of investigation. Taking supplements at the onset of a cold produced inconsistent results, and some of the trials where apparent benefits were reported used up to 8 g/day of vitamin C (i.e. 130 times the EU RDA and 40 times the average UK intake). A major report on the safety of large doses of micronutrients (FSA, 2003) concluded that doses of 1 g/day of vitamin C are unlikely to have any adverse effects, even in people who might potentially be more susceptible to harm from high intakes of the vitamin, and they noted that doses well in excess of this are widely used without any apparent ill-effects. At high doses absorption efficiency decreases, and as it is water soluble the vitamin is excreted in the urine. They noted the suggestion that high intakes may increase urinary oxalate excretion and increase the risk of kidney stones, although they noted that the evidence is conflicting and some claims may be due to experimental artefact.

8.7 Do vitamin D (and calcium) supplements improve bone health and have wider benefits?

Substantial numbers of British adults have poor biochemical status for vitamin D (see Table 8.1). Poor vitamin D status is also prevalent in elderly Britons, especially the institutionalised elderly and in children especially those of South Asian origin (Webb, 2011b). There is thus a strong prima facie case for widespread use of vitamin D supplements to improve vitamin D status of populations with limited access to good summer sunlight.

The main source of vitamin D for most people is from endogenous production in the skin when it is exposed to the correct wavelengths of UV light (summer sunlight at latitudes at or above those of the UK). A dehydrogenase in the skin produces 7-dehydrocholesterol from cholesterol and, when exposed to UV light, 7-dehydrocholesterol undergoes photochemical conversion to cholecalciferol or vitamin D_3 (Figure 8.1h). Ergosterol found in yeast and other fungi is converted to calciferol (vitamin D_2) when irradiated, and this has been used as a convenient source of vitamin D for supplements and food fortification. In the UK, no dietary standards are set for vitamin D for most adults and school age children because it was assumed by COMA (1991) that this endogenous skin production should produce sufficient amounts. RNI (range 7–10 μg/day) are set for babies, young children, pregnant and lactating women and the elderly.

Standards in the USA are set on the basis that exposure to sunlight is minimal and represent the estimated physiological need for the vitamin; they range from 15 μg/day for most children and adults, up to 20 μg/day for people over 70 years. Average UK dietary intakes are just 3 μg/day even though all margarine and some other foods are fortified with the vitamin. In the USA, most milk is fortified with vitamin D and daily intakes are around double those in the UK.

Plasma levels of 25-OH vitamin D are used as the biochemical indicator of vitamin D status. In Table 8.1, a level of <25 nmol/L was taken to indicate unsatisfactory status, but the US standards aim to achieve a plasma level of 50 nmol/L. The Endocrine Society in the USA has controversially suggested the following classification for plasma 25-OH vitamin D:

- <50 nmol/L – deficient
- 50–72.5 mmol/L – insufficient
- 100-150 mmol/L – optimal range.

A daily production or intake of 50 μg/day of vitamin D would be needed to achieve this optimum (discussed in Maxmen, 2011).

Vitamin D is a precursor of the renal hormone calcitriol (1, 25 dihydroxy-cholecalciferol). This hormone plays a key role in calcium homeostasis; it:

- Facilitates efficient intestinal calcium absorption
- Enables efficient renal re-absorption of filtered calcium
- Is vital for the formation of normal mineralised bone.

Deficiency of vitamin D causes rickets in children and osteomalacia in adults. Rachitic children do not grow normally and are very prone to infection; they have soft inadequately calcified bone, skeletal abnormalities and low plasma calcium concentration, which causes muscle weakness and even tetany. In the early twentieth century, rickets was prevalent in the industrial cities of northern Europe and parts of North America.

Vitamin D deficiency causes a compensatory secretion of parathyroid hormone, which stimulates bone mineral breakdown and maintains plasma calcium concentration. Osteoporosis is a gradual thinning and weakening of the bones in older people, especially women, which leads to an increased risk of fracture. Prolonged vitamin D insufficiency is a risk factor for osteoporosis (Lips *et al.*, 2006). The National Osteoporosis Society (NOS, 2006) estimated that 3 million people in the UK were affected by osteoporosis causing an annual toll of 70 000 hip fractures, 50 000 wrist fractures and 120 000 vertebral fractures. Hip fracture, where the neck of the femur shears off, is a major problem; many people die in the months immediately after the fracture and its surgical repair, and many more never regain full mobility.

Calcium is a major component of bone mineral, and so low dietary calcium intake was inevitably suspected as the major cause of osteoporosis and calcium supplements advocated for prevention. Poor vitamin D status impairs intestinal absorption of calcium, making it difficult to distinguish between the effects of vitamin D deficiency and low calcium intakes. High calcium intake might compensate for vitamin D insufficiency and optimal vitamin D status might ameliorate the effects of low calcium intake. Hegsted (1986) reported a positive correlation between calcium intake and incidence of hip fracture in nine countries. Despite the limitations of epidemiology in establishing cause and effect, this association between high calcium intake and osteoporosis risk make it unlikely that calcium deficiency per se is a major cause of osteoporosis.

In some clinical trials, vitamin D supplements, often given with calcium, reduced fracture risk in elderly people (e.g. Chapuy *et al.*, 1994). A meta-analysis of nine trials (c.25 000 elderly participants) of vitamin D supplements alone reported no significant effect of vitamin D upon fracture risk. Eight trials (47 000 participants) of combined vitamin D and calcium supplements indicated a significant reduction in hip fracture risk primarily due to the effect on frail, institutionalised elderly people (Avenell *et al.*, 2009). Dawson-Hughes (2006) in a review of seven clinical trials of vitamin D (with or without calcium) on non-vertebral fracture risk suggested that trials which had used at least 17.5 µg/day of vitamin D tended to produce positive results but those that used 10 µg/day or less did not. Avenell *et al.* (2009) did not separate studies according to vitamin D dose, but all of the vitamin D with calcium studies used 10–20 µg/day of vitamin D and 1000 mg/day of calcium. One large and thus heavily weighted study used 10 µg/day of vitamin D and showed only a trend for hip fracture risk. Like Dawson-Hughes (2006) they suggest that doses of vitamin D higher than 10 µg/day would appear to be more effective; recent increases in estimates of vitamin D requirements and adequacy criteria (Maxmen, 2011) suggests this apparent dose-effect needs to be carefully considered. Vitamin D deficiency is prevalent in the UK across the whole lifecycle even using a conservative criterion of adequacy. Prolonged vitamin D inadequacy may chronically impair bone health, and so improving the vitamin D status of the whole population may be more effective in reducing fracture risk than supplements given in old age. Vitamin D and calcium supplements seem to be ineffective in those who have already suffered a fracture (Record, 2005). Annual intramuscular injections of vitamin D have been tried as an alternative to oral dosing, and they would overcome any problems with patient compliance and intestinal absorption of the vitamin. A large meta-analysis published after this chapter was drafted found no evidence that vitamin D supplements given to healthy adults for an average of 2 years had any significant effect on bone density (Reid *et al.*, 2014).

Many cells that are not obviously involved in calcium metabolism have calcitriol receptors, including T and B-lymphocytes, monocytes, skin cells and many cultured tumour cell lines. The presence of receptors on many cells involved in immune and inflammatory responses suggests a role for calcitriol in regulating the immune system. The European Food Standards Authority (EFSA) concluded that there is sufficient evidence to support food labelling claims of a causal relationship between vitamin D intake and normal function of the immune system and a healthy inflammatory response. EFSA rejects the majority of such submissions to authorise claims.

Excessive exposure of the skin to UV radiation in sunlight causes acute sunburn and, more chronically, it increases signs of ageing and the risk of skin cancer and melanoma. Health promotion has thus tended to focus on protecting the skin from sunlight, and the potential benefits of sunlight exposure and vitamin D synthesis have been underplayed. A succession of studies and observations has suggested a range of possible beneficial effects of sunlight and/or vitamin D on a range of conditions unrelated to bone. Some of these potential benefits of vitamin D/sunlight are listed below:

- A protective effect against multiple sclerosis (MS) (discussed later).
- Reduced risk of type 1 diabetes (discussed later).
- Parker *et al.* (2010) in a review of 28 studies found that the highest levels of 25-OH vitamin D in serum were associated with a 40% reduction in cardio-metabolic disorders including cardiovascular diseases, type 2 diabetes and metabolic syndrome.
- Reduced blood pressure and less risk of hypertension. In many cross-sectional studies there is an inverse relationship between plasma 25-OH vitamin D and blood pressure. In a prospective cases-control study with 1500 women, Forman *et al.* (2008) reported that levels of 25-OH vitamin D were significantly lower in women who became hypertensive compared to those who did not. Calcitriol may reduce the output of renin from the juxtaglomerular cells in the kidney. Feelisch *et al.* (2010) have suggested that any beneficial cardiovascular effects of sunlight, including reduced blood pressure, may be independent of vitamin D production and due to the release of nitric oxide from skin, which exerts cardio-protective and anti-hypertensive effects.
- Sunlight and vitamin D supplements were used to treat tuberculosis in the pre-antibiotic era. Rachitic children are generally prone to infections, and vitamin D increases innate immune responses and reduces susceptibility to infection (Liu *et al.*, 2006; Holick and Chen, 2008). In a protocol for a meta-analysis of the role of vitamin D supplements in preventing infections in young children, Yakoob and Bhutta (2010) review the background to this question.
- Oral supplements of vitamin D have been used to treat psoriasis, but topical application of creams containing less toxic analogues are now accepted as an effective mode of treatment (Mason *et al.*, 2013).
- Some epidemiological studies have reported a reduced risk of some cancers in people with good vitamin D status. A major international report concluded that there is inconsistent evidence that good vitamin D status protects against colorectal cancer (WCRF/AICR, 2007).
- Vitamin D deficiency is associated with an increased risk of asthma and other atopic conditions (see Litonjua, 2013).

Increasingly, poor vitamin D status has been linked to increased risk of developing an autoimmune condition like type 1 diabetes or MS. Incidence of type 1 diabetes, MS, hypertension and some cancers increases with increasing latitude (i.e. reduced sunlight).

Vitamin D or calcitriol is said to reduce the incidence of diabetes in mice (NOD) with an inherited genetic susceptibility to type 1 diabetes (van Etten *et al.*, 2002). There is some support for a protective effect of early childhood vitamin supplementation and reduced risk of developing type 1 diabetes (Zipitis and Akobeng, 2008).

Good vitamin D status is associated with reduced risk of MS in several epidemiological studies. MS incidence increases with increasing latitude and, at any given latitude, high altitude (with stronger sunlight) is associated with reduced incidence. Migration studies tend to support a protective effect of solar radiation. In an experimental murine model of MS, vitamin D reduces the severity of the symptoms (see reviews by Hayes,

2000; Hanwell and Banwell, 2011; Smolders *et al.*, 2008). Ramagopolan *et al.* (2011) reported that being heterozygous for a gene mutation that leads to lowered levels of calcitriol in the blood is associated with increased risk of MS. This gene (CYP27B1) codes for the 1α-hydroxylase that activates vitamin D and being homozygous for this mutation causes vitamin D-dependent rickets (VDDR1). This is consistent with a role for vitamin D deficiency in the pathogenesis of MS. One of the co-authors of this study (Ebers) has suggested that the Scottish Government should fortify foods with vitamin D specifically to reduce the toll of MS; Scotland has one of the highest rates of MS in the world and one of the highest rates of vitamin D deficiency.

Measures designed to ensure good vitamin D status in all sectors of the population are clearly justified. Vitamin D deficiency is prevalent in the UK and in other populations across the world, especially those at living at high latitude. Holick and Chen (2008) describe vitamin D deficiency as a worldwide pandemic caused by insufficient skin exposure to sunlight. Improved vitamin D status should yield significant health benefits: improved bone health, improved immune function, and possibly reduced rates of hypertension, type 1 diabetes, MS and some cancers. Whilst the evidence for these putative benefits varies in strength, the overall case for improving vitamin D status is strong.

Natural food is unlikely to supply enough vitamin D to satisfy physiological needs for the vitamin. Ensuring adequate exposure of the skin to sunlight (without risking burning), dietary supplements, food fortification and bolus injections of vitamin D are the possible strategies for improving vitamin D status.

8.8 Can supplements of essential minerals reduce blood pressure?

High population salt (sodium chloride) intake raises average blood pressure and increases the incidence of hypertension. Individual salt reduction is one strategy used in the management of high blood pressure. There are also suggestions that relatively high intakes of potassium, magnesium or calcium may be protective against high blood pressure. Table 8.1 shows that average intakes of potassium and magnesium are relatively low compared to the UK dietary standard of adequacy (RNI), and many adults, especially young women, have intakes that are classified as inadequate.

There is inconsistent epidemiological evidence that high potassium intake is associated with reduced blood pressure and prevalence of hypertension. Diets rich in fruits and vegetables are high in potassium, and these are generally associated with lower blood pressure and may have some benefit in controlling hypertension. COMA (1994) in a report on nutrition and cardiovascular disease recommended that in order to reduce average blood pressure and hypertension incidence, salt intake should be substantially reduced and potassium intake increased by increasing fruit and vegetable intakes. A meta-analysis of controlled trials and cohort studies by Aburto *et al.* (2013) reported that increased potassium intake resulted in a significant reduction in blood pressure in those who were hypertensive, and that higher potassium intake reduced stroke incidence. Coupled with the low potassium intakes recorded in Table 8.1, this supports measures that would increase natural potassium intake and suggests that potassium should be a component of multi-nutrient supplements.

Dickinson *et al.* (2006a) review limited evidence that high magnesium intake may lower blood pressure. In a meta-analysis of controlled trials they found that magnesium supplements did produce an apparent small but significant reduction in diastolic but not systolic blood pressure. However, the quality of the reviewed trials was poor, and any apparent effect of magnesium may have been due to bias. A more recent meta-analysis by Kass *et al.* (2012) also reported a small blood pressure lowering effect of magnesium supplements. There is a need for large well-designed trials to clarify whether magnesium supplements have any clinically useful effect upon blood pressure.

Dickinson *et al.* (2006b) found no evidence to support the hypothesis that calcium supplements lower blood pressure in hypertensive adults. In this meta-analysis, supplements did apparently lead to a small reduction in systolic pressure, but the poor quality of the trials and the heterogeneity of results suggested that any effect was probably due to bias.

8.9 Should parents in areas without fluoridated water give their children fluoride supplements?

Fluoride is not classified as an essential nutrient in either the UK or USA, but it is on the approved list of substances that can be added to food supplements within the EU. It is regarded as a beneficial dietary constituent that reduces risk of tooth decay in children. Fluoride-only supplements are sold as medicines in the UK. In areas where the natural fluoride level in drinking water is around 1 mg/L, rates of tooth decay are relatively low and fluoridation of water to this level reduces rates of decayed, missing and filled teeth in children (WHO, 1970). Around two-thirds of Americans receive water that is fluoridated, but by 2005 only 10% of the UK population received fluoridated water.

Excess fluoride causes mottling of the teeth, which initially manifests as white flecks on the surface of the enamel, but they can become mottled with brown or yellow stains. This occurs where water fluoride levels exceed 10 mg/L. Large overdoses associated with drinking water from wells with very high fluoride concentrations can rarely cause skeletal fluorosis, which causes joint pain and osteoporosis and, in extreme cases, can lead to muscle wasting and neurological symptoms. Most toothpaste is now fluoridated, and this is credited with much of the reduction in dental caries that has occurred in western countries since the 1960s.

Some parents living in areas where water is not fluoridated choose to give their children fluoride tablets. The British Dental Association (BDA) recommends that these supplements should not be given prior to 6 months of age and that the dose should depend upon the age of the child and the concentration of fluoride in the local drinking water:

- No supplements should be given if the water concentration is above 700 µg/L.
- If the water concentration is <300 µg/L, then daily doses should be – 250 µg up to 3 years, 500 µg from 3 to 6 years and 1 mg from 6 years to puberty.
- If the water concentration is in the range 300–700 µg/L, then the daily dose should be 250 µg for 3–6 year olds and 500 µg from 6 years till puberty.

8.10 Do micronutrients improve immune function in the elderly?

Malnutrition has deleterious effects upon the functioning of the immune system. Malnourished people are more likely to develop infections, and the severity and duration are increased. The effects of both general energy-protein malnutrition and specific micronutrient deficiencies on immune function have been reviewed by Scrimshaw and SanGiovanni (1997). As an example, experimental vitamin A deficiency leads to reduced cell mediated and antibody mediated responses. There is reduced antibody formation, reduced numbers of natural killer cells and reduced ability of neutrophils to ingest and kill bacteria. Vitamin A deficiency leads to a loss of epithelial integrity, which increases vulnerability to infection.

There is also an age-related general decline in the functioning of both the innate and adaptive arms of the immune system – immunosenescence. Some of the well-documented changes in immune function in older people are summarised below (see Graham *et al.*, 2006). Ageing leads to:

- Involution of the thymus gland with reduced capacity to produce T-lymphocytes, especially naïve T-cells in response to a new infective challenge.
- Reduced functioning of B-lymphocytes, so the elderly respond less well to vaccination.
- Decline in natural killer cell function.
- Loss of integrity of the epithelial barrier to infection in the skin, lung and gut.

Poor micronutrient status in elderly people would be expected to exacerbate the normal age-related decline in immune function and might contribute to the weakened immune functioning of some older people. El-Kadiki and Sutton (2005) conducted a meta-analysis to evaluate the effectiveness of micronutrient supplements in reducing infection risk in the elderly. The included studies used different outcome measures, and so they did separate analyses for these different outcomes and two of these are summarised below:

- Three studies used "number of days suffering from an infection during a year" as their outcome measure. Combination of these studies showed a large and highly significant beneficial effect with an average of almost 18 less infected days during the year. El-Kadiki and Sutton (2005) noted the surprisingly small standard deviations in these studies for a measure expected to be very variable; all three studies were individually significant.
- Three studies used "likelihood of having an infection during the period", and these showed no significant effect of supplements, not even a non-significant trend towards reduced risk.

These analyses seem to be contradictory; micronutrient supplements greatly reduce the number of days with an infection but have no effect on the risk of infection. All three of the studies using the first outcome measure originate from the research group of Dr RK Chandra who has been accused in both the popular media and the scientific literature of fabricating clinical trial data (e.g. Smith, 2005). Chandra was for many years regarded as "the internationally recognised expert in nutrition and immunity" (Dickinson, 2002) and even dubbed "the father of nutritional immunology." He suggested that a causal relationship exists between under nutrition and impaired immunity and that this is usually a correctable abnormality – powerful justification for the use of supplements.

In 2000, Chandra submitted a paper to the *British Medical Journal* which purported to show that the same supplement used in the trials on immune function markedly improved cognitive function in the elderly. The *BMJ* rejected this paper, whose reviewer suggested that it "had all the hallmarks of having been entirely invented" (Smith, 2005). This paper was subsequently published in another journal (Chandra, 2001) where it attracted widespread criticism and doubts about its credibility (e.g. Shenkin *et al.* 2002). The paper was eventually retracted by the journal's editor (Meguid, 2005) who listed eight concerns about the paper which Chandra failed to address satisfactorily. Meguid refers to evidence that one of the most influential papers published by Chandra (1992) on the effects of supplements on infection risk may not have actually been conducted. Dr Chandra had previously been accused of fabricating trial data that purported to show that a brand of hypoallergenic milk could reduce allergies in susceptible babies—findings that have been used in the marketing of this product. He was accused of publishing the results of the study long before the recruitment of subjects was completed. He has been publicly accused of accepting sponsor's money to conduct the trial, but not actually conducting it (see O'Neill-Yates, 2006)

El-Kadiki and Sutton (2005) issued a correction to their initial analysis showing the results with and without the inclusion of data from Chandra's group. A meta-analysis by Stephen and Avenell (2006) addressed the same question and found no significant effects of micronutrient supplements on any outcome measures when results from Chandra's group were excluded. Several highly significant effects of supplements were found when data from Chandra's group were included in the analysis.

There may be theoretical grounds to suggest that micronutrient supplements might improve immune function in the elderly, but there is no trustworthy evidence from clinical trials to support this.

8.11 Conclusions

In the first half of the twentieth century, it was shown that increased intake of vitamins or minerals was able to prevent or cure several common, serious and sometimes fatal deficiency diseases such as pellagra, beriberi, cretinism and rickets. For example, from 1900 to 1950, there were three million cases and 100 000 deaths in the USA from pellagra caused by niacin (B_3) deficiency (Fletcher *et al.*, 2004). In 1924, prior to the use of iodised salt, incidence of endemic goitre caused by iodine deficiency was 39% in schools in Michigan (see Kimball, 1953).

Over the period 1929–1943, 11 people shared seven Nobel prizes in physiology, medicine or chemistry for vitamin-related work. These spectacular successes may have created a "legacy of expectation" about the ability of diet and micronutrient supplements to yield benefits beyond simply curing or preventing these specific deficiency diseases. However, despite a huge investment of research effort and resources, there is still no clear evidence that extra supplies of vitamins and minerals will yield general benefits in people whose intake from food already meets standards of adequacy. In some cases, the standards used to define adequacy are still disputed, notably for vitamin D.

Supplements certainly have the potential to improve vitamin and mineral adequacy, and this would have huge benefits for populations in developing countries where overt deficiency of some vitamins or minerals is still a major problem. Even in affluent industrialised countries, vitamin and mineral adequacy cannot be taken for granted. Overt clinical cases of deficiency diseases are usually uncommon in these countries (except iron deficiency anaemia) but many people have unsatisfactory intakes from food or show biochemical indications of poor nutritional status for one or more micronutrients. There are also a limited number of examples of situations where extra vitamins or minerals may help specified groups of people. A clear example is the ability of surplus peri-conceptual amounts of folic acid to reduce the risk of women having a baby affected by a NTD. Even where they could be beneficial, supplements have had limited practical impact because they do not reach or are not taken by those likely to benefit from them.

When large clinical trials of micronutrient supplements are conducted using random samples of industrialised populations, most of the sample will already be receiving adequate amounts of the substance(s) being tested. A lack of significant effect of the supplement may simply reflect the already good status of most of the sample. If initial status was measured at the outset of the study, this would allow the effect of the supplement to be determined in those with less than ideal initial status. Of course this would not detract from the argument that supplements generally produce only measurable benefits in those whose intake or status is unsatisfactory.

References

Aburto, N.J., Hanson, S., Gutierrez, H., Hooper, C., Elliot, P. and Capuccio, F.P. (2013) Effect of increased potassium intake on cardiovascular risk factors and disease: systematic review and meta-analyses. *British Medical Journal* 346, 378. Available from: http://www.bmj.com/content/346/bmj.f1378?view=long&pmid=23558164.

Andersson, M., de Benoist, B., Darnton-Hill, I. and Delange, F. (2007) Iodine deficiency in Europe: a continuing public health problem. Geneva, World Health Organisation (with UNICEF). Available from: http://www.who.int/nutrition/publications/VMNIS_Iodine_deficiency_in_Europe.pdf.

Arbelovic, S., Sam, G., Dallal, G.E., Jacques, P.F., Selhub, J., Rosenberg, I.H. and Robenhoff, R. (2007) Preliminary evidence shows that folic acid fortification of the food supply is associated with higher methotrexate dosing in patients with rheumatoid arthritis. *Journal of the American College of Nutrition*, 26, 453–455. Available from: http://www.jacn.org/content/26/5/453.long.

Avenell, A., Gillespie, W.J., Gillespie, L.D. and O'Connell, D. (2009) Vitamin D and vitamin D analogues for preventing fractures associated with involutional and post-menopausal osteoporosis. *Cochrane Database of Systematic Reviews* 2009, Issue 2. Art. No.: CD000227. DOI: 10.1002/14651858.CD000227.pub3. Available from: http://onlinelibrary.wiley.com/doi/10.1002/14651858.CD000227.pub3/full.

Bailey, R.L., Mills, J.L., Yetley, E.A., Gahche, J.J., Pfeiffer, C.M., Dwyer, J.T., Dodd, K.N., Sempos, C.T., Betz, J.N. and Picciano, M.F. (2010) Unmetabolized serum folic acid and its relation to folic acid intake from diet and supplements in a nationally representative sample of adults aged > or =60 y in the United States. *American Journal of Clinical Nutrition*, 92, 383–389. Available from: http://www.ajcn.org/content/92/2/383.long.

Bath, S.C., Steer, C.D., Golding, L., Emmett, P. and Rayman, M.P. (2013) Effect of inadequate iodine status in UK pregnant women on cognitive outcomes in their children: results from the Avon Longitudinal Study of Parents and Children (ALSPAC). *Lancet*, 382, 331–337. Available from: http://www.sciencedirect.com/science/article/pii/S0140673613604365.

Bjelakovic, G., Nikolova, D., Gluud, L.L., Simonetti, R.G. and Gluud, C. (2008) Antioxidant supplements for prevention of mortality in healthy participants and patients with various diseases. *Cochrane Database of Systematic Reviews* 2008, Issue 2. Art. No.: CD007176. DOI: 10.1002/14651858.CD007176. Available from: http://onlinelibrary.wiley.com/doi/10.1002/14651858.CD007176/abstract;jsessionid=608BF080C4B6C5440D21A8BE164F0B39.d01t03.

Botto, L.D., Lisi, A., Robert-Gnansia, E., Erickson, J.D., Vollset, S.C., Mastroiacovo, P. Botting, B., Cochi, C., de Vigan, C., de Walle, H., Feifoo, M., Irgens, M., McDonnell, B., Merlob, P., Ritauven, A., Scarano, G., Siffel, C., Metueki, J., Stoll, C., Smithells, R. And Goujard, J. (2005) International retrospective cohort study of neural tube defects in relation to folic acid recommendations: are the recommendations working? *British Medical Journal*, 330, 571. Available from: https://www.ncbi.nlm.nih.gov/pmc/articles/PMC554029/.

Branch, J.D. (2003) Effect of creatine supplementation on body composition and performance: a meta-analysis. *International Journal of Sport Nutrition and Exercise Metabolism*, 13, 198–226.

Broad, E.M., Maughan, R.J. and Galloway, S.D. (2005) Effects of four weeks L-carnitine L-tartrate ingestion on substrate utilization during prolonged exercise. *International Journal of Sport Nutrition and Exercise Metabolism*, 15, 665–679.

Carmel, R. (2006) Folic acid In Shils, M.E., Shike, M., Ross, A.C., Caballero, B.J. and Cousins, R.J. *Modern Nutrition in Health and Disease* 10th edn. Philadelphia, Lippincott, Williams and Wilkins, 470–481.

Chandra, R.K. (1992) Effect of vitamin and trace-element supplementation on immune responses and infection in elderly subjects. *Lancet*, 340, 1124–1126.

Chandra, R.K. (2001) (RETRACTED) Effect of vitamin and trace-element supplementation on cognitive function in elderly subjects. *Nutrition*, 17, 709–712. Available from: http://www.sciencedirect.com/science/article/pii/S0899900701006104.

Chapuy, M.C., Arlot, M.E., Delmas, P.D. and Meunier, P.J. (1994) Effects of calcium and cholecalciferol treatment for three years on hip fractures in elderly women. *British Medical Journal*, 308, 1081–1082. Available from: http://www.bmj.com/content/308/6936/1081?view=long&pmid=8173430.

COMA (1991) Dietary reference values for food energy and nutrients for the United Kingdom: report no. 41 of the Committee on Medical Aspects of Food Policy. London, HMSO.

COMA (1994). Nutritional aspects of cardiovascular disease: report no. 46 of the Committee on Medical Aspects of Food Policy. London, HMSO.

Clarke, R., Daly, L., Robinson, K., Naughtan, E., Cahalane, S., Fowler, B. and Graham, I. (1991) Hyperhomocysteinemia: an independent risk factor for vascular disease. *New England Journal of Medicine*, 324, 1149–1155. Available from: http://www.nejm.org/doi/full/10.1056/NEJM199104253241701.

Czeizel, A.E. (2009) Periconceptual folic acid and multivitamin supplementation for the prevention of neural tube defects and other congenital abnormalities. *Birth Defects Research Part A: Clinical and Molecular Teratology*, 85, 260–268. http://onlinelibrary.wiley.com/doi/10.1002/bdra.20563/full.

Dawson-Hughes, B. (2006) Osteoporosis In Shils, M.E., Ross, A.C., Caballero, B.J. and Cousins, R.J. *Modern Nutrition in Health and Disease* 10th edn. Philadelphia, Lippincott, Williams and Wilkins, 1339–1352.

De Benoist, B., McLean, E., Andersson, M. and Rogers, L. (2008) Iodine deficiency in 2007: global progress since 2003. *Food and Nutrition Bulletin*, 29, 195–202. Available from: http://www.who.int/nutrition/publications/micronutrients/FNBvol29N3sep08.pdf.

De-Regil, L.M., Fernández-Gaxiola, A.C., Dowswell, T. and Peña-Rosas, J.P. (2010) Effects and safety of periconceptional folate supplementation for preventing birth defects. *Cochrane Database of Systematic Reviews* 2010, Issue 10. Art. No.: CD007950. DOI: 10.1002/14651858.CD007950.pub2. Available from: http://onlinelibrary.wiley.com/doi/10.1002/14651858.CD007950.pub2/full.

De Wals, P., Tairou, F., Van Allen, M.I., Lowry, R.B., Evans, J.A., Van den Hoff, M.C., Crowley, M., Uh, S-H., Zimmer, P., Sibbald, B., Fernandez, B., Lee, N.S. and Niyonsenga, T. (2008) Spina bifida before and after folic acid fortification in Canada. *Birth Defect Research Part A Clinical and Molecular Teratology*, 82, 622–626. Available from: http://onlinelibrary.wiley.com/doi/10.1002/bdra.20485/full.

DH (1992) Folic acid and the prevention of Neural Tube Defects. Report from an expert working group. London, Department of Health.

Dickinson, A. (2002) Benefits of nutritional supplements: immune function in the elderly. In The benefits of nutritional supplements Washington DC, Council for Responsible Nutrition. Available from: http://www.crnusa.org/benpdfs/CRN009benefits_elderly.pdf.

Dickinson, H.O., Nicolson, D., Campbell, F., Cook, J.V., Beyer, F.R., Ford, G.A. and Mason, J. (2006a) Magnesium supplementation for the management of primary hypertension in adults. *Cochrane Database of Systematic Reviews* 2006, Issue 3. Art. No.: CD004640. DOI: 10.1002/14651858.CD004640.pub2. Available from: http://onlinelibrary.wiley.com/doi/10.1002/14651858.CD004640.pub2/full.

Dickinson, H.O., Nicolson, D., Cook, J.V., Campbell, F., Beyer, F.R., Ford, G.A. and Mason, J. (2006b) Calcium supplementation for the management of primary hypertension in adults. *Cochrane Database of Systematic Reviews* 2006, Issue 2. Art. No.: CD004639. DOI: 10.1002/14651858.CD004639.pub2. Available from: http://onlinelibrary.wiley.com/doi/10.1002/14651858.CD004639.pub2/full.

El-Kadiki, A. and Sutton, A.J. (2005) Role of multivitamins and mineral supplements in preventing infections in elderly people: systematic review and meta-analysis of randomised controlled trials. *British Medical Journal*, 330, 871. Available from: http://www.bmj.com/content/330/7496/871?view=long&pmid=15805125.

Feelisch, M., Kolb-Bachofen, V., Liu, D., Lundberg, J.O., Revelo, C.P., Suschek, C.V. and Weller, R.B. (2010) Is sunlight good for our heart? *European Heart Journal*, 31, 1041–1045. Available from: http://eurheartj.oxfordjournals.org/content/31/9/1041.long.

Finch, S., Doyle, W., Lowe, C., Bates, C.J., Prentice, A., Smithers, G and Clarke, P.C. (1998) National diet and nutrition survey: people aged 65 years and over. London, The Stationery Office.

Fletcher, R.J., Bell, I.P. and Lambert, J.P. (2004) Public health aspects of food fortification: a question of balance. *Proceedings of the Nutrition Society*, 63, 605–614. Available from: http://journals.cambridge.org/action/displayAbstract?fromPage=online&aid=902204.

Forman, J.P., Curhan, G.C. and Taylor, E.N. (2008) Plasma 25-hydroxyvitamin D levels and risk of incident hypertension among young women. *Hypertension*, 52, 828–832. Available from: http://hyper.ahajournals.org/content/52/5/828.long.

FSA (2003) Food Standards Agency. Safe upper levels for vitamins and minerals. Report of the Expert Group on Vitamins and minerals, The Stationary Office, London. Available from: http://www.food.gov.uk/multimedia/pdfs/vitmin2003.pdf .

Gey, K.F., Puska, P., Jordan, P. and Moser, U.K. (1991) Inverse correlation between plasma vitamin E and mortality from ischemic heart disease in cross-cultural epidemiology. *American Journal of Clinical Nutrition*, 53, 326S–334S. Available from: http://www.ajcn.org/content/53/1/326S.long.

Graham, J.E., Christian, L.M. and Kiecolt-Glaser, J.K. (2006) Stress, age and immune function: toward a lifespan approach. *Journal of Behavioural Medicine*, 29, 389–400. Available from: http://www.ncbi.nlm.nih.gov/pmc/articles/PMC2805089/

Hanwell, HE and Banwell, B. (2011) Assessment of evidence for a protective role of vitamin D in multiple sclerosis. *Biochimica et Biophysica Acta*, 1812, 202–212. Available from: http://www.sciencedirect.com/science/article/pii/S0925443910001547.

Hardy, M., Coulter, I., Morton, S.C., Favreau, J., Venturupalli, S., Chiapelli, F., Rossi, F., Orschansky, G., Jungvig, L.K., Roth, E.A., Suttorp, M.J. and Shekelle, P. (2002) S-Adenosyl-L-Methionine for Treatment of Depression, Osteoarthritis, and Liver Disease. Evidence Report/Technology Assessment Number 64. AHRQ Publication No. 02-E034. Rockville, MD, Agency for Healthcare Research and Quality. Available from: http://www.ncbi.nlm.nih.gov/books/bv.fcgi?rid=hstat1a.chapter.2159.

Harman, D. (1972) Free radical theory of aging: nutritional implications. *American Journal of Clinical Nutrition* 25, 839–843. Available from: http://www.ajcn.org/content/25/8/839.long.

Harper, A.E. (1999) Defining the essentiality of nutrients. In Shils, M.E. *et al. Modern Nutrition in Health and Disease* 9th edn. Philadelphia, Lippincott, Williams and Wilkins, 3–10.

Harris, R.C., Soderlund, K. and Hultman, E. (1992) Elevation of creatine in resting and exercised muscle of normal subjects by creatine supplementation. *Clinical Science*, 83, 367–374.

Hayes, C.E. (2000) Vitamin D: a natural inhibitor of multiple sclerosis. *Proceedings of the Nutrition Society*, 59, 531–535. Available from: http://journals.cambridge.org/action/displayAbstract?fromPage=online&aid=796900.

Hegsted, D.M. (1986) Calcium and osteoporosis. *Journal of Nutrition*, 116, 2316–2319. Available from: http://jn.nutrition.org/content/116/11/2316.long.

Hemila, H. and Chalker, E. (2013) Vitamin C for preventing and treating the common cold. *Cochrane Database of Systematic Reviews* 2013, Issue 1. Art. No.: CD000980. DOI: 10.1002/14651858.CD000980.pub4. Available from: http://onlinelibrary.wiley.com/doi/10.1002/14651858.CD000980.pub4/full.

Heseker, H.B., Mason, J.B., Sahib, J., Rosenber, I.H. and Jacques, P.F. (2009) Not all cases of neural-tube defect can be prevented by increasing the intake of folic acid. *British Journal of Nutrition*, 102, 173–180. Available from: http://journals.cambridge.org/action/displayAbstract?fromPage=online&aid=5905772.

Higgins, J.P.T. and Flicker, L. (2000) Lecithin for dementia and cognitive impairment. *Cochrane Database of Systematic Reviews* 2000, Issue 4. Art. No.: CD001015. DOI: 10.1002/14651858.CD001015. Available from: http://onlinelibrary.wiley.com/doi/10.1002/14651858.CD001015/full.

Hoare, J., Henderson, L., Bates, C.J., Prentice, A., Birch, M., Swan, G. and Farron, M. (2004) National Diet & Nutrition Survey: adults aged 19 to 64 years. Volume 5: Summary report. London, The Stationery Office. Available from: http://www.food.gov.uk/multimedia/pdfs/ndns5full.pdf.

Holick, M.F. and Chen, T.C. (2008) Vitamin D deficiency: a worldwide problem with health consequences. *American Journal of Clinical Nutrition*, 87(suppl), 1080S–1086S. Available from: http://www.ajcn.org/content/87/4/1080S.long.

Ionescu-Ittu, R., Marelli, A.J., Mackie, A.S. and Pilote, L. (2009) Prevalence of severe congenital heart disease after folic acid fortification of grain products: a time trend analysis in Quebec, Canada. *British Medical Journal* 338, b1673. Available from: http://www.bmj.com/content/338/bmj.b1673.long.

Kass, L., Weekes, J. and Carpenter, L. (2012) Effect of magnesium supplementation on blood pressure: a meta-analysis. *European Journal of Clinical Nutrition*, 66, 411–418.

Kimball, O.P. (1953) History of the prevention of endemic goitre. *Bulletin of the World Health Organization*, 9, 241–248. Available from: http://whqlibdoc.who.int/bulletin/1953/Vol9/Vol9-No2/bulletin_1953_9(2)_241-248.pdf.

Klugman, A., Sauer, J., Tabet, N. and Howard, R. (2004) Alpha lipoic acid for dementia. *Cochrane Database of Systematic Reviews* 2004, Issue 1. Art. No.: CD004244. DOI: 10.1002/14651858.CD004244.pub2. Available from: http://onlinelibrary.wiley.com/doi/10.1002/14651858.CD004244.pub2/full.

Lips, P., Hosking, D., Lippuner, K., Norquist, J.M., Wehren, L., Maalouf, G., Ragi-Eis, S. and Chandler, J. (2006) The prevalence of vitamin D inadequacy amongst women with osteoporosis: an international epidemiological investigation. *Journal of Internal Medicine*. 260, 245–254. Available from: http://onlinelibrary.wiley.com/doi/10.1111/j.1365-2796.2006.01685.x/pdf.

Litonuja, A.A. (2013) Vitamin D and corticosteroids in asthma: synergy, interaction and potential therapeutic effects. *Expert Review in Respiratory Medicine*, 7, 101–104. Available from: http://www.expert-reviews.com/doi/full/10.1586/ers.12.85.

Liu, P.T., Stenger, S., Li, H., Wenzell, L., Tan, B.H., Krutzik, K., Ochoa, M.T., Schauber, J., Wu, K., Meinken, C., Kaman, D.L., Zugel, U., Gallo, R.L., Eisenberg, D., Hewison, M., Hollis, B.W., Adams, J.S., Bloom, S.R. and Modlin, R.L.. (2006) Toll-like receptor triggering of a vitamin D-mediated human antimicrobial response. *Science*, 311, 1770–1773. Available from: http://www.sciencemag.org/content/311/5768/1770.long.

Lopez-Camelo, J.S., Castilla, E.E. and Orioli, I.M. (2010) Folic acid fortification: impact on the frequencies of 52 congenital anomaly types in three South American countries. *American Journal of Medical Genetics. Part A*. 152A, 2444–2458. Available from: http://onlinelibrary.wiley.com/doi/10.1002/ajmg.a.33479/full.

Malouf, R. and Grimley Evans, J. (2008) Folic acid with or without vitamin B12 for the prevention and treatment of healthy elderly and demented people. *Cochrane Database of Systematic Reviews* 2008, Issue4. Art. No.: CD004514.DOI: 10.1002/14651858.CD004514.pub2. Available from: http://onlinelibrary.wiley.com/o/cochrane/clsysrev/articles/CD004514/frame.html.

Marcoff, L. and Thompson, P.D. (2007) The role of coenzyme Q10 in statin-associated myopathy: a systematic review. *Journal of the American College of Cardiology*, 49, 2231–2237. Available from: http://www.sciencedirect.com/science/article/pii/S0735109707010546.

Mason, A.R., Mason, J., Cork, M. et al. (2013) Topical treatments for chronic plaque psoriasis. *Cochrane Database of Systematic Reviews* 2013, Issue 3. Art. No.: CD005028. DOI: 10.1002/14651858.CD005028.pub3. Available from: http://onlinelibrary.wiley.com/doi/10.1002/14651858.CD005028.pub3/full.

Mason, J.B., Dickstein, A., Jacques, P.F., Haggarty, P., Selhub, J., Dallal, G. and Rosenberg, I.H. (2007) A temporal association between folic acid fortification and an increase in colorectal cancer rates may be illuminating important biological principles: a hypothesis. *Cancer Prevention, Epidemiology and Biomarkers*, 16, 1325–1329. Available from: http://cebp.aacrjournals.org/content/16/7/1325.long.

Mathers, J.C. (2009) Folate intake and bowel cancer risk. *Genes and Nutrition*, 4, 173–178. Available from: http://www.springerlink.com/content/2v57m28125721j09/.

Maxmen, A. (2011) Nutrition advice: the vitamin D-lemma. *Nature*, 475, 23–25. http://www.nature.com/news/2011/110706/full/475023a.html.

Mayo-Wilson, E., Imdad, A., Herzer, K., Yakoob, M.Y. and Bhutta, Z.A. (2011) Vitamin A supplements for preventing mortality, illness, and blindness in children under 5: Systematic review and meta-analysis. *British Medical Journal*, 343: d5294. Available from: http://www.bmj.com/content/343/bmj.d5094?view=long&pmid=21868478.

Meguid, M. (2005) Retraction of: Chandra RK, Nutrition 2001: 17; 709–12. *Nutrition* 21, 286. http://www.sciencedirect.com/science/article/pii/S0899900704003089.

Mintel (2009) Vitamins and supplements – UK – May 2009. London, Mintel International Group Limited.

MRC (1991) The MRC Vitamin Study Group. Prevention of neural tube defects: results of the Medical Research Council Vitamin Study. *Lancet*, 338, 131–137.

Myung, S.K., Ju, W., Cho, B., Oh, S-W., Park, S.M., Koo, B-K. and Park, B-J. (2013) Efficacy of vitamin and antioxidant supplements in prevention of cardiovascular disease: a systematic review and meta-analysis of randomised controlled trials. *British Medical Journal*, 346, f10. http://www.bmj.com/content/346/bmj.f10?view=long&pmid=23335472.

NOS (2006) National osteoporosis Society. Osteoporosis facts and figures. Available from: http://www.nos.org.uk/page.aspx?pid=328&srcid=328.

Omenn, G.S., Goodman, G.E., Thornquist, M.D., Balmes, J., Cullen, M.R., Glass, A., Keogh, J.P., Meyskens, F.L., Valanais, B., Williams, J.H., Barnhart, S. and Hammar, S. (1996) Combination of beta-carotene and vitamin A on lung cancer and cardiovascular disease. *New England Journal of Medicine*, 334, 1150–1155. Available from: http://www.nejm.org/doi/full/10.1056/NEJM199605023341802.

O'Neill-Yates, C. (2006) (TV documentary) The secret life of Dr Chandra (part 1, transcript CBC's The National). Available from: http://www.infactcanada.ca/Chandra_Jan30_2006.htm.

Oosthuizen, W., Virster, H.H., Vermaak, W.J., Smuts, C.M., Jerling, J.C., Veldman, F.J. and Burger, H.M. (1998) Lecithin has no effect on serum lipoprotein, plasma fibrinogen and macro molecular protein complex levels in hyperlipidaemic men in a double-blind controlled study. *European Journal of Clinical Nutrition*, 52, 419–424.

Parker, J., Hashmi, O., Dutton, D., Mavrodaris, A., Stranges, S., Kandala, N.B., Clarke, A. and Franco, O.H. (2010) Levels of vitamin D and cardiometabolic disorders: systematic review and meta-analysis. *Maturitas*, 65, 225–236.

Pitkin, R.M. (2007) Folate and neural tube defects. *American Journal of Clinical Nutrition*, 85, 285S–288S. Available from: http://www.ajcn.org/content/85/1/285S.long.

Prey, S. and Paul, C. (2009) Effect of folic or folinic acid supplementation on methotrexate associated safety and efficacy in inflammatory disease: a systematic review. *British*

Journal of Dermatology, 160, 622–628. Available from: http://onlinelibrary.wiley.com/doi/10.1111/j.1365-2133.2008.08876.x/full.

Ramagopolan, S.V., Dyment, D.A., Cader, M.Z., Morrisom, K.M., Disanto, G., Morahan, J.M., Berlanga-Tayloer, A.J., Handel, A., De Luca, G.G., Sadovnick, A.D., Lepage, P., Montpetit, A. and Ebers, G.C. (2011a) Rare variants in the CYP27B1 gene are associated with multiple sclerosis. *Annals of Neurology*, 70, 881–886. Available from: http://onlinelibrary.wiley.com/doi/10.1002/ana.22678/full.

Ramagopalan, S.V., Handel, A.E., Giovanni, G., Siegel, S.R., Ebers, G.C. and Chaplin, G. (2011b) Relationship of UV exposure to prevalence of multiple sclerosis in England. *Neurology*, 76, 1410–1414. Available from: http://www.ncbi.nlm.nih.gov/pmc/articles/PMC3087404/?tool=pubmed.

Rambaldi, A. and Gluud, C. (2006) S-adenosyl-L-methionine for alcoholic liver diseases. *Cochrane Database of Systematic Reviews* 2006, Issue 2. Art. No.: CD002235. DOI: 10.1002/14651858.CD002235.pub2. Available from: http://onlinelibrary.wiley.com/doi/10.1002/14651858.CD002235.pub2/full.

Record Trial Group (2005) Oral vitamin D3 and calcium for secondary prevention of low-trauma fractures in elderly people (Randomised Evaluation of Calcium Or Vitamin S, RECORD): a randomised placebo-controlled trial. *Lancet*, 365, 1621–1628. Available from: http://www.sciencedirect.com/science/article/pii/S0140673605630139.

Reid, I.R., Bolland, M.J. and Grey, A. (2014) Effects of vitamin D supplements on bone mineral density: a systematic review and meta-analysis. *Lancet*, 383, 146–155. Available from: http://www.sciencedirect.com/science/article/pii/S0140673613616475.

Rimm, E.B., Stampfer, M.J., Ascheirio, A., Giovanucci, K.M., Colditz, G.A. and Willett, W.C. (1993) Vitamin E consumption and the risk of coronary heart disease in men. *New England Journal of Medicine*, 328, 1450–1455. Available from: http://www.nejm.org/doi/full/10.1056/NEJM199305203282004.

Roswall, N., Olsen, A., Christensen, J., Dragsted, L.O., Dragsted, L.O., Overad, K. and Tjonneland, A.. (2010) Micronutrient intake and risk of colon and rectal cancer in a Danish cohort. *Cancer Epidemiology*, 34, 40–46. Available from: http://www.sciencedirect.com/science/article/pii/S187778210900191X.

Rutjes, A.W.S., Nüesch, E., Reichenbach, S. and Jüni, P. (2009) S-Adenosylmethionine for osteoarthritis of the knee or hip. *Cochrane Database of Systematic Reviews* 2009, Issue 4. Art. No.: CD007321. DOI: 10.1002/14651858.CD007321.pub2. Available from: http://onlinelibrary.wiley.com/doi/10.1002/14651858.CD007321.pub2/full.

Scrimshaw, N.S. and Sangiovanni, J.P. (1997) Synergism of nutrition, infection, and immunity: an overview. *American Journal of Clinical Nutrition*, 66, 464S–477S. Available from: http://www.ajcn.org/content/66/2/464S.long.

SEARCH collaborative group (2010) Study of the effectiveness of additional reductions in cholesterol and homocysteine (SEARCH) collaborative Group. 2010 Effects of homocysteine-lowering with folic acid plus vitamin B12 vs placebo on mortality and major morbidity in myocardial infarction survivors: a randomized trial. *Journal of the American Medical Association*, 303, 2486–2494.Available from: http://jama.ama-assn.org/content/303/24/2486.long.

Shea, B., Swinden, M.V., Tanjong Ghogomu, E., Ortiz, Z., Katchamart, W., Rader, T., Bombardier, C., Wells, G.A. and Tugwell, P. (2013) Folic acid and folinic acid for reducing side effects in patients receiving methotrexate for rheumatoid arthritis. *Cochrane Database of Systematic Reviews* 2013, Issue 5. Art. No.: CD000951. DOI: 10.1002/14651858.CD000951.pub2. Available from: http://onlinelibrary.wiley.com/doi/10.1002/14651858.CD000951.pub2/full.

Shekelle, P., Morton, S. and Hardy, M. (2003a) Effect of the Supplemental Use of Antioxidants Vitamin C, Vitamin E, and the Coenzyme Q10 for the Prevention and Treatment of Cancer. Summary, Evidence Report/Technology Assessment: Number 75. AHRQ Publication Number 04 -E002, October 2003.Rockville, MD, Agency for Healthcare Research and Quality. Available from: http://archive.ahrq.gov/clinic/tp/aoxcardtp.htm.

Shekelle, P., Morton, S. and Hardy, M. (2003b) Effect of supplemental antioxidants vitamin C, vitamin E, and coenzyme Q10 for the prevention and treatment of cardiovascular disease. Evidence report/technology assessment No.83. Rockville M,: Agency for Health care Research and Quality. Available from: http://www.ncbi.nlm.nih.gov/books/bv.fcgi?rid=hstat1a.chapter.16082.

Shenkin, S.D., Whiteman, M.C., Pattie, A. and Deary, I.J. (2002) Supplementation and the elderly: dramatic results? *Nutrition*, 18, 364. Available from: http://www.sciencedirect.com/science/article/pii/S0899900702007682.

Smith, W.A., Fry, A.C., Tschume, L.C. and Bloomer, R.J. (2008a) Effect of glycine propionyl-L-carnitine on aerobic and anaerobic exercise performance. *International Journal of Sport Nutrition and Exercise Metabolism*, 18, 19–36.

Smith, A.D., Kim, Y.I. and Refsum, H. (2008b) Is folic acid good for everyone? *American Journal of Clinical Nutrition*, 87, 517–533. Available from: http://www.ajcn.org/cgi/content/full/87/3/517

Smith, R. (2005) Investigating the previous studies of a fraudulent author. *British Medical Journal*, 331, 288–291. Available from: http://www.bmj.com/content/331/7511/288?view=long&pmid=16052023.

Smolders, J., Damoiseeaux, J., Menheere, P. and Hupperts, R. (2008) Vitamin D as an immune regulator in multiple sclerosis, a review. *Journal of Neuroimmunology*, 194, 7–17. http://www.sciencedirect.com/science/article/pii/S0165572807004316.

Solomons, N.W. (2007) Food fortification with folic acid: has the other shoe dropped? *Nutrition Reviews*, 65, 512–515.

Stampfer, M.J., Hennekens, C.H., Manson, J.E., Colditz, G.A., Rosner, B. and Willett, W.C. (1993) Vitamin E consumption and the risk of coronary disease in women. *New England Journal of Medicine*, 328, 1444–1449. http://www.nejm.org/doi/full/10.1056/NEJM199305203282003.

Stephen, A.I. and Avenell, A. (2006) A systematic review of multivitamin and multimineral supplementation for infection. *Journal of Human Nutrition and Dietetics*, 19, 179–190.

Thal, L.J., Calvani, M., Amato, A. and Carta, A. (2000) A 1-year controlled trial of acetyl-l-carnitine in early-onset AD. *Neurology*, 55, 805–810.

Thal, L.J., Carta, A., Clarke, W.R., Ferris, S.H., Friedland, R.P., Petersen, R.C., Pettegrew, J.W., Pfeiffer, E., Raskind, M.A., Sano, M., Tuszynski, M.H. and Woolson, R.F. (1996) A 1-year multicenter placebo-controlled study of acetyl-L-carnitine in patients with Alzheimer's disease. *Neurology*, 47, 705–711.

Van der Linden, I.J., Afman, L.A., Heil, S.G. and Blom, H.J. (2006) Genetic variation in genes of folate metabolism and neural-tube defect risk. *Proceedings of the Nutrition Society*, 65, 204–215. Available from: http://journals.cambridge.org/download.php?file=%2FPNS%2FPNS65_02%2FS0029665106000267a.pdf&code=28d2b847b67a9fd0c3e652438a6bb5dd.

Vanderpump, P.J., Lazarus, J.H., Smyth, P.P., Laurberg, P., Holder, R.L., Boelaerd, K. and Franklyn, J.A. (2011) Iodine status of UK schoolgirls: a cross-sectional survey. *Lancet*, 377, 2007–2012. Available from: http://www.sciencedirect.com/science/article/pii/S0140673611606934.

Van Etten, E., Decallonne, B. and Mathieu, C. (2002) 1,25-dihydroxycholecalciferol: endocrinology meets the immune system. *Proceedings of the Nutrition Society*, 61, 375–380.

Vivekanathan, D.P., Penn, M.S., Sapp, S.K., Hsu, A. and Topol, E.J. (2003) Use of antioxidant vitamins for the prevention of cardiovascular disease: meta-analysis of randomised trials. *Lancet*, 361, 2017–2023. Available from: http://www.sciencedirect.com/science/article/pii/S0140673603136379.

Vollset, S.E., Clarke, R., Lewington, S., Ebbing, M., Halsey, J., Lonn, E., Armitage, J., Manson, J.E., Hankey, G.J., Spence, J.D., Golan, P., Bonn, K.H., Jamison, R., Gaziano, J.M., Guarino, P., Baron, J.A., Logan, R.F.A., Giovanucci, E.L., den Heijer, M., Ueland, P.M., Bennett, D., Collins, R. and Peto, R. (2013) Effects of folic acid supplementation on overall and site-specific cancer incidence during the randomised trials: meta-analysis of data on 50 000 individuals. *Lancet*, 381, 1029–1036. Available from: http://www.sciencedirect.com/science/article/pii/S0140673612620017.

WCRF/AICR 2007 World Cancer Research Fund/ American Institute for Cancer Research. Food, nutrition, physical activity, and the prevention of cancer: a global perspective. Washington DC, AICR.

Webb, G.P. (2007) Nutritional supplements and conventional medicine; what should the physician know? *Proceedings of the Nutrition Society*, 66, 471–478. Available from: http://journals.cambridge.org/download.php?file=%2FPNS%2FPNS66_04%2FS0029665107005782a.pdf&code=b582cdc20b951a8b3a840b894cced959.

Webb, G.P. (2011a) *Dietary Supplements and Functional Foods* 2nd edition. Oxford, Wiley-Blackwell.

Webb, G.P. (2011b) Vitamin fortification of foods: a critical review. Food Science and Technology *Bulletin: Functional Foods*, 8(1) 1–10.

Webb, G.P. (2012) *Nutrition: Maintaining and Improving Health*. 4th edition. London, Hodder Education.

WHO (1970) Fluorides and human health. World Health Organization monographs series No 59, Geneva, WHO. Available from: http://whqlibdoc.who.int/monograph/WHO_MONO_59_(part1).pdf.

Wilcox, A.J., Lie, R.T., Solvoll, K., Taylor, J., McConnaughey, D.R., Abyholm, F., Vindenes, H., Vollset, S.E. and Drevan, C.A. (2007) Folic acid supplements and risk of facial clefts: national population based case-control study. *British Medical Journal*, 334, 433–434. Available from: http://www.bmj.com/content/334/7591/464?view=long&pmid=17259187.

Wright, A.J., Dainty, J.R. and Finglas, P.M. (2007) Folic acid metabolism in human subjects revisited: potential implications for proposed mandatory folic acid fortification in the UK. *British Journal of Nutrition*, 98, 667–675.

Yakoob, M.Y. and Bhutta, Z.A. (2010) Vitamin D supplementation for preventing infections in children less than five years of age (Protocol). *Cochrane Database of Systematic Reviews* 2010, Issue 11. Art. No.: CD008824. DOI: 10.1002/14651858.CD008824. Available from: http://onlinelibrary.wiley.com/doi/10.1002/14651858.CD008824/full.

Ziegler, R.G. (1991) Vegetables, fruits and carotenoids and the risk of cancer. American Journal of Clinical *Nutrition*. 53, 251S–259S. Available from: http://www.ajcn.org/content/53/1/251S.long.

Zimmerman, M. and Delange, F. (2004) Iodine supplements of pregnant women in Europe: a review and recommendations. *European Journal of Clinical Nutrition*, 58, 979–984. Available from: http://www.nature.com/ejcn/journal/v58/n7/full/1601933a.html.

Zipitis, C.S. and Akobeng, A.K. (2008) Vitamin D supplementation in early childhood and risk of type 1 diabetes: a systematic review and meta-analysis. *Archives of Disease in Childhood* 93, 512–517. Available from: http://adc.bmj.com/content/93/6/512.long.

Reviewing clinical studies of probiotics as dietary supplements: probiotics for gastrointestinal disorders, *Helicobacter* eradication, lactose malabsorption and inflammatory bowel disease (IBD)

M. Lunder
University of Ljubljana, Ljubljana, Slovenia

9.1 Introduction

The use of microorganisms to promote health is very ancient and can even be traced back to classical Roman literature where food fermented with microorganisms was used as a therapeutic agent (Plinius Secundus Maior G. *Naturalis historiae* AD 77). The modern idea of probiotics, prebiotics and synbiotics is to produce food or food supplements which, after ingestion, augment healthy intestinal microbiota, by either adding probiotic microorganisms, indigestible but fermentable prebiotic carbohydrates, or both constituents combined in synbiotics. However, many professed probiotic products have not been properly characterized, documented, proven clinically effective and manufactured under good manufacturing practices. To provide consumers with reliable and effective probiotic products, establishment of standards and guidelines represent a necessary first step (FAO/WHO, 2002). Since even closely related probiotic strains can have different clinical effects, reliable identification of organisms at the strain level is essential for clinical studies. Beneficial effects observed in one strain cannot be assumed to occur in other strains (FAO/WHO, 2001).

9.1.1 Gut microbiota

The human body is colonized by various microorganisms, and the human gut is considered the most densely populated ecosystem on Earth. Average human gastrointestinal tract with length of approximately 6.5 m and surface area of 200–300 m^2 offers a home for 10^{13-14} bacteria of 400 different species and subspecies (Hao and Lee, 2004).

The longitudinal distribution of intestinal microorganisms increases in density progressing from the small bowel to colon, with bacterial load 10^{12} organisms per gram of faecal material in the large intestine (Marchesi and Shanahan, 2007).

Colonization by commensal bacteria occurs immediately after birth and continues throughout the first year of life (Arboleya et al., 2012). Acquisition and development of gut microbiota can be influenced primarily by mode of delivery, maternal microbiota as well as genetic factors of the host and later by breastfeeding and other environmental factors (Azad and Kozyrskyj, 2012; Bisgaard et al., 2009; Fallani et al., 2010; Penders et al., 2006). The human intestinal microbiota represents the most significant microbial exposure for the developing infant. It begins as a dynamic ecosystem, dominated by bifidobacteria that stabilizes during the first 2–3 years. During life the microbial composition increases in both diversity and richness (Scholtens et al., 2012). In healthy adults, 80% of the identified faecal microbiota can be classified into three dominant phyla: *Bacteroidetes, Firmicutes* and *Actinobacteria* (Lay et al., 2005). Near the end of adolescence final composition is achieved, which displays a high stability in healthy adults (Franks et al., 1998). Despite relatively stable microbiota, recent studies have indicated that modifications occur in the composition, especially in elderly individuals (Mariat et al., 2009).

Intestinal microflora exerts several functions. Synthesis and excretion of vitamins (vitamin K, vitamin B12) in excess of their own needs provides nutrients for their hosts. Competing for attachment sites or essential nutrients prevents colonization of pathogens. Microflora stimulates the development of several tissues, that is the caecum and certain lymphatic tissues (Peyer's patches) in the gastrointestinal tract. They stimulate the production of antibodies and produce a variety of substances, ranging from relatively non-specific fatty acids and peroxides to highly specific bacteriocins that inhibit or kill other bacteria (Iannitti and Palmieri, 2010).

The gut microbiota is now virtually recognized as a complex whole organ consisting of an incredible amount of bacteria of different species. The collective genome of the entire gut microbiota, designated as "microbiome," exceeds the human nuclear genome by at least 100 times (Qin et al., 2010). Over the last 5 years, an intense research effort has been made to understand the crucial role of gut microbiota in health and disease by various metagenomic and metabolomic studies using high throughput sequencing technologies, mass and nuclear magnetic resonance (NMR) spectroscopy that has enabled in-depth analysis of gut microbial compositional changes, structural elements and metabolites in host physiology and metabolism under different conditions (Fischer et al., 2012; Gerritsen et al., 2011; Martin et al., 2011).

9.1.2 Definition of probiotics

Fermented foods have been an important food component during man's history, and still remain a key component of the diet in many cultures. The idea of suppressing and displacing harmful bacteria in the intestine by orally administering "beneficial" ones and thus improving microbial balance, health and longevity, was born a century ago by Carre (Carre, 1887), Tissier (Tissier, 1906), and Metchnikoff (Metchnikoff, 1907).

The term "probiotic" derives from the Greek/Latin word "pro" and "bios," meaning for life. It was created in the 1950s by W. Kollath to describe various components of food, essential for healthy development of life, also considered to be the opposite of antibiotics (Kollath, 1953). In 1965 Lilly and Stillwell used this term for live bacteria and spores in animal feed supplements that were supposed to reduce the use of antibiotics in animal farming. They defined probiotic as "a substance produced by one microorganism stimulating the growth of another microorganism" (Lilly and Stillwell, 1965). The first generally accepted definition was given by Fuller in 1989. He defined a probiotic as "a live microbial feed supplement which beneficially affects the host animal by improving its intestinal microbial balance" (Fuller, 1989). Broader definition provided by the World Health Organization (WHO) and the Food and Agriculture Organization of the United Nations defines probiotics as "live microorganisms, which, when administered in adequate amounts, confer a health benefit on the host."

According to most definitions, probiotic microorganisms must be viable and must exert scientifically proven health effects. However, neither "viability" nor "survivability" during the gastrointestinal transit is an indispensable quality of health-promoting microorganisms, since dead cells and cell components may also exert some physiological effects (Sanders, 2003).

Together with chapters 10 and 11, this chapter reviews the available clinical studies for the therapeutic role of probiotics in a range of medical conditions and diseases. This chapter reviews studies on the use of probiotics in the treatment of gastrointestinal disorders, *Helicobacter* eradication, lactose malabsorption and inflammatory bowel disease (IBD).

9.2 Probiotics for gastrointestinal disorders

This section will examine the evidence for probiotics in the management of a broad range of gastrointestinal disorders, ranging from diarrhoea to constipation.

9.2.1 Acute diarrhoea

Diarrhoea is defined by the WHO as three or more loose or watery stools in a 24-h period. Diarrhoea is acute if the illness started less than 14 days previously, and persistent if the episode has lasted 14 days or more. Infectious diarrhoea is an episode of diarrhoea that is caused by an infectious agent (Allen *et al.*, 2010). More than 20 viruses, bacteria and parasites are associated with acute diarrhoea. Worldwide, rotavirus is the most common cause of severe diarrhoea and diarrhoea mortality in children. Other important viral pathogens are astrovirus, human caliciviruses (norovirus and sapovirus) and enteric adenoviruses. Important bacterial pathogens are diarrhoeagenic *Escherichia coli*, *Salmonella*, *Shigella*, *Yersinia*, *Campylobacter*, and *Vibrio cholerae.* The main parasitic causes of diarrhoea are *Cryptosporidium* and *Giardia* (O'Ryan *et al.*, 2005). Acute diarrhoea is frequent among travellers, in whom enterotoxigenic *E. coli* is particularly common (Black, 1986). Chemotherapy and radiation can also cause acute diarrhoea.

The rationale for using probiotics in infectious diarrhoea is that they act against enteric pathogens by competing for available nutrients and binding sites, making the gut contents acidic, producing a variety of chemicals, and increasing specific and non-specific immune responses (Goldin, 1998). The use of probiotic microorganisms lowers dependence on antibiotics, is relatively inexpensive, and is well tolerated, even for prolonged use (Mcfarland, 2007).

A number of randomized controlled trials have been done to determine whether probiotics are beneficial in acute infectious diarrhoea; most of them have been carried out on the effectiveness of probiotics in children's diarrhoea. A number of systematic reviews and meta-analyses have been published. In a meta-analysis of trials using yeast probiotic *Saccharomyces boulardii* for treating acute diarrhoea in children, Szajewska *et al.* reported significant reduction in the duration of diarrhoea, risk of diarrhoea, the number of stools per day, and length of hospitalization (Szajewska *et al.*, 2007). The results of two older meta-analyses on children's diarrhoea also confirmed the benefit of bacterial probiotic in reducing the duration of diarrhoea by approximately 1 day (Huang *et al.*, 2002; Van Niel *et al.*, 2002). A recent meta-analysis by Salari *et al.* included 19 studies on children that used different types of probiotics, differing in their function in the gut. The authors concluded that probiotics decrease the duration of children's diarrhoea, depending on the dose and type of probiotic, with no adverse effects (Salari *et al.*, 2012).

Moreover, results of published randomized controlled trials indicate that there is modest benefit in giving probiotics to prevent acute infectious diarrhoea in healthy infants and children (Hatakka *et al.*, 2001; Oberhelman *et al.*, 1999; Pedone *et al.*, 2000; Saavedra *et al.*, 2004; Szajewska *et al.*, 2001; Thibault *et al.*, 2004; Weizman *et al.*, 2005). Most of the studies were conducted in child care centres, where rotavirus is the most common cause of acute diarrhoea. The strains of probiotics used included *Lactobacillus rhamnosus* GG, *Streptococcus thermophilus*, *Lactobacillus casei*, *Bifidobacterium lactis*, or *Lactobacillus reuteri* mixed with milk or infant formula or given as an oral supplement. The results of a meta-analysis indicate that approximately seven children would need to have been given *L. rhamnosus* GG to prevent one child from developing nosocomial rotavirus gastroenteritis in a child care centre setting (Szajewska *et al.*, 2001). So far, data do not support routine use for prevention. However, there may be special circumstances in healthcare facilities or in childcare centres in which routine use may be beneficial (Thomas and Greer, 2010).

To assess the effects of probiotics in proven or presumed acute infectious diarrhoea in both children and adults, Allen *et al.* (Allen *et al.*, 2010) meta-analysed randomized and quasi-randomized controlled trials comparing a specified probiotic agent with a placebo or no probiotic. Sixty-three studies met the inclusion criteria, with a total of 8014 participants. Most of the trials (56) recruited infants and young children. The trials were undertaken in a wide range of different settings and also varied greatly in probiotic organisms, dosage, participants' characteristics and also in quality. Despite the high level of quantitative heterogeneity, beneficial effect of probiotics was consistent across the different diarrhoea outcomes and was statistically significant in many trials. The authors showed a pattern and an important effect. Using a random effects approach, probiotics reduced the mean duration of diarrhoea (mean difference 24.76 h; 95% confidence interval 15.9–33.6 h; n = 4555, trials = 35), diarrhoea lasting ≥ 4 days (risk ratio 0.41; 0.32–0.53; n = 2853, trials = 29) and stool frequency on day 2 (mean difference 0.80; 0.45–1.14; n = 2751, trials = 20). The differences in these analyses are an average across all studies with quantitative heterogeneity, demonstrating that probiotics have a substantive and significant effect, rather than being a precise estimate of the size of the effect. With the exception of possible mild hypersensitivity to *E. coli* strain, Nissle reported in one participant (Henker *et al.*, 2008), no trial reported adverse events attributable to probiotics. The authors could not assess the efficacy of probiotics according to participants' age, since less than three studies reported the same diarrhoea outcome in adults (Allen *et al.*, 2010).

Although some studies focus attention on the possibilities of probiotic therapy of adults' diarrhoea, amoebiasis, diarrhoea in HIV positive patients, radiation-induced diarrhoea, and chemotherapy-induced diarrhoea, this is a more neglected area of research. Salari *et al.* critically reviewed those studies, and the efficacy of probiotics is less convincing (Salari *et al.*, 2012).

9.2.2 Traveller's diarrhoea

Traveller's diarrhoea is a common health disorder among travellers. Travel destination is the most significant risk factor. Rates of diarrhoea occurrence can range from 5% to over 50%. Food and water contaminated with faecal matter are the main sources of infection (Yates, 2005).

Meta-analysis of probiotics for the prevention of traveller's diarrhoea included 12 randomized controlled studies (Mcfarland, 2007). Six trials reported significant prevention of diarrhoea for the probiotic in their trial, with two trials having multiple treatment arms (Black *et al.*, 1989; Hilton *et al.*, 1997; Kollaritsch *et al.*, 1993, 1989) One study found a trend (p = 0.07) for efficacy (Oksanen *et al.*, 1990) and five other treatments found no significant difference between probiotic and control groups, with two trials having multiple treatment arms (De Dios Pozo-Olano *et al.*, 1978; Katelaris *et al.*, 1995; Kollaritsch *et al.*, 1989). Contradictory results may arise from differences in study populations, type of probiotic being investigated or differences in probiotic doses and duration of treatment. For traveller's diarrhoea, additional factors, such as trip destination, probiotic potency during travel, medication compliance and behaviours of the traveller, may influence the results. However, the advantage of selecting a non-restrictive study population is that they may represent tourists in general. The ten trials that presented data on adverse reactions reported no serious side effects. One study reported abdominal cramping associated with two per cent of the subjects taking *L. rhamnosus* GG (Hilton *et al.*, 1997). Grouped by the type of probiotic and adjusted for differences in study sample size, three (75%) of the *S. boulardii* treatment arms were significantly protective of traveller's diarrhoea, but only one (13%) of the Lactobacilli trials was protective. Whether this was due to the type of probiotic chosen or other influences is not clear. Inconsistent efficacy results may also be due to the viability and stability of the probiotic product. Lyophilized probiotics are stable at room temperature; however, products that require refrigeration may represent a difficulty for travellers. McFarland concluded that several probiotics (*S. boulardii* and a mixture of *Lactobacillus acidophilus* and *Bifidobacterium bifidum*) had significant efficacy and may offer a safe and effective method to prevent traveller's diarrhoea.

The efficacy of a non-viable probiotic preparation for preventing traveller's diarrhoea was investigated in a randomized, double-blind, controlled trial by Briand et al. (Briand et al., 2006). Travellers (147) were randomized to receive either non-viable *L. acidophilus* or a placebo twice daily from 1 day before their departure to 3 days after their return. There was no beneficial effect of treatment with non-viable probiotic.

9.2.3 Antibiotic associated and Clostridium difficile associated diarrhoea (CDAD)

The use of antibiotics that disturb the gastrointestinal flora is associated with clinical symptoms of diarrhoea, which occurs in about 5–30% of patients, either early during antibiotic therapy or up to 2 months after the end of the treatment. Almost all antibiotics, particularly those that act on anaerobes, can cause diarrhoea, but the risk is higher with broad-spectrum antibiotics, which have a low degree of absorption from the intestinal tract. Host factors for antibiotic associated diarrhoea (AAD) include age over 65, immunosuppression, being in an intensive care unit, and prolonged hospitalization (Barbut and Meynard, 2002). Clinical presentations of AAD range from mild diarrhoea, which is the most frequent result, to fulminant pseudomembranous. The latter is characterized by watery diarrhoea, fever (in 80% of cases), leucocytosis (80%), and the presence of pseudomembranes on endoscopic examination. Severe complications include toxic megacolon, perforation, and shock. A specific type of AAD is *CDAD*. The anaerobic bacterium *Clostridium difficile* is an important nosocomial pathogen, the most commonly diagnosed cause of infectious hospital diarrhoea. *Clostridium difficile* infection has a wide clinical range, from asymptomatic carriage, to mild self-limiting diarrhoea, and more severe pseudomembranous colitis. About a third of AAD cases are caused by *Clostridium difficile* (Avadhani and Miley, 2011).

There is an increasing interest in probiotic interventions and evidence for the effectiveness of probiotics in preventing or treating AAD and CDAD is accumulating. To determine the efficacy of probiotics in preventing antibiotic associated and *Clostridium difficile* associated diarrhoea in hospitalized adult populations, Avadhani et al. meta-analysed eight studies that met the inclusion criteria (Avadhani and Miley, 2011). Total number of participants across the studies was 1220. The results were in favour of treatment with probiotics. The use of probiotics decreased the incidence of AAD by 44% and CDAD for 71%.

Videlock *et al.* estimated the reduction in risk of AAD, irrespective of the presence of *Clostridium difficile* (Videlock and Cremonini, 2012). Meta-analysis of 34 randomized, double-blinded, placebo-controlled trials included 4138 patients treated with antibiotics and administered a probiotic for at least the duration of the antibiotic treatment. The preventive effect of probiotic administration was present across different probiotic species; it was observed equally in children and adults, and appears to be independent of the concomitant antibiotics used and of the indication for the antibiotic treatment. When including all studies on adult and paediatric populations, probiotics resulted in a pooled risk ratio of AAD of 0.53 (95% CI 0.44–0.63) compared to placebo. This risk reduction corresponded to the average number needed to treat eight (95% CI 7–11). This and other (Hempel *et al.*, 2012; Johnston *et al.*, 2011, 2012) recent meta-analyses confirm earlier results supporting the preventive effects of probiotics in antibiotic associated and CDAD.

9.2.4 Constipation

Chronic constipation is a very common and heterogeneous condition characterized by unsatisfying defecation associated with infrequent stools, difficult stool passage, or both (Anon, 2005). Chronic constipation has been reported in 15–25% of the general population. In the vast majority of cases, no underlying organic cause is found and functional constipation is diagnosed (Rasquin *et al.*, 2006). Even though traditional treatment is well established and safe, for many patients it does not provide satisfying improvement, prompting interest in other therapeutic strategies (Bongers *et al.*, 2009).

Probiotics are increasingly being used in the management of constipation. The rationale for their use comes from data demonstrating differences in the intestinal microbiota between healthy individuals and those with chronic constipation (Zoppi *et al.*, 1998). Whether dysbiosis is secondary manifestation of constipation, or a factor contributing to constipation, remains to be answered. Probiotics lower the pH in the colon due to the bacterial production of short-chain fatty acids (butyric acid, propionic acid, and lactic acid). They also release metabolites that contribute to increased colonic osmotic pressure, drawing water into the colon and enhancing peristalsis (Salminen and Salminen, 1997), which may decrease the colonic transit time. This was confirmed in studies involving the administration of *B. lactis* DN-173 010 or *B. lactis* HN019, where gut transit times were improved, both in a healthy population (Bouvier *et al.*, 2001; Marteau *et al.*, 2002; Meance *et al.*, 2003; Waller *et al.*, 2011) and in constipated patients (Agrawal *et al.*, 2009).

To evaluate the efficacy and safety of using probiotics for the treatment of constipation in both paediatric and adult populations, recently Chmielewska *et al.* systematically reviewed data from randomized controlled trials (Chmielewska and Szajewska, 2010). Five trials including a total of 377 subjects met inclusion criteria. The authors concluded that adults with constipation might benefit from ingestion of *B. lactis* DN-173 010, *L. casei* Shirota, and *E. coli* Nissle 1917, which were shown to increase defecation frequency and improve stool consistency (Koebnick *et al.*, 2003;

Mollenbrink and Bruckschen, 1994; Yang et al., 2008). Although the results were statistically significant, the overall effects were clinically modest. For example, compared with placebo, *B. lactis* DN-173 010 increased the number of stools per week by only one (Yang et al., 2008). More studies with positive results include adults. In children, the administration of *L. rhamnosus* GG was not effective (Banaszkiewicz and Szajewska, 2005), while the administration of *L. casei rhamnosus* Lcr35 augmented the number of stools and reduced the number of hard stools (Bu et al., 2007). No adverse effects were noted in any of the included studies.

Additional clinical trials have been performed on adults (Cassani et al., 2011; De Milliano et al., 2012; Del Piano et al., 2010; Riezzo et al., 2012) and children (Coccorullo et al., 2010; Guerra et al., 2011; Tabbers et al., 2011) that were not included in the review of Chmielewska et al. Only one study found no difference in stool frequency in probiotic and control group (Tabbers et al., 2011).

Small numbers of participants and methodological limitations call for great caution when drawing conclusions. While more studies are needed, especially repeat studies with the probiotic strains that have been proven effective, probiotics hold promise for helping relieve constipation.

9.2.5 Irritable bowel syndrome (IBS)

IBS is the most common functional digestive disorder, and may affect 11–20% of the adult population in industrialized countries. It often overlaps with chronic constipation (Basilisco and Coletta, 2013). IBS involves abdominal pain and bowel habit disturbance, which are not explained by structural or biochemical abnormalities. Several hypotheses attempt to account for the pathophysiology of IBS, but the aetiology still remains uncertain or obscure, and most probably multifactorial (Longstreth et al., 2006). Preliminary evidence suggests alterations in intestinal microbiota in patients with IBS; however, it remains to be determined if these alterations are a cause or a consequence of altered gut motility and secretion (Jeffery et al., 2012; Rhee et al., 2009).

Meta-analyses vary in their conclusions on the effectiveness, in part because of inadequate sample size, poor study design and use of various probiotic strains in the reviewed studies. A thorough meta-analysis of 20 randomized controlled trials (1404 subjects) shows that the use of probiotics was associated with overall improvement in IBS (RR = 0.77) and a reduction in abdominal pain episodes (RR = 0.78) (Mcfarland and Dublin, 2008). Similar conclusions were reached in a meta-analysis that identified 19 randomized controlled trials published between 1966 and 2008 (Moayyedi et al., 2010). Both claim that probiotics are beneficial in the treatment of IBS, but the extent of the benefit and the most effective species (or combinations) are still uncertain. Recently, Clarke et al. reviewed 42 randomized controlled trials of the effect of lactic acid bacteria probiotics on IBS symptoms. Thirty-four of these trials reported benefit in at least one of the end points studied (Clarke et al., 2012), although with tremendous variation in both the magnitude of effect and the choice of outcome under consideration.

Brenner et al. evaluated 16 strictly selected randomized controlled trials and found 11 that were inadequately blinded, of too short duration, of too small sample size, and/or lacked intention to treat analysis (Brenner et al., 2009). The authors concluded that only two of appropriately designed studies showed significant improvements in abdominal pain/discomfort, bloating/distension and/or bowel movements compared with placebo. In both studies *Bifidobacterium infantis* 35624 was used (O'Mahony et al., 2005; Whorwell et al., 2006).

Given the controversies in IBS pathophysiology, patient heterogeneity, or lack of clear, reproducible evidence for gut microbiota abnormalities in patients with IBS, additional randomized controlled trials with appropriate end points and design are needed to determine the extent to which (and in which IBS subpopulations) certain probiotics represent useful therapeutic strategy.

9.3 Probiotics for *Helicobacter* eradication

When the mucosal integrity has been compromised by environmental factors such as increased acid production, pharmaceutical agents, dietary toxins, or stress, *Helicobacter pylori* colonizes the gastrointestinal lining. In up to 20% of infected individuals, colonization leads to ulcerations in the mucosal lining and causes peptic ulcer disease (Starzynska and Malfertheiner, 2006). In developing countries, 70–90% of the population carry *H. pylori*. In developed countries, the prevalence of infection is lower (Dunn et al., 1997). One of the main treatment goals for peptic ulcer disease is *H. pylori* eradication. It consists of triple or quadruple therapy that includes antimicrobials and acid suppressive therapy with a proton pump inhibitor, histamine receptor antagonist, and bismuth (Malfertheiner et al., 2007). Such therapy is not recommended in "healthy" asymptomatic carriers and in dyspeptic subjects without ulcers (Lesbros-Pantoflickova et al., 2007). However, permanent or long-term suppression of *H. pylori* could decrease the risk of developing related diseases (Blaser, 1999). There is thus a great interest in developing low-cost, large-scale solutions to prevent or decrease *H. pylori* colonization. In this respect, probiotics may close the gap. It has been suggested that the intake of probiotics strengthens the barrier by producing antimicrobial substances. Moreover, probiotics compete with *H. pylori* for adhesion receptors, stimulate mucin production, and stabilize the gut mucosal barrier (Lesbros-Pantoflickova et al., 2007).

In a recent meta-analysis, Wang et al. investigated whether *Lactobacillus* and *Bifidobacterium* containing probiotic preparation could improve *H. pylori* eradication rates and reduce side effects (Wang et al., 2013). Ten parallel controlled trials comparing probiotic supplementation to control (no probiotic administration) during *H. pylori* eradication therapy were included in meta-analysis. The authors concluded that probiotics have beneficial effects on eradication rate and incidence of total side effects. Earlier meta-analysis by Tong et al. also showed that supplementation with probiotics is effective in increasing eradication rates of *H. pylori* (Tong et al., 2007). Trials in the mentioned meta-analyses used multiple probiotic strains. Both meta-analyses showed that effect of *Lactobacillus* GG was dominant; effects of other probiotics were limited. Since the predominant probiotic in the human stomach is *Lactobacillus*, Zou *et al.* (2009) presumed that *Lactobacillus* probiotics are essential for the inhibitory effect on *H. pylori* and concluded in meta-analysis that adding *Lactobacilli* to *H. pylori* eradication regimens improves eradication rates for first-treated patients and reduces side-effects such as diarrhoea, bloating and taste disturbances during treatment.

Szajewska *et al.* meta-analysed the effects of yeast probiotic *Saccharomyces boulardii* as supplementation to standard triple therapy on *H. pylori* eradication rates and therapy associated side effects (Szajewska *et al.*, 2010b). Five randomized clinical trials involving a total of 1307 participants (among them 90 children) met the inclusion criteria. Addition of *S. boulardii* compared with placebo or no intervention improved eradication rates, reduced overall therapy-related adverse effects, and decreased some individual symptoms such as diarrhoea. Results may be applicable only to the adult population, since the majority of patients included were adults. There were no significant differences between groups in the risk of adverse effects.

According to these meta-analyses, there is evidence to recommend the use of yeast such as *S. boulardii* as well as bacterial probiotics (*Lactobacillus* and *Bifidobacterium*), along with standard triple therapy, as an option for increasing the eradication rates and decreasing overall therapy-related side effects, particularly diarrhoea.

9.4 Probiotics for lactose malabsorption

Lactose intolerance is lactose maldigestion accompanied by clinical symptoms such as bloating, flatulence, nausea, diarrhoea, and abdominal pain. These symptoms are caused by undigested lactose in the large intestine, where the lactose serves as a fermentable substrate for the bacterial flora and osmotically increases water flow into the lumen (de Vrese *et al.*, 2001). In primary or adult-type lactose malabsorption, lactase activity is high at birth, decreases in childhood and adolescence, and remains low in adulthood. With the exception of the population of Northern and Central Europe and its offspring in America and Australia, 70–100% of adults worldwide are lactose malabsorbers. Lactose-intolerant people can ingest a certain amount of lactose without having adverse symptoms. Most of these people tolerate nine to 12 g (equivalent to 200 mL of milk) (Johnson *et al.*, 1993).

Numerous studies summarized by de Vrese (de Vrese *et al.*, 2001) showed that fermented milk products such as yogurt can efficiently improve lactose digestion in lactose malabsorbers and are well tolerated by most lactose-intolerant subjects. Possible reasons for these effects are based mainly on the fact that fermented milk products with live bacteria contain microbial β-galactosidase that survives the passage through the stomach and is liberated in the small intestine to support lactose hydrolysis (Oozeer *et al.*, 2002). However, depending on the definition of "probiotic" this is not a specific probiotic effect, because it does not depend on the survival of the bacteria in the small intestine. Furthermore, primary or adult-type lactose malabsorption is not a disease, but rather a normal physiological situation.

9.5 Probiotics for inflammatory bowel disease (IBD) and associated conditions

IBD consists of chronic and relapsing inflammatory diseases of the intestine, comprising two similar yet distinct subtypes: ulcerative colitis (UC) and Crohn's disease (CD). They differ by the intestinal localization and features of the inflammation (Bousvaros *et al.*, 2007). The proposed mechanisms in the genetically susceptible host that lead towards aggressive cellular immune responses to components of the microbiota include loss of epithelial cell barrier function, overexpression of pro-inflammatory mediators in different effector T lymphocyte subsets, deficient protective and regulatory signals, and/or abnormal antigen presentation (Clavel and Haller, 2007; Sartor, 2006). The conventional treatments for IBD have focused on targeting inflammation and suppressing the enhanced immune response with steroids, aminosalicylates, and anti-tumour necrosis factor antibodies. Though these agents have reasonable efficacy, they may produce significant side effects associated with chronic immune suppression (malignancy and serious infections) (Veerappan *et al.*, 2012). Recently, attempts to modify intestinal flora using probiotics have gained attention. The addition of beneficial bacteria to this complex microenvironment may have a number of effects, for example, on the immunological reaction of the host, on the mucosal barrier function to lessen interaction with the host immune system, on the displacement of deleterious microbes from luminal-mucosal interface, or on the metabolic end products of the microbiota (Mack, 2011; Szajewska *et al.*, 2006).

9.5.1 Ulcerative colitis (UC)

Probiotics have been used in patients with UC, both for treatment of active inflammation and as maintenance therapy. Several studies suggest that selected probiotics have a positive effect for induction (Bibiloni *et al.*, 2005; Guslandi *et al.*, 2003; Kato *et al.*, 2004; Rembacken *et al.*, 1999; Sood *et al.*, 2009; Tursi *et al.*, 2004, 2010) and maintenance of remission (Huynh *et al.*, 2009; Kruis *et al.*, 2004, 1997; Rembacken *et al.*, 1999; Zocco *et al.*, 2006). Two small studies also support probiotic use for induction and maintenance of remission in paediatric patients (Huynh *et al.*, 2009; Miele *et al.*, 2009). However, the data are based on relatively small studies, which are not sufficient to determine the benefits and harms implicated.

A Cochrane review examined probiotics' role in inducing remission in UC. Four studies (Furrie *et al.*, 2005; Kato *et al.*, 2004; Rembacken *et al.*, 1999; Tursi *et al.*, 2004) were analysed including a total of 244 patients. The review concluded that adding probiotics to conventional treatment did not improve the overall remission rates in mild to moderate UC, but it was possible to obtain a slight benefit in decreasing disease activity (Mallon *et al.*, 2007).

Zigra *et al.* systematically reviewed randomized controlled trials and compared the effect of probiotics to the effect of anti-inflammatory drugs or placebo for the induction and maintenance of remission (Zigra *et al.*, 2007). Nine studies (Cui *et al.*, 2004; Furrie *et al.*, 2005; Ishikawa *et al.*, 2003; Kato *et al.*, 2004; Kruis *et al.*, 2004,

1997; Rembacken et al., 1999; Tursi et al., 2004; Zocco et al., 2006) met the inclusion criteria and provided data on 972 subjects. Three studies estimated induction of remission as an outcome measure. One of them reported significantly improved remission (Furrie et al., 2005) for the probiotics, and the other two studies had a trend for increased efficacy (Kato et al., 2004; Tursi et al., 2004). The pooled relative risk was 2.27 (95% CI 1.00–5.14, $p = 0.049$), showing a significant difference between probiotic and control group. Six randomized, controlled studies provided adequate data for the maintenance of remission. Two of them reported significantly higher remission in UC for the probiotics compared with the control group (Cui et al., 2004; Ishikawa et al., 2003). The other four trials did not find any significant difference between the probiotic and control group.

Trials assessing induction of remission as an outcome measure give better results for patients receiving probiotics than the trials assessing maintenance of remission. The authors hypothesized that the type of probiotic (most of the trials assessing induction of remission as outcome measure used bifidobacteria) may be related to this finding. Furthermore, trials that compared the effects of probiotics with the effect of placebo gave better results than studies that compared the effect of probiotics with the effect of anti-inflammatory drugs. Among five randomized, controlled studies comparing probiotics with anti-inflammatory drugs, one trial showed a trend for increased efficacy (Tursi et al., 2004). The other four studies did not find any significant difference between probiotics and anti-inflammatory agents (Kruis et al., 2004, 1997; Rembacken et al., 1999; Zocco et al., 2006).

Meta-analysis concluded that, despite many methodological differences and a significant heterogeneity of studies, probiotics do not differ significantly from anti-inflammatory drugs for efficacy and safety in achieving UC remission. This finding is most likely related to a similar effectiveness of probiotics and anti-inflammatory drugs, and not to a lower effectiveness of the specific probiotics used in these trials.

Recently, a Cochrane Database Review by Naidoo and colleagues evaluated four studies with a total of 587 patients that compared probiotics to any other therapy in the maintenance of remission for UC. Overall, there was no significant difference in efficacy or safety between probiotics or 5-aminosalicylic acid (Naidoo et al., 2011).

Use of probiotics in UC is provocative and suggests potential for benefit in some patients; however, concerns remain regarding proof from trials. For those 5-aminosalicylate intolerant patients, specific probiotic products appear to have more potential for a modest effect in maintaining remission of mild to moderate disease activity (Mack, 2011).

9.5.2 Crohn's disease (CD)

Limited studies are available on probiotic use for inducing remission, maintaining remission, and preventing postoperative relapse in CD. For inducing remission, there is one randomized placebo-controlled trial (Schultz et al., 2004) and a few open labelled studies (Fujimori et al., 2007; Gupta et al., 2000). Studies included in total 25 patients. Based on insufficient data, probiotics shows no role in inducing remission of active CD.

More literature exists regarding probiotics for maintaining remission in CD (Bousvaros *et al.*, 2005; Guslandi *et al.*, 2000; Malchow, 1997). In the largest maintenance trial to date, Bousvaros *et al.* reported no significant difference in probiotic efficacy in those receiving *L. rhamnosus* GG (2×10^{10} CFU) compared with a placebo. Two meta-analyses suggest that probiotics are not a therapeutic option for maintaining CD remission (Rahimi *et al.*, 2008; Rolfe *et al.*, 2006).

Data are even more robust on preventing relapse following surgical intervention, but again probiotics (Marteau *et al.*, 2006; Prantera *et al.*, 2002; Van Gossum *et al.*, 2007) or synbiotics (Chermesh *et al.*, 2007) fail to prevent endoscopic or clinical recurrence. A meta-analysis of different interventions for preventing postoperative recurrence of CD suggests that the effect of probiotics was no better than placebo (Doherty *et al.*, 2009).

There is no evidence that patients with CD will benefit from ingestion of probiotics for any aspect of their disease, whether it is for treating active disease, maintaining remission, or preventing postoperative recurrence of disease. The lack of treatment effect may be due to the transmural nature of this disease, the poor design of the studies, or other as-yet unidentified factors.

9.5.3 Pouchitis

In some patients with UC, proctocolectomy with ileal pouch–anal anastomosis may be required because their disease is medically intractable or they have developed secondary dysplasia or cancer. The most common complication of the surgery is pouchitis or inflammation of the ileal reservoir created during the procedure, which occurs in 15–50% of patients. Although the exact aetiology is not clear, host genetic factors, local pouch issues and the microbiota contained within the pouch are thought to be involved (Pardi *et al.*, 2009). Thus, alteration of the microbiota by addition of probiotics is considered for preventing and treating pouchitis.

Trials for treating mild/moderate pouchitis are few with small numbers of adult participants (Gionchetti *et al.*, 2007; Kuisma *et al.*, 2003; Laake *et al.*, 2005). Thus, there is limited evidence supporting a role for probiotics as monotherapy for mild to moderate pouchitis at the present time.

For preventing pouchitis two trials have studied whether there is an advantage in initiating probiotics immediately following ileal pouch–anal anastomosis, and both found delay in the onset of pouchitis (Gionchetti *et al.*, 2003; Holubar *et al.*, 2010). Regarding maintenance of remission, two clinical trials reported a remarkable effect in preventing recurrent pouchitis in patients with antibiotic-dependent pouchitis (Gionchetti *et al.*, 2000; Mimura *et al.*, 2004). Both used probiotic blend VSL#3. It is a commercially available probiotic cocktail containing eight strains of lactic acid bacteria: *Lactobacillus plantarum*, *Lactobacillus delbrueckii* subsp. *Bulgaricus*, *Lactobacillus paracasei*, *L. acidophilus*, *Bifidobacterium breve*, *Bifidobacterium longum*, *B. infantis*, and *Streptococcus salivarius* subsp. *Thermophilus*. The number needed to treat with oral probiotic therapy to prevent one additional relapse was 2 (Holubar *et al.*, 2010). In contrast, an open label trial by Shen (Shen *et al.*, 2005) reported fewer responses. Whether this is due to some difference in the patient populations and their microflora, patient adherence, or other factors is so far unknown.

While further study is certainly reasonable, it is safe to say that a subset of patients with pouchitis may benefit from using most extensively studied probiotic mixture VSL#3, most likely due to an increase in microflora biodiversity leading to a less inflammatory milieu at the mucosal interface. At present the data support its use in prophylaxis and maintenance of remission and not for treatment of pouchitis (Veerappan et al., 2012).

9.5.4 Necrotizing enterocolitis (NEC)

Preterm infants frequently have delayed and aberrant acquisition of the "normal" digestive microflora, most likely due to restricted enteral feeding and frequent use of antibiotics (Penders et al., 2006). The immature intestine of preterm infants is especially prone to inflammation and loss of epithelial integrity (Cotten et al., 2009). Necrotizing enterocolitis (NEC) is associated with 30% mortality, despite extensive medical and surgical efforts, and with severe and costly consequences if the patient survives. The disease can be difficult to diagnose before intestinal perforation occurs (Nanthakumar et al., 2000). Enhanced risk of NEC gives rationale for the use of probiotic supplements.

Several systematic reviews and meta-analyses on the subject have been published in recent years (Alfaleh and Bassler, 2008; Alfaleh et al., 2010, 2011; Bernardo et al., 2013; Deshpande et al., 2010; Guthmann et al., 2010; Wang et al., 2012) and similarly showed the benefits of probiotic supplementation. Meta-analyses of probiotic studies using strains of *Bifidobacterium*, *Lactobacillus*, *Saccharomyces* and/or *S. thermophilus* to prevent NEC show reduction in frequency and overall mortality.

Despite the evidence that probiotics prevent NEC in very-low-birth-weight infants, more studies to clarify the effective dose and strain of probiotic before issuing clinical recommendations are necessary (Mihatsch et al., 2012; Thomas and Greer, 2010). For example, one systematic review of three randomized clinical trials (RCTs) evaluating *Bifidobacterium animalis* CNCM I-3446 in 293 preterm babies reported only a trend towards preventing NEC, suggesting that this treatment regimen may not be as effective as others (Szajewska et al., 2010a). Others consider available evidence sufficient to support a change in practice (Alfaleh et al., 2011; Deshpande et al., 2010). This opinion is based on the lack of treatment options for NEC and the strength of evidence that probiotics can prevent severe NEC and all-cause mortality in preterm infants (Sanders et al., 2013).

9.6 Safety of probiotics

The safety of probiotics is supported by the fact that many strains have a long history of safe use and moreover are normal commensals of human origin. Nevertheless, side effects have been reported, including extremely rare systemic infections (Cannon *et al.*, 2005; Henriksson *et al.*, 2005; Ledoux *et al.*, 2006; Oggioni *et al.*, 1998). There are some theoretical concerns regarding the safety of probiotics due to the risk of bacteraemia or endocarditis in immuno-compromised patients, due to potential toxic or metabolic effects in the gastrointestinal tract and due to the potential for transfer of antibiotic resistance to other microorganisms (Snydman, 2008). To establish safety guidelines for probiotic organisms, the FAO and WHO recommended characterization of probiotic strains with a series of tests, including antibiotic resistance patterns, metabolic activities, toxin production, haemolytic activity, infectivity in immuno-compromised animal models, side effects in humans, and adverse incidents in consumers (FAO/WHO, 2002).

Hempel *et al.* catalogued what is known about the safety of interventions containing organisms from six different genera used as probiotic agents (*Lactobacillus, Bifidobacterium, Saccharomyces, Streptococcus, Enterococcus,* and *Bacillus*), alone or in combination, used to reduce the risk of, prevent, or treat disease in research studies. Six hundred and twenty-two studies with 24 615 participants taking a probiotic product were included in the review (Hempel *et al.*, 2011). Two hundred and thirty-five studies made only non-specific safety statements, for example "the intervention was well tolerated," without indicating what kind of adverse events were monitored. The remaining 387 studies reported the presence or absence of one or more specific adverse events. The most commonly reported adverse events were of gastrointestinal nature, followed by infections and infestations associated with administered probiotic organisms. The study showed no indication that participants using probiotic organisms experienced statistically significantly more gastrointestinal infections, or other adverse events, compared to control group participants. Moreover, there was also no statistically increased risk of adverse events in medium health-compromised participants and critically ill patients compared with control group participants with similar patient characteristics. Nonetheless, case studies most often report serious adverse events potentially caused by probiotic organisms for health-compromised, not generally healthy, participants. The authors concluded that probiotic intervention studies lack assessment and systematic reporting of adverse events, yet available evidence does not indicate an increased risk (Hempel *et al.*, 2011).

Despite increased probiotic use, the incidence of bacteraemia attributable to probiotic strains remains extremely low (Salminen *et al.*, 2002). However, there are patients, for whom caution might be warranted, such as premature infants, elderly patients, the immuno-compromised, those with short bowel syndrome, those with central venous catheters, and those with cardiac valve disease. Nevertheless, the presence of any of these factors may not necessarily preclude a clinical trial (Snydman, 2008).

9.7 Conclusions and future trends

Awareness of the intestinal microbiota's role in nutrition, health, and disease has increased significantly. Recently developed technology has been used to explore the transcriptional profiles and genome differences of a variety of microorganisms, allowing a better understanding of their composition and activity in the gut. The appropriate selection of probiotic strains forms the basis for further development of supplements and food products, as well as for planning future clinical trials.

Wherever bacteria thrive, bacteriophages also exist and they undoubtedly influence ecosystems such as human intestine. Under stress conditions they can extensively alter microbial composition and may be an important biological aspect behind the "non-responders" in clinical trials. The role of phages in the human intestine has received little attention so far, and consequently knowledge of their functionality and diversity is limited (Mills et al., 2013). Influence of phage on bacterial balance in the gut remains to be elucidated and taken into account.

The current and proposed uses of probiotics cover a wide range of diseases and conditions. Only a few have significant research to back up the claims. Proven benefits of probiotics include the treatment of acute diarrhoea and AAD. Applications with substantial evidence include prevention of atopic eczema, prevention of traveller's diarrhoea, increased eradication of *H. pylori*, alleviating chronic constipation in adults and prevention of NEC. Promising applications include maintenance of remission in UC and pouchitis.

Before bringing probiotics into routine usage, proper evaluation of these products is essential. Ensuring identity and potency of probiotic products utilizing molecular techniques is vital. The concerns of regulatory agencies should be considered in the trial design. The use of international standards for probiotic trials on human health may facilitate the comparison of results from different probiotic products and allow meta-analyses and systematic reviews to strengthen the power of such studies.

With increasing development of molecular biology, genetic modification of probiotics has been undertaken to increase certain physiological or immunological properties within the organism, and to use the probiotic as a mucosal delivery system or a vaccine vector. Probiotics, especially those belonging to a group of lactic acid bacteria, are gaining importance as vehicles for the delivery of proteins to the mucosal surfaces. Delivered proteins may interact with the immune system, and have been shown to be effective, either as vaccines or as tolerance-inducing, anti-allergy agents (Berlec and Strukelj, 2009; Ravnikar et al., 2010). Recombinant lactic acid bacteria expressing proteins with biological functions that could be used in therapy have already made it to clinical trials (Steidler et al., 2004). However, as such they must be considered as medicaments and not as food supplements.

References

Agrawal, A., Houghton, L. A., Morris, J., Reilly, B., Guyonnet, D., Goupil Feuillerat, N., Schlumberger, A., Jakob, S. and Whorwell, P. J. (2009) "Clinical trial: the effects of a fermented milk product containing Bifidobacterium lactis DN-173 010 on abdominal distension and gastrointestinal transit in irritable bowel syndrome with constipation" *Aliment Pharmacol Ther*, 29, 104–114.

Alfaleh, K., Anabrees, J. and Bassler, D. (2010) "Probiotics reduce the risk of necrotizing enterocolitis in preterm infants: a meta-analysis" *Neonatology,* 97, 93–99.

Alfaleh, K., Anabrees, J., Bassler, D. and Al-Kharfi, T. (2011) "Probiotics for prevention of necrotizing enterocolitis in preterm infants" *Cochrane Database of Systematic Reviews.*

Alfaleh, K. and Bassler, D. (2008) "Probiotics for prevention of necrotizing enterocolitis in preterm infants" *Cochrane Database of Systematic Reviews.*

Allen, S. J., Martinez, E. G., Gregorio, G. V. and Dans, L. F. (2010) "Probiotics for treating acute infectious diarrhoea" *Cochrane Database Syst Rev,* CD003048.

Anon. (2005) "An evidence-based approach to the management of chronic constipation in North America" *Am J Gastroenterol,* 100, Suppl 1, S1–S4.

Arboleya, S., Binetti, A., Salazar, N., Fernandez, N., Solis, G., Hernandez-Barranco, A., Margolles, A., De Los Reyes-Gavilan, C. G. and Gueimonde, M. (2012) "Establishment and development of intestinal microbiota in preterm neonates" *FEMS Microbiol Ecol,* 79, 763–772.

Avadhani, A. and Miley, H. (2011) "Probiotics for prevention of antibiotic-associated diarrhea and Clostridium difficile-associated disease in hospitalized adults--a meta-analysis" *J Am Acad Nurse Pract,* 23, 269–274.

Azad, M. B. and Kozyrskyj, A. L. (2012) "Perinatal programming of asthma: the role of gut microbiota" *Clin Dev Immunol,* 2012, 932072.

Banaszkiewicz, A. and Szajewska, H. (2005) "Ineffectiveness of Lactobacillus GG as an adjunct to lactulose for the treatment of constipation in children: A double-blind, placebo-controlled randomized trial" *J Pediatr,* 146, 364–369.

Barbut, F. and Meynard, J. L. (2002) "Managing antibiotic associated diarrhoea" *BMJ,* 324, 1345–1346.

Basilisco, G. and Coletta, M. (2013) "Chronic constipation: A critical review" *Dig Liver Dis,* 45(11), 886–893.

Berlec, A. and Strukelj, B. (2009) "Novel applications of recombinant lactic acid bacteria in therapy and in metabolic engineering" *Recent Pat Biotechnol,* 3, 77–87.

Bernardo, W. M., Aires, F. T., Carneiro, R. M., Sa, F. P., Rullo, V. E. and Burns, D. A. (2013) "Effectiveness of probiotics in the prophylaxis of necrotizing enterocolitis in preterm neonates: a systematic review and meta-analysis" *J Pediatr (Rio J),* 89, 18–24.

Bibiloni, R., Fedorak, R. N., Tannock, G. W., Madsen, K. L., Gionchetti, P., Campieri, M., De Simone, C. and Sartor, R. B. (2005) "VSL#3 probiotic-mixture induces remission in patients with active ulcerative colitis" *Am J Gastroenterol,* 100, 1539–1546.

Bisgaard, H., Halkjaer, L. B., Hinge, R., Giwercman, C., Palmer, C., Silveira, L. and Strand, M. (2009) "Risk analysis of early childhood eczema" *J Allergy Clin Immunol,* 123, 1355–1360 e1355.

Black, F., Andersen, P., Ørskov, J., Ørskov, F., Gaarslev, K. and Laulund, S. (1989). Prophylactic efficacy of lactobacilli on traveler's diarrhea. In: *Travel Medicine.* R. Steffen, H. Lobel, J. Haworth and D.J. Bradley (eds), Springer, Berlin Heidelberg.

Black, R. E. (1986) "Pathogens that cause travelers' diarrhea in Latin America and Africa" *Rev Infect Dis,* 8, S131–S135.

Blaser, M. J. (1999) "Hypothesis: the changing relationships of Helicobacter pylori and humans: implications for health and disease" *J Infect Dis,* 179, 1523–1530.

Bongers, M. E. J., Benninga, M. A., Maurice-Stam, H. and Grootenhuis, M. A. (2009) "Health-related quality of life in young adults with symptoms of constipation continuing from childhood into adulthood" *Health and Quality of Life Outcomes,* 7.

Bousvaros, A., Antonioli, D. A., Colletti, R. B., Dubinsky, M. C., Glickman, J. N., Gold, B. D., Griffiths, A. M., Jevon, G. P., Higuchi, L. M. and Hyams, J. S. (2007) "Differentiating ulcerative colitis from Crohn disease in children and young adults: report of a working group of the North American Society for Pediatric Gastroenterology, Hepatology, and Nutrition and the Crohn's and Colitis Foundation of America" *J Pediatr Gastroenterol Nutr,* 44, 653.

Bousvaros, A., Guandalini, S., Baldassano, R. N., Botelho, C., Evans, J., Ferry, G. D., Goldin, B., Hartigan, L., Kugathasan, S., Levy, J., Murray, K. F., Oliva-Hemker, M., Rosh, J. R., Tolia, V., Zholudev, A., Vanderhoof, J. A. and Hibberd, P. L. (2005) "A randomized, double-blind trial of Lactobacillus GG versus placebo in addition to standard maintenance therapy for children with Crohn's disease" *Inflamm Bowel Dis,* 11, 833–839.

Bouvier, M., Meance, S., Bouley, C., Berta, J.-L. and Grimaud, J.-C. (2001) "Effects of consumption of a milk fermented by the probiotic strain Bifidobacterium animalis DN-173 010 on colonic transit times in healthy humans" *Biosci Microflora,* 20, 43–48.

Brenner, D. M., Moeller, M. J., Chey, W. D. and Schoenfeld, P. S. (2009) "The utility of probiotics in the treatment of irritable bowel syndrome: a systematic review" *Am J Gastroenterol,* 104, 1033–1049; quiz 1050.

Briand, V., Buffet, P., Genty, S., Lacombe, K., Godineau, N., Salomon, J., Vandemelbrouck, E., Ralaimazava, P., Goujon, C., Matheron, S., Fontanet, A. and Bouchaud, O. (2006) "Absence of efficacy of nonviable Lactobacillus acidophilus for the prevention of traveler's diarrhea: a randomized, double-blind, controlled study" *Clin Infect Dis,* 43, 1170–1175.

Bu, L. N., Chang, M. H., Ni, Y. H., Chen, H. L. and Cheng, C. C. (2007) "Lactobacillus casei rhamnosus Lcr35 in children with chronic constipation" *Pediatr Int,* 49, 485–490.

Cannon, J. P., Lee, T. A., Bolanos, J. T. and Danziger, L. H. (2005) "Pathogenic relevance of Lactobacillus: a retrospective review of over 200 cases" *Eur J Clin Microbiol Infect Dis,* 24, 31–40.

Carre, C. (1887) "Ueber Antagonisten unter den Bacterien.' *Correspondenz-Blatt Schweiz Aerzte,* 385–392.

Cassani, E., Privitera, G., Pezzoli, G., Pusani, C., Madio, C., Iorio, L. and Barichella, M. (2011) "Use of probiotics for the treatment of constipation in Parkinson's disease patients" *Minerva Gastroenterol e dietol,* 57, 117.

Chermesh, I., Tamir, A., Reshef, R., Chowers, Y., Suissa, A., Katz, D., Gelber, M., Halpern, Z., Bengmark, S. and Eliakim, R. (2007) "Failure of Synbiotic 2000 to prevent postoperative recurrence of Crohn's disease" *Dig Dis Sci,* 52, 385–389.

Chmielewska, A. and Szajewska, H. (2010) "Systematic review of randomised controlled trials: probiotics for functional constipation" *World J Gastroenterol,* 16, 69–75.

Clarke, G., Cryan, J. F., Dinan, T. G. and Quigley, E. M. (2012) "Review article: probiotics for the treatment of irritable bowel syndrome – focus on lactic acid bacteria" *Aliment Pharmacol Ther,* 35, 403–413.

Clavel, T. and Haller, D. (2007) "Bacteria- and host-derived mechanisms to control intestinal epithelial cell homeostasis: implications for chronic inflammation" *Inflamm Bowel Dis,* 13, 1153–1164.

Coccorullo, P., Strisciuglio, C., Martinelli, M., Miele, E., Greco, L. and Staiano, A. (2010) "Lactobacillus reuteri (DSM 17938) in infants with functional chronic constipation: a double-blind, randomized, Placebo-Controlled Study" *J Pediat,* 157, 598–602.

Cotten, C. M., Taylor, S., Stoll, B., Goldberg, R. N., Hansen, N. I., Sánchez, P. J., Ambalavanan, N. and Benjamin, D. K. (2009) "Prolonged duration of initial empirical antibiotic treatment is associated with increased rates of necrotizing enterocolitis and death for extremely low birth weight infants" *Pediatrics,* 123, 58–66.

Cui, H. H., Chen, C. L., Wang, J. D., Yang, Y. J., Cun, Y., Wu, J. B., Liu, Y. H., Dan, H. L., Jian, Y. T. and Chen, X. Q. (2004) "Effects of probiotic on intestinal mucosa of patients with ulcerative colitis" *World J Gastroenterol*, 10, 1521–1525.

De Dios Pozo-Olano, J., Warram Jr, J., Gomez, R. and Cavazos, M. (1978) "Effect of a lactobacilli preparation on traveler's diarrhea. A randomized, double blind clinical trial" *Gastroenterology*, 74, 829.

De Milliano, I., Tabbers, M. M., Van Der Post, J. A. and Benninga, M. A. (2012) "Is a multi-species probiotic mixture effective in constipation during pregnancy?' A pilot study" *Nutr J*, 11, 1–6.

De Vrese, M., Stegelmann, A., Richter, B., Fenselau, S., Laue, C. and Schrezenmeir, J. (2001) "Probiotics – compensation for lactase insufficiency" *Am J Clin Nutr*, 73, 421s–429s.

De Vrese, M., Winkler, P., Rautenberg, P., Harder, T., Noah, C., Laue, C., Ott, S., Hampe, J., Schreiber, S., Heller, K. and Schrezenmeir, J. (2006) "Probiotic bacteria reduced duration and severity but not the incidence of common cold episodes in a double blind, randomized, controlled trial" *Vaccine*, 24, 6670–6674.

Del Piano, M., Carmagnola, S., Anderloni, A., Andorno, S., Ballarè, M., Balzarini, M., Montino, F., Orsello, M., Pagliarulo, M. and Sartori, M. (2010) "The use of probiotics in healthy volunteers with evacuation disorders and hard stools: a double-blind, randomized, placebo-controlled study" *J Clin Gastroenterol*, 44, S30–S34.

Deshpande, G., Rao, S., Patole, S. and Bulsara, M. (2010) "Updated meta-analysis of probiotics for preventing necrotizing enterocolitis in preterm neonates" *Pediatrics*, 125, 921–930.

Doherty, G., Bennett, G., Patil, S., Cheifetz, A. and Moss, A. C. (2009) "Interventions for prevention of post-operative recurrence of Crohn's disease" *Cochrane Database Syst Rev*, CD006873.

Dunn, B. E., Cohen, H. and Blaser, M. J. (1997) "Helicobacter pylori" *Clin Microbiol Rev*, 10, 720–741.

FAO/WHO (2002), *Guidelines for the evaluation of probiotics in food: report of a joint FAO/WHO Working Group* London Ontario, Canada. Available from: ftp://ftp.fao.org/es/esn/food/wgreport2.pdf [Accessed 28 August 2013]

FAO/WHO (2001), *Evaluation of health and nutritional properties of powder milk and live lactic acid bacteria Food and Agriculture Organization of the United Nations and World Health Organization Report* Available from: http://www.who.int/foodsafety/publications/fs_management/en/probiotics.pdf [Accessed 28 August 2013]

Fallani, M., Young, D., Scott, J., Norin, E., Amarri, S., Adam, R., Aguilera, M., Khanna, S., Gil, A., Edwards, C. A. and Dore, J. (2010) "Intestinal microbiota of 6-week-old infants across Europe: geographic influence beyond delivery mode, breast-feeding, and antibiotics" *J Pediatr Gastroenterol Nutr*, 51, 77–84.

Fischer, A., Whiteson, K., Lazarevic, V., Hibbs, J., Francois, P. and Schrenzel, J. (2012) "Infant gut microbial colonization and health: recent findings from metagenomics studies" *J Integr OMICS*, 2, 1–16.

Franks, A. H., Harmsen, H. J., Raangs, G. C., Jansen, G. J., Schut, F. and Welling, G. W. (1998) "Variations of bacterial populations in human feces measured by fluorescent in situ hybridization with group-specific 16S rRNA-targeted oligonucleotide probes" *Appl Environ Microbiol*, 64, 3336–3345.

Fujimori, S., Tatsuguchi, A., Gudis, K., Kishida, T., Mitsui, K., Ehara, A., Kobayashi, T., Sekita, Y., Seo, T. and Sakamoto, C. (2007) "High dose probiotic and prebiotic cotherapy for remission induction of active Crohn's disease" *J Gastroenterol Hepatol*, 22, 1199–1204.

Fuller, R. (1989) "Probiotics in man and animals" *J Appl Bacteriol*, 66, 365–378.

Furrie, E., Macfarlane, S., Kennedy, A., Cummings, J. H., Walsh, S. V., O'Neil D, A. and Macfarlane, G. T. (2005) "Synbiotic therapy (Bifidobacterium longum/Synergy 1) initiates resolution of inflammation in patients with active ulcerative colitis: a randomised controlled pilot trial" *Gut,* 54, 242–249.

Gerritsen, J., Smidt, H., Rijkers, G. T. and De Vos, W. M. (2011) "Intestinal microbiota in human health and disease: the impact of probiotics" *Genes Nutr,* 6, 209–240.

Gionchetti, P., Rizzello, F., Helwig, U., Venturi, A., Lammers, K. M., Brigidi, P., Vitali, B., Poggioli, G., Miglioli, M. and Campieri, M. (2003) "Prophylaxis of pouchitis onset with probiotic therapy: a double-blind, placebo-controlled trial" *Gastroenterology,* 124, 1202–1209.

Gionchetti, P., Rizzello, F., Morselli, C., Poggioli, G., Tambasco, R., Calabrese, C., Brigidi, P., Vitali, B., Straforini, G. and Campieri, M. (2007) "High-dose probiotics for the treatment of active pouchitis" *Dis Colon Rectum,* 50, 2075–2082; discussion 2082-2074.

Gionchetti, P., Rizzello, F., Venturi, A., Brigidi, P., Matteuzzi, D., Bazzocchi, G., Poggioli, G., Miglioli, M. and Campieri, M. (2000) "Oral bacteriotherapy as maintenance treatment in patients with chronic pouchitis: a double-blind, placebo-controlled trial" *Gastroenterology,* 119, 305–309.

Goldin, B. R. (1998) "Health benefits of probiotics" *Br J Nutr,* 80, S203-207.

Guerra, P. V., Lima, L. N., Souza, T. C., Mazochi, V., Penna, F. J., Silva, A. M., Nicoli, J. R. and Guimarães, E. V. (2011) "Pediatric functional constipation treatment with Bifidobacterium-containing yogurt: a crossover, double-blind, controlled trial" *World J gastroenter: WJG,* 17, 3916.

Gupta, P., Andrew, H., Kirschner, B. S. and Guandalini, S. (2000) "Is lactobacillus GG helpful in children with Crohn's disease? Results of a preliminary, open-label study" *J Pediatr Gastroenterol Nutr,* 31, 453–457.

Guslandi, M., Giollo, P. and Testoni, P. A. (2003) "A pilot trial of Saccharomyces boulardii in ulcerative colitis" *Eur J Gastroenterol Hepatol,* 15, 697–698.

Guslandi, M., Mezzi, G., Sorghi, M. and Testoni, P. A. (2000) "Saccharomyces boulardii in maintenance treatment of Crohn's disease" *Dig Dis Sci,* 45, 1462–1464.

Guthmann, F., Kluthe, C. and Buhrer, C. (2010) "Probiotics for prevention of necrotising enterocolitis: an updated meta-analysis" *Klin Padiatr,* 222, 284–290.

Hao, W. L. and Lee, Y. K. (2004) "Microflora of the gastrointestinal tract: a review" *Methods Mol Biol,* 268, 491–502.

Hatakka, K., Savilahti, E., Ponka, A., Meurman, J. H., Poussa, T., Nase, L., Saxelin, M. and Korpela, R. (2001) "Effect of long term consumption of probiotic milk on infections in children attending day care centres: double blind, randomised trial" *BMJ,* 322, 1327.

Helin, T., Haahtela, S. and Haahtela, T. (2002) "No effect of oral treatment with an intestinal bacterial strain, Lactobacillus rhamnosus (ATCC 53103), on birch-pollen allergy: a placebo-controlled double-blind study" *Allergy,* 57, 243–246.

Hempel, S., Newberry, S., Ruelaz, A., Wang, Z., Miles, J. N., Suttorp, M. J., Johnsen, B., Shanman, R., Slusser, W., Fu, N., Smith, A., Roth, B., Polak, J., Motala, A., Perry, T. and Shekelle, P. G. (2011) "Safety of probiotics used to reduce risk and prevent or treat disease" *Evid Rep Technol Assess (Full Rep),* 1–645.

Hempel, S., Newberry, S. J., Maher, A. R., Wang, Z., Miles, J. N. V., Shanman, R., Johnsen, B. and Shekelle, P. G. (2012) "Probiotics for the prevention and treatment of antibiotic-associated diarrhea: a systematic review and meta-analysis" *Jama-J Am Med Assoc,* 307, 1959–1969.

Henker, J., Laass, M. W., Blokhin, B. M., Maydannik, V. G., Bolbot, Y. K., Elze, M., Wolff, C., Schreiner, A. and Schulze, J. (2008) "Probiotic Escherichia coli Nissle 1917 versus placebo for treating diarrhea of greater than 4 days duration in infants and toddlers" *Pediatr Infect Dis J,* 27, 494–499.

Henriksson, A., Borody, T. and Clancy, R. (2005) "Probiotics under the regulatory microscope" *Expert Opin Drug Saf,* 4, 1135–1143.

Hilton, E., Kolakowski, P., Singer, C. and Smith, M. (1997) "Efficacy of Lactobacillus GG as a diarrheal preventive in travelers" *J Travel Med,* 4, 41–43.

Holubar, S. D., Cima, R. R., Sandborn, W. J. and Pardi, D. S. (2010) "Treatment and prevention of pouchitis after ileal pouch-anal anastomosis for chronic ulcerative colitis" *Cochrane Database Syst Rev,* CD001176.

Huang, J. S., Bousvaros, A., Lee, J. W., Diaz, A. and Davidson, E. J. (2002) "Efficacy of probiotic use in acute diarrhea in children – A meta-analysis" *Digestive Diseases and Sciences,* 47, 2625–2634.

Huynh, H. Q., Debruyn, J., Guan, L., Diaz, H., Li, M., Girgis, S., Turner, J., Fedorak, R. and Madsen, K. (2009) "Probiotic preparation VSL#3 induces remission in children with mild to moderate acute ulcerative colitis: a pilot study" *Inflamm Bowel Dis,* 15, 760–768.

Iannitti, T. and Palmieri, B. (2010) "Therapeutical use of probiotic formulations in clinical practice" *Clin Nutr,* 29, 701–725.

Ishikawa, H., Akedo, I., Umesaki, Y., Tanaka, R., Imaoka, A. and Otani, T. (2003) "Randomized controlled trial of the effect of bifidobacteria-fermented milk on ulcerative colitis" *Journal of the American College of Nutrition,* 22, 56–63.

Jeffery, I. B., Quigley, E. M., Ohman, L., Simren, M. and O'Toole, P. W. (2012) "The microbiota link to irritable bowel syndrome: an emerging story" *Gut Microbes,* 3, 572–576.

Johnson, A. O., Semenya, J. G., Buchowski, M. S., Enwonwu, C. O. and Scrimshaw, N. S. (1993) "Adaptation of lactose maldigesters to continued milk intakes" *Am J Clin Nutr,* 58, 879–881.

Johnston, B. C., Goldenberg, J. Z., Vandvik, P. O., Sun, X. and Guyatt, G. H. (2011) "Probiotics for the prevention of pediatric antibiotic-associated diarrhea" *Cochrane Database Syst Rev,* CD004827.

Johnston, B. C., Ma, S. S., Goldenberg, J. Z., Thorlund, K., Vandvik, P. O., Loeb, M. and Guyatt, G. H. (2012) "Probiotics for the prevention of Clostridium difficile-associated diarrhea: a systematic review and meta-analysis" *Ann Intern Med,* 157, 878–888.

Katelaris, P. H., Salam, I. and Farthing, M. J. (1995) "Lactobacilli to prevent traveler's diarrhea?" *New Engl J Med,* 333, 1360–1361.

Kato, K., Mizuno, S., Umesaki, Y., Ishii, Y., Sugitani, M., Imaoka, A., Otsuka, M., Hasunuma, O., Kurihara, R., Iwasaki, A. and Arakawa, Y. (2004) "Randomized placebo-controlled trial assessing the effect of bifidobacteria-fermented milk on active ulcerative colitis" *Aliment Pharmacol Ther,* 20, 1133–1141.

Koebnick, C., Wagner, I., Leitzmann, P., Stern, U. and Zunft, H. J. (2003) "Probiotic beverage containing Lactobacillus casei Shirota improves gastrointestinal symptoms in patients with chronic constipation" *Can J Gastroenterol,* 17, 655–659.

Kollaritsch, H., Holst, H., Grobara, P. and Wiedermann, G. (1993) "Prevention of traveler's diarrhea with Saccharomyces boulardii. Results of a placebo controlled double-blind study" *Fortschr Med,* 111, 152–156.

Kollaritsch, H., Kremsner, P., Wiedermann, G. and Scheiner, O. (1989) "Prevention of traveller's diarrhea: comparison of different non-antibiotic preparations" *Travel Med Int,* 11, 9–17.

Kollath, W. (1953) "Nutrition and the tooth system; general review with special reference to vitamins" *Dtsch Zahnarztl Z,* 8, Suppl 7–16.

Kruis, W., Fric, P., Pokrotnieks, J., Lukas, M., Fixa, B., Kascak, M., Kamm, M. A., Weismueller, J., Beglinger, C., Stolte, M., Wolff, C. and Schulze, J. (2004) "Maintaining remission of

ulcerative colitis with the probiotic Escherichia coli Nissle 1917 is as effective as with standard mesalazine" *Gut,* 53, 1617–1623.
Kruis, W., Schutz, E., Fric, P., Fixa, B., Judmaier, G. and Stolte, M. (1997) "Double-blind comparison of an oral Escherichia coli preparation and mesalazine in maintaining remission of ulcerative colitis" *Aliment Pharmacol Ther,* 11, 853–858.
Kuisma, J., Mentula, S., Jarvinen, H., Kahri, A., Saxelin, M. and Farkkila, M. (2003) "Effect of Lactobacillus rhamnosus GG on ileal pouch inflammation and microbial flora" *Aliment Pharmacol Ther,* 17, 509–515.
Laake, K. O., Bjorneklett, A., Aamodt, G., Aabakken, L., Jacobsen, M., Bakka, A. and Vatn, M. H. (2005) "Outcome of four weeks' intervention with probiotics on symptoms and endoscopic appearance after surgical reconstruction with a J-configurated ileal-pouch-anal-anastomosis in ulcerative colitis" *Scand J Gastroenterol,* 40, 43–51.
Lay, C., Sutren, M., Rochet, V., Saunier, K., Dore, J. and Rigottier-Gois, L. (2005) "Design and validation of 16S rRNA probes to enumerate members of the Clostridium leptum subgroup in human faecal microbiota" *Environ Microbiol,* 7, 933–946.
Ledoux, D., Labombardi, V. J. and Karter, D. (2006) "Lactobacillus acidophilus bacteraemia after use of a probiotic in a patient with AIDS and Hodgkin's disease" *Int J Std Aids,* 17, 280–282.
Lesbros-Pantoflickova, D., Corthesy-Theulaz, I. and Blum, A. L. (2007) "Helicobacter pylori and probiotics" *J Nutr,* 137, 812S-818S.
Lilly, D. M. and Stillwell, R. H. (1965) "Probiotics: Growth-promoting factors produced by microorganisms" *Science,* 147, 747–748.
Liu, Z., Qin, H., Yang, Z., Xia, Y., Liu, W., Yang, J., Jiang, Y., Zhang, H., Wang, Y. and Zheng, Q. (2011) "Randomised clinical trial: the effects of perioperative probiotic treatment on barrier function and post-operative infectious complications in colorectal cancer surgery – a double-blind study" *Aliment Pharmacol Ther,* 33, 50–63.
Liu, Z. H., Huang, M. J., Zhang, X. W., Wang, L., Huang, N. Q., Peng, H., Lan, P., Peng, J. S., Yang, Z., Xia, Y., Liu, W. J., Yang, J., Qin, H. L. and Wang, J. P. (2013) "The effects of perioperative probiotic treatment on serum zonulin concentration and subsequent post-operative infectious complications after colorectal cancer surgery: a double-center and double-blind randomized clinical trial" *Am J Clin Nutr,* 97, 117–126.
Longstreth, G. F., Thompson, W. G., Chey, W. D., Houghton, L. A., Mearin, F. and Spiller, R. C. (2006) "Functional Bowel Disorders" *Gastroenterology,* 130, 1480–1491.
Mack, D. R. (2011) "Probiotics in inflammatory bowel diseases and associated conditions" *Nutrients,* 3, 245–264.
Malchow, H. A. (1997) "Crohn's disease and Escherichia coli. A new approach in therapy to maintain remission of colonic Crohn's disease?" *J Clin Gastroenterol,* 25, 653–658.
Malfertheiner, P., Megraud, F., O'Morain, C., Bazzoli, F., El-Omar, E., Graham, D., Hunt, R., Rokkas, T., Vakil, N. and Kuipers, E. J. (2007) "Current concepts in the management of Helicobacter pylori infection: the Maastricht III Consensus Report" *Gut,* 56, 772–781.
Mallon, P., Mckay, D., Kirk, S. and Gardiner, K. (2007) "Probiotics for induction of remission in ulcerative colitis" *Cochrane Database Syst Rev,* CD005573.
Marchesi, J. and Shanahan, F. (2007) "The normal intestinal microbiota" *Curr Opin Infect Dis,* 20, 508–513.
Mariat, D., Firmesse, O., Levenez, F., Guimaraes, V., Sokol, H., Dore, J., Corthier, G. and Furet, J. P. (2009) "The Firmicutes/Bacteroidetes ratio of the human microbiota changes with age" *BMC Microbiol,* 9, 123.
Marteau, P., Cuillerier, E., Meance, S., Gerhardt, M., Myara, A., Bouvier, M., Bouley, C., Tondu, F., Bommelaer, G. and Grimaud, J. (2002) "Bifidobacterium animalis strain

DN-173 010 shortens the colonic transit time in healthy women: a double-blind, randomized, controlled study" *Aliment Pharmacol Therap,* 16, 587–593.
Marteau, P., Lemann, M., Seksik, P., Laharie, D., Colombel, J. F., Bouhnik, Y., Cadiot, G., Soule, J. C., Bourreille, A., Metman, E., Lerebours, E., Carbonnel, F., Dupas, J. L., Veyrac, M., Coffin, B., Moreau, J., Abitbol, V., Blum-Sperisen, S. and Mary, J. Y. (2006) "Ineffectiveness of Lactobacillus johnsonii LA1 for prophylaxis of postoperative recurrence in Crohn's disease: a randomised, double blind, placebo controlled GETAID trial" *Gut,* 55, 842–847.
Martin, F. P. J., Collino, S. and Rezzi, S. (2011) "1H NMR-based metabonomic applications to decipher gut microbial metabolic influence on mammalian health" *Magn Reson Chem,* 49, S47–S54.
Mcfarland, L. V. (2007) "Meta-analysis of probiotics for the prevention of traveler's diarrhea" *Travel Med Infect Dis,* 5, 97–105.
Mcfarland, L. V. and Dublin, S. (2008) "Meta-analysis of probiotics for the treatment of irritable bowel syndrome" *World J Gastroenterol,* 14, 2650–2661.
Meance, S., Cayuela, C., Raimondi, A., Turchet, P., Lucas, C. and Antoine, J.-M. (2003) "Recent advances in the use of functional foods: effects of the commercial fermented milk with Bifidobacterium animalis strain DN-173 010 and yoghurt strains on gut transit time in the elderly" *Microb Ecol Health Dis,* 15, 15–22.
Metchnikoff, E. (1907). Lactic acid as inhibiting intestinal putrefaction. In: *The Prolongation of Life: Optimistic Studies* P. Chalmers Mitchell (ed.), London, Heinemann.
Miele, E., Pascarella, F., Giannetti, E., Quaglietta, L., Baldassano, R. N. and Staiano, A. (2009) "Effect of a probiotic preparation (VSL#3) on induction and maintenance of remission in children with ulcerative colitis" *Am J Gastroenterol,* 104, 437–443.
Mihatsch, W. A., Braegger, C. P., Decsi, T., Kolacek, S., Lanzinger, H., Mayer, B., Moreno, L. A., Pohlandt, F., Puntis, J., Shamir, R., Stadtmuller, U., Szajewska, H., Turck, D. and Van Goudoever, J. B. (2012) "Critical systematic review of the level of evidence for routine use of probiotics for reduction of mortality and prevention of necrotizing enterocolitis and sepsis in preterm infants" *Clin Nutr,* 31, 6–15.
Mills, S., Shanahan, F., Stanton, C., Hill, C., Coffey, A. and Ross, R. P. (2013) "Movers and shakers: influence of bacteriophages in shaping the mammalian gut microbiota" *Gut Microbes,* 4, 4–16.
Mimura, T., Rizzello, F., Helwig, U., Poggioli, G., Schreiber, S., Talbot, I., Nicholls, R., Gionchetti, P., Campieri, M. and Kamm, M. (2004) "Once daily high dose probiotic therapy (VSL# 3) for maintaining remission in recurrent or refractory pouchitis" *Gut,* 53, 108–114.
Moayyedi, P., Ford, A. C., Talley, N. J., Cremonini, F., Foxx-Orenstein, A. E., Brandt, L. J. and Quigley, E. M. (2010) "The efficacy of probiotics in the treatment of irritable bowel syndrome: a systematic review" *Gut,* 59, 325–332.
Mollenbrink, M. and Bruckschen, E. (1994) "[Treatment of chronic constipation with physiologic Escherichia coli bacteria. Results of a clinical study of the effectiveness and tolerance of microbiological therapy with the E. coli Nissle 1917 strain (Mutaflor)]" *Med Klin (Munich),* 89, 587–593.
Naidoo, K., Gordon, M., Fagbemi, A. O., Thomas, A. G. and Akobeng, A. K. (2011) "Probiotics for maintenance of remission in ulcerative colitis" *Cochrane Database Syst Rev,* CD007443.
Nanthakumar, N. N., Fusunyan, R. D., Sanderson, I. and Walker, W. A. (2000) "Inflammation in the developing human intestine: A possible pathophysiologic contribution to necrotizing enterocolitis" *Proc Natl Acad Sci U S A,* 97, 6043–6048.

O'Mahony, L., Mccarthy, J., Kelly, P., Hurley, G., Luo, F., Chen, K., O'Sullivan, G. C., Kiely, B., Collins, J. K., Shanahan, F. and Quigley, E. M. (2005) "Lactobacillus and bifidobacterium in irritable bowel syndrome: symptom responses and relationship to cytokine profiles" *Gastroenterology*, 128, 541–551.

O'Ryan, M., Prado, V. and Pickering, L. K. (2005). A millennium update on pediatric diarrheal illness in the developing world. *Semin Pediatr Infect Dis*, 16(2), 125–136.

Oberhelman, R. A., Gilman, R. H., Sheen, P., Taylor, D. N., Black, R. E., Cabrera, L., Lescano, A. G., Meza, R. and Madico, G. (1999) "A placebo-controlled trial of Lactobacillus GG to prevent diarrhea in undernourished Peruvian children" *J Pediatr*, 134, 15–20.

Oggioni, M. R., Pozzi, G., Valensin, P. E., Galieni, P. and Bigazzi, C. (1998) "Recurrent septicemia in an immunocompromised patient due to probiotic strains of Bacillus subtilis" *J Clin Microbiol*, 36, 325–326.

Oksanen, P. J., Salminen, S., Saxelin, M., Hamalainen, P., Ihantola-Vormisto, A., Muurasniemi-Isoviita, L., Nikkari, S., Oksanen, T., Porsti, I., Salminen, E., Siitonen, S. Stuckey, H. Toppila, A. and Vapaatalo, H. (1990) "Prevention of travellers' diarrhoea by Lactobacillus GG" *Ann Med*, 22, 53–56.

Oozeer, R., Goupil-Feuillerat, N., Alpert, C. A., Van De Guchte, M., Anba, J., Mengaud, J. and Corthier, G. (2002) "Lactobacillus casei is able to survive and initiate protein synthesis during its transit in the digestive tract of human flora-associated mice" *Appl Environ Microbiol*, 68, 3570–3574.

Pardi, D. S., D'haens, G., Shen, B., Campbell, S. and Gionchetti, P. (2009) "Clinical guidelines for the management of pouchitis" *Inflamm Bowel Dis*, 15, 1424–1431.

Pedone, C. A., Arnaud, C. C., Postaire, E. R., Bouley, C. F. and Reinert, P. (2000) "Multicentric study of the effect of milk fermented by Lactobacillus casei on the incidence of diarrhoea" *Int J Clin Pract*, 54, 568–571.

Penders, J., Thijs, C., Vink, C., Stelma, F. F., Snijders, B., Kummeling, I., Van Den Brandt, P. A. and Stobberingh, E. E. (2006) "Factors influencing the composition of the intestinal microbiota in early infancy" *Pediatrics*, 118, 511–521.

Prantera, C., Scribano, M. L., Falasco, G., Andreoli, A. and Luzi, C. (2002) "Ineffectiveness of probiotics in preventing recurrence after curative resection for Crohn's disease: a randomised controlled trial with Lactobacillus GG" *Gut*, 51, 405–409.

Qin, J. J., Li, R. Q., Raes, J., Arumugam, M., Burgdorf, K. S., Manichanh, C., Nielsen, T., Pons, N., Levenez, F., Yamada, T., Mende, D. R., Li, J. H., Xu, J. M., Li, S. C., Li, D. F., Cao, J. J., Wang, B., Liang, H. Q., Zheng, H. S., Xie, Y. L., Tap, J., Lepage, P., Bertalan, M., Batto, J. M., Hansen, T., Le Paslier, D., Linneberg, A., Nielsen, H. B., Pelletier, E., Renault, P., Sicheritz-Ponten, T., Turner, K., Zhu, H. M., Yu, C., Li, S. T., Jian, M., Zhou, Y., Li, Y. R., Zhang, X. Q., Li, S. G., Qin, N., Yang, H. M., Wang, J., Brunak, S., Dore, J., Guarner, F., Kristiansen, K., Pedersen, O., Parkhill, J., Weissenbach, J., Bork, P., Ehrlich, S. D., Wang, J. and Consortium, M. (2010) "A human gut microbial gene catalogue established by metagenomic sequencing" *Nature*, 464, 59-U70.

Rahimi, R., Nikfar, S., Rahimi, F., Elahi, B., Derakhshani, S., Vafaie, M. and Abdollahi, M. (2008) "A meta-analysis on the efficacy of probiotics for maintenance of remission and prevention of clinical and endoscopic relapse in Crohn's disease" *Dig Dis Sci*, 53, 2524–2531.

Rasquin, A., Di Lorenzo, C., Forbes, D., Guiraldes, E., Hyams, J. S., Staiano, A. and Walker, L. S. (2006) "Childhood functional gastrointestinal disorders: Child/adolescent" *Gastroenterology*, 130, 1527–1537.

Ravnikar, M., Strukelj, B., Obermajer, N., Lunder, M. and Berlec, A. (2010) "Engineered lactic acid bacterium Lactococcus lactis capable of binding antibodies and tumor necrosis factor alpha" *Appl Environ Microbiol*, 76, 6928–6932.

Rembacken, B. J., Snelling, A. M., Hawkey, P. M., Chalmers, D. M. and Axon, A. T. (1999) "Non-pathogenic Escherichia coli versus mesalazine for the treatment of ulcerative colitis: a randomised trial" *Lancet,* 354, 635–639.

Rhee, S. H., Pothoulakis, C. and Mayer, E. A. (2009) "Principles and clinical implications of the brain-gut-enteric microbiota axis" *Nat Rev Gastroenterol Hepatol,* 6, 306–314.

Riezzo, G., Orlando, A., D'attoma, B., Guerra, V., Valerio, F., Lavermicocca, P., Candia, S. and Russo, F. (2012) "Randomised clinical trial: efficacy of Lactobacillus paracasei-enriched artichokes in the treatment of patients with functional constipation–a double-blind, controlled, crossover study" *Aliment Pharmacol Therap,* 35, 441–450.

Rolfe, V. E., Fortun, P. J., Hawkey, C. J. and Bath-Hextall, F. (2006) "Probiotics for maintenance of remission in Crohn's disease" *Cochrane Database Syst Rev,* CD004826.

Saavedra, J. M., Abi-Hanna, A., Moore, N. and Yolken, R. H. (2004) "Long-term consumption of infant formulas containing live probiotic bacteria: tolerance and safety" *Am J Clin Nutr,* 79, 261–267.

Salari, P., Nikfar, S. and Abdollahi, M. (2012) "A meta-analysis and systematic review on the effect of probiotics in acute diarrhea" *Inflamm Allergy Drug Targets,* 11, 3–14.

Salminen, M. K., Tynkkynen, S., Rautelin, H., Saxelin, M., Vaara, M., Ruutu, P., Sarna, S., Valtonen, V. and Jarvinen, A. (2002) "Lactobacillus bacteremia during a rapid increase in Probiotic use of Lactobacillus rhamnosus GG in Finland" *Clin Infect Dis,* 35, 1155–1160.

Salminen, S. and Salminen, E. (1997) "Lactulose, lactic acid bacteria, intestinal microecology and mucosal protection" *Scand J Gastroenterol Suppl,* 222, 45–48.

Sanders, M. E. (2003) "Probiotics: considerations for human health' *Nutr Rev,* 61, 91–99.

Sanders, M. E., Guarner, F., Guerrant, R., Holt, P. R., Quigley, E. M. M., Sartor, R. B., Sherman, P. M. and Mayer, E. A. (2013) "An update on the use and investigation of probiotics in health and disease" *Gut,* 62, 787–796.

Sartor, R. B. (2006) "Mechanisms of disease: pathogenesis of Crohn's disease and ulcerative colitis" *Nat Clin Pract Gastroenterol Hepatol,* 3, 390–407.

Scholtens, P. A., Oozeer, R., Martin, R., Amor, K. B. and Knol, J. (2012) "The early settlers: intestinal microbiology in early life" *Annu Rev Food Sci Technol,* 3, 425–447.

Senok, A. C., Verstraelen, H., Temmerman, M. and Botta, G. A. (2009) "Probiotics for the treatment of bacterial vaginosis" *Cochrane Database Syst Rev,* CD006289.

Shen, B., Brzezinski, A., Fazio, V. W., Remzi, F. H., Achkar, J. P., Bennett, A. E., Sherman, K. and Lashner, B. A. (2005) "Maintenance therapy with a probiotic in antibiotic-dependent pouchitis: experience in clinical practice" *Aliment Pharmacol Ther,* 22, 721–728.

Snydman, D. R. (2008) "The safety of probiotics" *Clin Infect Dis,* 46 Suppl 2, S104–S111; discussion S144-151.

Sood, A., Midha, V., Makharia, G. K., Ahuja, V., Singal, D., Goswami, P. and Tandon, R. K. (2009) "The probiotic preparation, VSL#3 induces remission in patients with mild-to-moderately active ulcerative colitis" *Clin Gastroenterol Hepatol,* 7, 1202–1209, 1209 e1201.

Starzynska, T. and Malfertheiner, P. (2006) "Helicobacter and digestive malignancies" *Helicobacter,* 11 Suppl 1, 32–35.

Steidler, L., Remaut, E. and Fiers, W., (Vlaams Interuniversitair Instituut voor Biotechnologie VZW) 2004. *Use of a cytokine-producing lactococcus strain to treat colitis.* US patent 6746671, 2004-Jun-08.

Szajewska, H., Guandalini, S., Morelli, L., Van Goudoever, J. B. and Walker, A. (2010a) "Effect of Bifidobacterium animalis subsp lactis supplementation in preterm infants: a systematic review of randomized controlled trials" *J Pediatr Gastroenterol Nutr,* 51, 203–209.

Szajewska, H., Horvath, A. and Piwowarczyk, A. (2010b) "Meta-analysis: the effects of Saccharomyces boulardii supplementation on Helicobacter pylori eradication rates and side effects during treatment" *Aliment Pharmacol Ther,* 32, 1069–1079.

Szajewska, H., Kotowska, M., Mrukowicz, J. Z., Armanska, M. and Mikolajczyk, W. (2001) "Efficacy of Lactobacillus GG in prevention of nosocomial diarrhea in infants" *J Pediatr,* 138, 361–365.

Szajewska, H., Setty, M., Mrukowicz, J. and Guandalini, S. (2006) "Probiotics in gastrointestinal diseases in children: hard and not-so-hard evidence of efficacy" *J Pediatr Gastroenterol Nutr,* 42, 454–475.

Szajewska, H., Skorka, A. and Dylag, M. (2007) "Meta-analysis: Saccharomyces boulardii for treating acute diarrhoea in children" *Aliment Pharmacol Ther,* 25, 257–264.

Tabbers, M. M., Chmielewska, A., Roseboom, M. G., Crastes, N., Perrin, C., Reitsma, J. B., Norbruis, O., Szajewska, H. and Benninga, M. A. (2011) "Fermented Milk Containing Bifidobacterium lactis DN-173 010 in Childhood Constipation: A Randomized, Double-Blind, Controlled Trial" *Pediatrics,* 127, E1392-E1399.

Thibault, H., Aubert-Jacquin, C. and Goulet, O. (2004) "Effects of long-term consumption of a fermented infant formula (with Bifidobacterium breve c50 and Streptococcus thermophilus 065) on acute diarrhea in healthy infants" *J Pediatr Gastroenterol Nutr,* 39, 147–152.

Thomas, D. W. and Greer, F. R. (2010) "Probiotics and prebiotics in pediatrics" *Pediatrics,* 126, 1217–1231.

Tissier, H. (1906) "Traitement des infections intestinales par la méthode de la flore bactérienne de l'intestin." *CR Soc Biol,* 359–361.

Tong, J. L., Ran, Z. H., Shen, J., Zhang, C. X. and Xiao, S. D. (2007) "Meta-analysis: the effect of supplementation with probiotics on eradication rates and adverse events during Helicobacter pylori eradication therapy" *Aliment Pharmacol Ther,* 25, 155–168.

Tursi, A., Brandimarte, G., Giorgetti, G. M., Forti, G., Modeo, M. E. and Gigliobianco, A. (2004) "Low-dose balsalazide plus a high-potency probiotic preparation is more effective than balsalazide alone or mesalazine in the treatment of acute mild-to-moderate ulcerative colitis" *Med Sci Monit,* 10, PI126–PI131.

Tursi, A., Brandimarte, G., Papa, A., Giglio, A., Elisei, W., Giorgetti, G. M., Forti, G., Morini, S., Hassan, C., Pistoia, M. A., Modeo, M. E., Rodino, S., D'amico, T., Sebkova, L., Sacca, N., Di Giulio, E., Luzza, F., Imeneo, M., Larussa, T., Di Rosa, S., Annese, V., Danese, S. and Gasbarrini, A. (2010) "Treatment of relapsing mild-to-moderate ulcerative colitis with the probiotic VSL#3 as adjunctive to a standard pharmaceutical treatment: a double-blind, randomized, placebo-controlled study" *Am J Gastroenterol,* 105, 2218–2227.

Van De Pol, M. A., Lutter, R., Smids, B. S., Weersink, E. J. and Van Der Zee, J. S. (2011) "Synbiotics reduce allergen-induced T-helper 2 response and improve peak expiratory flow in allergic asthmatics" *Allergy,* 66, 39–47.

Van Gossum, A., Dewit, O., Louis, E., De Hertogh, G., Baert, F., Fontaine, F., Devos, M., Enslen, M., Paintin, M. and Franchimont, D. (2007) "Multicenter randomized-controlled clinical trial of probiotics (Lactobacillus johnsonii, LA1) on early endoscopic recurrence of Crohn's disease after Ileo-caecal resection" *Inflamm Bowel Dis,* 13, 135–142.

Van Niel, C. W., Feudtner, C., Garrison, M. M. and Christakis, D. A. (2002) "Lactobacillus therapy for acute infectious diarrhea in children: a meta-analysis" *Pediatrics,* 109, 678–684.

Van Nimwegen, F. A., Penders, J., Stobberingh, E. E., Postma, D. S., Koppelman, G. H., Kerkhof, M., Reijmerink, N. E., Dompeling, E., Van Den Brandt, P. A., Ferreira, I., Mommers, M.

and Thijs, C. (2011) "Mode and place of delivery, gastrointestinal microbiota, and their influence on asthma and atopy" *J Allergy Clin Immunol,* 128, 948–955 e941-943.

Veerappan, G. R., Betteridge, J. and Young, P. E. (2012) "Probiotics for the treatment of inflammatory bowel disease" *Curr Gastroenterol Rep,* 14, 324–333.

Videlock, E. J. and Cremonini, F. (2012) "Meta-analysis: probiotics in antibiotic-associated diarrhoea" *Aliment Pharmacol Ther,* 35, 1355–1369.

Villena, J., Oliveira, M. L., Ferreira, P. C., Salva, S. and Alvarez, S. (2011) "Lactic acid bacteria in the prevention of pneumococcal respiratory infection: future opportunities and challenges" *Int Immunopharmacol,* 11, 1633–1645.

Waller, P. A., Gopal, P. K., Leyer, G. J., Ouwehand, A. C., Reifer, C., Stewart, M. E. and Miller, L. E. (2011) "Dose-response effect of Bifidobacterium lactis HN019 on whole gut transit time and functional gastrointestinal symptoms in adults" *Scand J Gastroenterol,* 46, 1057–1064.

Wang, Q. Z., Dong, J. and Zhu, Y. M. (2012) "Probiotic supplement reduces risk of necrotizing enterocolitis and mortality in preterm very low-birth-weight infants: an updated meta-analysis of 20 randomized, controlled trials" *J Pediatr Sur,* 47, 241–248.

Wang, Z. H., Gao, Q. Y. and Fang, J. Y. (2013) "Meta-analysis of the efficacy and safety of Lactobacillus-containing and Bifidobacterium-containing probiotic compound preparation in Helicobacter pylori eradication therapy" *J Clin Gastroenterol,* 47, 25–32.

Weizman, Z., Asli, G. and Alsheikh, A. (2005) "Effect of a probiotic infant formula on infections in child care centers: comparison of two probiotic agents" *Pediatrics,* 115, 5–9.

Whorwell, P. J., Altringer, L., Morel, J., Bond, Y., Charbonneau, D., O'Mahony, L., Kiely, B., Shanahan, F. and Quigley, E. M. (2006) "Efficacy of an encapsulated probiotic Bifidobacterium infantis 35624 in women with irritable bowel syndrome" *Am J Gastroenterol,* 101, 1581–1590.

Yang, Y. X., He, M., Hu, G., Wei, J., Pages, P., Yang, X. H. and Bourdu-Naturel, S. (2008) "Effect of a fermented milk containing Bifidobacterium lactis DN-173010 on Chinese constipated women" *World J Gastroenterol,* 14, 6237–6243.

Yates, J. (2005) "Traveler's diarrhea" *Am Fam Physician,* 71, 2095–2100.

Zigra, P. I., Maipa, V. E. and Alamanos, Y. P. (2007) "Probiotics and remission of ulcerative colitis: a systematic review" *Neth J Med,* 65, 411–418.

Zocco, M. A., Dal Verme, L. Z., Cremonini, F., Piscaglia, A. C., Nista, E. C., Candelli, M., Novi, M., Rigante, D., Cazzato, I. A., Ojetti, V., Armuzzi, A., Gasbarrini, G. and Gasbarrini, A. (2006) "Efficacy of Lactobacillus GG in maintaining remission of ulcerative colitis" *Aliment Pharmacol Ther,* 23, 1567–1574.

Zoppi, G., Cinquetti, M., Luciano, A., Benini, A., Muner, A. and Bertazzoni Minelli, E. (1998) "The intestinal ecosystem in chronic functional constipation" *Acta Paediatr,* 87, 836–841.

Zou, J., Dong, J. and Yu, X. (2009) "Meta-analysis: Lactobacillus containing quadruple therapy versus standard triple first-line therapy for Helicobacter pylori eradication" *Helicobacter,* 14, 97–107.

Reviewing clinical studies of probiotics as dietary supplements: probiotics for atopic and allergic disorders, urinary tract and respiratory infections

M. Lunder
University of Ljubljana, Ljubljana, Slovenia

10.1 Introduction

As noted in Chapter 9, the modern concept of probiotics, prebiotics and synbiotics is to produce food or food supplements which, after ingestion, augment healthy intestinal microbiota, by adding probiotic microorganisms, indigestible but fermentable prebiotic carbohydrates, or both constituents combined in synbiotics. However, many professed probiotic products have not been properly characterized, documented, proven clinically effective and manufactured under good manufacturing practice.

Together with chapters 9 and 11, this chapter reviews clinical studies of the effectiveness of probiotics in treating a number of diseases and medical conditions. This chapter reviews the use of probiotics in:

- Atopic and allergic disorders (including eczema and asthma).
- Urogenital infections (bacterial vaginosis, candidal vaginitis (CV) and urinary tract infections (UTI)).
- Respiratory tract infections (including the common cold).

The chapter provides detailed references to allow further investigation of the therapeutic role of probiotics in treating or alleviating these conditions.

10.2 Probiotics for atopic and allergic disorders

Over the past few decades the prevalence of allergic disease has increased dramatically. Twenty to thirty per cent of individuals living in Western countries suffer at least one form of allergic disease (Zuercher *et al.*, 2006). Reduced exposure to microbes in early life (commonly referred to as the "hygiene hypothesis") is considered to be the main mechanism. A relationship between intestinal microbiota and allergic disease is well established (Van Nimwegen *et al.*, 2011). Several epidemiological studies have reported that microbiota differences exist between allergic and non-allergic infants, as well as between countries with high or low allergy prevalence rates (Bjorksten *et al.*, 2001; Watanabe *et al.*, 2003).

Infants from non-allergic parents are more frequently colonized by healthy lactobacilli, suggesting a role for maternal microbiota in protection from allergic disease (Johansson *et al.*, 2011). Healthy infants are usually colonized with infant-type *Bifidobacteruim longum* and *Bifidobacterium breve* species, while infants with eczema are more frequently colonized with adult-type *Bifidobacterium adolescentis* (Ouwehand *et al.*, 2001). Reduced microbial diversity, accompanied with lower numbers of lactobacilli and bifidobacteria, and early life colonization by *Staphylococcus aureus* and *Clostridium difficile* are associated with the development of allergic disease later in life (Penders *et al.*, 2007). Prophylactic or therapeutic strategies that target intestinal microbiota have been the subject of intense scientific research.

A number of studies have examined the clinical benefit of probiotics for the prevention or treatment of allergic diseases. Most of them have focused on eczema, since this is frequently the first manifestation of allergic disease, while a few studies have looked at other outcomes, such as asthma and food allergy. So far at least 15 intervention studies for the treatment of eczema have been reported (Toh *et al.*, 2012), significantly differing in the study populations and in the selection of probiotic strains used. Some report improved clinical symptoms, reduced SCORing Atopic Dermatitis (SCORAD) – a clinical tool for assessing the severity of atopic dermatitis as objectively as possible – and changes in immunological parameters; others report no difference with the placebo group. Systematic reviews and meta-analyses (Boyle *et al.*, 2008; Lee *et al.*, 2008; Tang *et al.*, 2010) that have evaluated the beneficial effect of probiotics in the treatment of eczema gave inconclusive answers. The Cochrane meta-analysis found no significant reduction in eczema symptoms or severity by probiotics compared to placebo and suggests that probiotics are not an effective treatment for eczema. Heterogeneity between studies could explain the lack of a probiotic treatment effect. Pooled analyses may mask the activity of potentially beneficial probiotic strains. Therefore, the ability of probiotics to improve eczema outcomes cannot be completely excluded.

Probiotics have also been investigated in food allergic individuals (Majamaa and Isolauri, 1997; Pelto *et al.*, 1998). The few studies that have examined whether probiotic treatment can modify the course of food allergy have not demonstrated an effect (Hol *et al.*, 2008; Viljanen *et al.*, 2005). At present, evidence suggests that probiotics cannot induce clinical tolerance to food antigens.

There is also limited and conflicting data on the effect of probiotic treatment for asthma. Most reported studies do not support the use of probiotics (Giovannini *et al.*, 2007; Helin *et al.*, 2002; Van De Pol *et al.*, 2011; Wheeler *et al.*, 1997). However, one study of children with asthma/allergic rhinitis treated with *Lactobacillus gasseri* showed significant improvements in clinical symptoms as well as reduced allergic cytokine levels such as IL-13 (Chen *et al.*, 2010).

While the evidence for the use of probiotics in the treatment of allergic disease remains mainly inconclusive, several clinical trials have been successful in the prevention of allergic disease. So far at least 14 randomized controlled trials evaluating various probiotics have been reported, mostly involving infants of families with a history of allergic disease (Abrahamsson et al., 2007; Boyle et al., 2011; Dotterud et al., 2010; Huurre et al., 2008; Kalliomaki et al., 2001; Kim et al., 2010; Kopp et al., 2008; Kukkonen et al., 2007; Niers et al., 2009; Rautava et al., 2006; Soh et al., 2009; Taylor et al., 2007; West et al., 2009; Wickens et al., 2008). Nine of them involved both a prenatal and postnatal intervention period, four studies evaluated only postnatal, and one study examined only a prenatal approach. For the combined prenatal–postnatal probiotic studies, six (Dotterud et al., 2010; Kalliomaki et al., 2001; Kim et al., 2010; Kukkonen et al., 2007; Niers et al., 2009; Wickens et al., 2008) of the nine published trials showed a significant reduction in the cumulative incidence of eczema and/or IgE-associated eczema by the age of 2.

No beneficial effects on eczema or sensitization were found in three of the four studies using a postnatal treatment approach (Rautava et al., 2006; Soh et al., 2009; Taylor et al., 2007). Moreover, one study that used *Lactobacillus acidophilus* LAVRI-A1 demonstrated an increased risk of both IgE-associated eczema and atopic sensitization at 1 year of age (Taylor et al., 2007). The remaining study found a reduced cumulative incidence of eczema at 13 months with *Lactobacillus paracasei* F19 (West et al., 2009). The only study to date that has evaluated a prenatal-only probiotic approach (using *Lactobacillus rhamnosus* GG) showed no evidence for a beneficial effect on eczema or sensitization at 12 months (Boyle et al., 2011). These studies suggest that a prenatal intervention or a postnatal probiotic treatment alone may be insufficient in reducing the clinical symptoms of allergic disease, and highlights the fact that the importance of the early life period in modulating microbiota and/or immune function begins prior to birth.

A recent meta-analysis based on the 14 studies provided evidence in support of a moderate role of probiotics in the prevention of atopic dermatitis and IgE-associated atopic dermatitis in infants and, on the contrary, demonstrated that the favourable effect was similar regardless of the time of probiotic use (pregnancy or early life) and the subject(s) receiving probiotics (mother, child or both) (Pelucchi et al., 2012).

Regarding the selection of probiotic species and strains, meta-analysis of the impact of maternal probiotic supplementation on eczema development found a significantly reduced risk in children by 2–7 years of age with the use of lactobacilli but not with other probiotic species and strains compared to placebo treatment (Doege et al., 2012). Since probiotics elicit unique biological activities, selection of probiotic species and strain should be carefully considered.

Despite the generally beneficial effects of probiotics, some studies reported increased risks of asthma-like symptoms at 2 years (Kopp et al., 2008) and at 7 years (Kalliomaki et al., 2007), suggesting that it will be critical to follow these cohorts for several years to determine any long-term impact (beneficial or otherwise) of the probiotic effect.

Several variables can have an impact on the potential beneficial effects, including the probiotic species and strain, dose, and duration of administration, as well as geographical and other differences in the populations studied. These differences make drawing conclusions about the effectiveness of probiotics complicated. Further studies are therefore required to determine the optimal dose, bacterial strain and timing for intervention as well as patient populations that would provide optimal effects in the prevention or treatment of allergic disease.

10.3 Probiotics for urogenital infections

This section provides critical assessment of the efficacy of probiotics in prevention or treatment of three major urogenital infections: bacterial vaginosis, vulvovaginal candidiasis, and urinary tract infection.

10.3.1 Bacterial vaginosis (BV)

BV is a common bacterial infection of the vagina. It may arise and remit spontaneously, but often appears as a chronic or recurrent disease. While the symptoms are usually mild, it can have severe consequences during pregnancy (Manns-James, 2011). It is characterized by an overgrowth of predominantly anaerobic organisms in the vagina, leading to a replacement of lactobacilli. Lactobacilli dominate the healthy flora and are believed to protect the host against infections by several mechanisms, such as tight adhesion to the epithelium, stabilization of a low pH, and the production of antimicrobial substances such as hydrogen peroxide, acids and bacteriocins, the degradation of polyamines or the production of surfactants, which inhibit the adhesion of pathogens (Reid, 2001). Therefore, probiotic lactobacilli seem an obvious choice to restore an imbalanced flora.

Evidence for the use of probiotic preparations either alone or in conjunction with antibiotics for the treatment of BV was meta-analysed by Senok (Senok *et al.*, 2009). The current research does not provide conclusive evidence that probiotics are superior to or enhance the effectiveness of antibiotics in the treatment of BV. Regarding the prevention of recurrent BV, the Cochrane review focused on the effect of probiotics in preventing urogenital tract infections in pregnant women or in women planning pregnancy (Othman *et al.*, 2007). Although the studies were too small to draw firm conclusions, pooled results showed an 81% reduction in the risk of genital infection with the use of probiotics. So far, there is insufficient evidence to recommend the use of probiotics either before, during or after antibiotic treatment as a means of ensuring successful treatment or to reduce recurrence.

10.3.2 Candidal vaginitis (CV)

The second most common cause of vaginal inflammation after BV is CV, an infection of the vagina's mucous membranes by *Candida albicans* (Sobel, 1985). It afflicts an estimated 75% of sexually active women at least once in their life and of these approximately 50% will develop a second episode, with 5% suffering recurrent episodes (Ferrer, 2000). Although the pathogenesis of CV remains a controversial issue, it seems that when the balance between the microorganisms existing in the vaginal microbiota is disrupted, the overgrowth of *Candida* is facilitated (Jeavons, 2003). There are some *in vitro* experiments which show that some lactobacilli strains can inhibit the adherence and/or the growth of *C. albicans* (Boris *et al.*, 1998; Osset *et al.*, 2001; Reid and Bruce, 2001; Strus *et al.*, 2005). Since the physiological or pathophysiological mechanisms occurring *in vivo* are far more complicated, these results do not necessarily apply to treatment and prevention of vaginitis.

It has been shown in some studies that orally or (Reid *et al.*, 2001a, 2001b, 2003) intravaginally (Hilton *et al.*, 1995; Williams *et al.*, 2001) administered lactobacilli have the ability to colonize the vagina and/or reduce the vaginal colonization and infection by *Candida*. On the other hand, there are some studies that do not support a role for probiotics in the prevention of recurrent CV (Pirotta *et al.*, 2004; Shalev *et al.*, 1996).

Falagas *et al.* tried to sum up the existing clinical data regarding the potential use of probiotics for the prevention of CV (Falagas *et al.*, 2006) and found that most of clinical studies have important methodological shortcomings. In the majority of the studies, only a small sample of women was included or completed the study, and CV was either not confirmed or was self-diagnosed; moreover, some studies were not placebo-controlled. There were also differences among the trials regarding the strain of the tested probiotic, its dosage and duration of treatment. Consequently, it is difficult to draw reliable conclusions from the existing studies. Probiotics, especially *L. acidophilus*, *L. rhamnosus* GR-1 and *Lactobacillus fermentum* RC-14, may be considered potential experimental preventive agents in women who suffer from frequent episodes of CV (more than three episodes per year), since adverse effects are uncommon. Such treatment is rational, particularly when the use of antifungal agents is contraindicated or is associated with adverse effects (Falagas *et al.*, 2006).

It is still controversial whether probiotics can actually prevent recurrence of CV, since lactobacilli have frequently been found to co-exist with *Candida* in the vaginal epithelium of women with CV, and are not significantly reduced as in the case of BV (Sobel and Chaim, 1996). However, the composition of lactobacilli species and strains is different between healthy women and those with CV. Therefore, more randomized, double-blind, placebo-controlled trials with larger sample sizes should be carried out to elucidate whether probiotics can be used efficiently and safely for the prophylaxis of recurrent CV.

10.3.3 Urinary tract infections (UTI)

Around 50–60% of women experience at least one UTI during their lifetime, and 25–30% of these have a recurrence within 3–4 months of the initial infection (Finer and Landau, 2004; Rahn, 2008). Recurrent UTI (rUTI) (usually defined as three episodes in the last 12 months or two episodes in the last 6 months) can have a considerable impact on a woman's quality of life. Almost 95% of UTI cases are caused by bacteria, which multiply at the proximal part of the urethra and enter the bladder (the ascending route). *Escherichia coli* has been found to be the most common causative organism (Kurutepe *et al.*, 2005). Continuous antibiotic prophylaxis or postcoital prophylaxis, if there is close correlation with sexual intercourse, are most effective in preventing rUTI (Wagenlehner *et al.*, 2013).

A recent meta-analysis (Grin *et al.*, 2013) compiled results of existing randomized clinical trials to determine the efficacy of using a *Lactobacillus* prophylactic against rUTI in premenopausal adult women. After excluding studies using ineffective strains and studies testing for safety, data from 127 patients in two studies were included. A statistically significant decrease in rUTI was found in patients given *Lactobacillus*, represented by the pooled risk ratio of 0.51 (95% confidence interval 0.26–0.99, $p = 0.05$) with no statistical heterogeneity. The authors concluded that probiotic strains of *Lactobacillus* are safe and effective in preventing rUTI in adult women and could potentially replace low-dose, long-term antibiotics as a safer prophylactic agent. Nevertheless, more studies are required before a definitive recommendation can be made, since the patient population contributing data to this meta-analysis was small (Grin *et al.*, 2013).

10.4 Probiotics for respiratory tract infections

Recent studies have centred on whether probiotics might sufficiently stimulate the common mucosal immune system to provide protection to other mucosal sites. There is gradually increasing evidence that orally delivered probiotics are able to regulate immune responses outside the gastrointestinal tract, including the respiratory mucosa, which would increase resistance to infections, even in immuno-compromised hosts (Forsythe, 2011; Villena *et al.*, 2011). Gluck *et al.* showed that regular oral intake of probiotic fermented milk (*Lactobacillus* GG) can reduce nasal colonization with potentially pathogenic bacteria (*S. aureus*, *Streptococcus pneumoniae*, beta-haemolytic streptococci, and *Haemophilus influenzae*). The mechanisms underlying this further indicate a linkage of the lymphoid tissue between the gut and the upper respiratory tract (Gluck and Gebbers, 2003).

Administration of probiotics has been associated with lower incidence of ventilator-associated pneumonia (Morrow *et al.*, 2010; Schultz and Haas, 2011; Siempos *et al.*, 2010); however, a recent meta-analysis failed to confirm this (Gu *et al.*, 2012). The authors concluded that probiotics show no beneficial effect in patients who are mechanically ventilated; thus, probiotics should not be recommended for routine clinical application (Gu *et al.*, 2012). However, the results of this meta-analysis should be interpreted with caution because of the heterogeneity among study designs.

Next, probiotics reduced respiratory infections in healthy and hospitalized children (Hatakka *et al.*, 2001b; Hojsak *et al.*, 2010) and elderly (Makino *et al.*, 2010), and reduced the duration of the common cold infection (De Vrese *et al.*, 2006). A recent meta-analysis assessed the effectiveness and safety of probiotics for preventing acute upper respiratory tract infections. Data from ten randomized controlled trials were extracted, which involved 3451 participants, including infants, children and adults aged around 40 years. They found that probiotics were better than placebo in reducing the number of participants experiencing episodes of acute upper respiratory tract infections and the rate ratio (calculated to compare the rate of events occurring at any given point in time) of episodes. Three of the trials showed that live microorganisms can reduce the prescription of antibiotics. There was no difference in the mean duration of an episode of acute upper respiratory tract infection. Side effects of probiotics were minor, and gastrointestinal symptoms were the most common (Hao et al., 2011).

The common cold, or upper respiratory tract infection, is one of the leading reasons for physician visits. It is generally caused by viruses and is treated symptomatically. It should be noted that in addition to causing morbidity and mortality directly, there is evidence that respiratory infections, particularly viral infections, are a contributing factor, not only to the exacerbation of asthma, but also to development of the disease (Holtzman et al., 2009).Therefore, there is a need for further examination of the therapeutic potential of commensal-induced modulation of the mucosal immune response.

10.5 Conclusions

As noted in Chapter 9, awareness of the intestinal microbiota's role in nutrition, health, and disease has increased significantly. The current and proposed uses of probiotics cover a wide range of diseases and conditions. Only a few have significant research to back up the claims. Applications with substantial evidence discussed in this chapter include prevention of atopic eczema and prevention of respiratory infections in children. Promising applications also discussed in this chapter include prevention of recurrent urogenital infections.

References

Abrahamsson, T. R., Jakobsson, T., Bottcher, M. F., Fredrikson, M., Jenmalm, M. C., Bjorksten, B. and Oldaeus, G. (2007) "Probiotics in prevention of IgE-associated eczema: a double-blind, randomized, placebo-controlled trial" *J Allergy Clin Immunol*, 119, 1174–1180.

Bjorksten, B., Sepp, E., Julge, K., Voor, T. and Mikelsaar, M. (2001) "Allergy development and the intestinal microflora during the first year of life" *J Allergy Clin Immunol*, 108, 516–520.

Boris, S., Suarez, J. E., Vazquez, F. and Barbes, C. (1998) "Adherence of human vaginal lactobacilli to vaginal epithelial cells and interaction with uropathogens" *Infect Immun*, 66, 1985–1989.

Boyle, R. J., Bath-Hextall, F. J., Leonardi-Bee, J., Murrell, D. F. and Tang, M. L. (2008) "Probiotics for treating eczema" *Cochrane Database Syst Rev*, CD006135.

Boyle, R. J., Ismail, I. H., Kivivuori, S., Licciardi, P. V., Robins-Browne, R. M., Mah, L. J., Axelrad, C., Moore, S., Donath, S., Carlin, J. B., Lahtinen, S. J. and Tang, M. L. K. (2011) "Lactobacillus GG treatment during pregnancy for the prevention of eczema: a randomized controlled trial" *Allergy*, 66, 509–516.

Cui, H. H., Chen, C. L., Wang, J. D., Yang, Y. J., Cun, Y., Wu, J. B., Liu, Y. H., Dan, H. L., Jian, Y. T. and Chen, X. Q. (2004) "Effects of probiotic on intestinal mucosa of patients with ulcerative colitis" *World J Gastroenterol*, 10, 1521–1525.

De Dios Pozo-Olano, J., Warram Jr, J., Gomez, R. and Cavazos, M. (1978) "Effect of a lactobacilli preparation on traveler's diarrhea. A randomized, double blind clinical trial" *Gastroenterology*, 74, 829.

De Milliano, I., Tabbers, M. M., Van Der Post, J. A. and Benninga, M. A. (2012) "Is a multispecies probiotic mixture effective in constipation during pregnancy?"A pilot study' *Nutr J*, 11, 1–6.

De Vrese, M., Stegelmann, A., Richter, B., Fenselau, S., Laue, C. and Schrezenmeir, J. (2001) "Probiotics – compensation for lactase insufficiency" *Am J Clin Nutr*, 73, 421s-429s.

De Vrese, M., Winkler, P., Rautenberg, P., Harder, T., Noah, C., Laue, C., Ott, S., Hampe, J., Schreiber, S., Heller, K. and Schrezenmeir, J. (2006) "Probiotic bacteria reduced duration and severity but not the incidence of common cold episodes in a double blind, randomized, controlled trial" *Vaccine*, 24, 6670–6674.

Doege, K., Grajecki, D., Zyriax, B. C., Detinkina, E., Zu Eulenburg, C. and Buhling, K. J. (2012) "Impact of maternal supplementation with probiotics during pregnancy on atopic eczema in childhood – a meta-analysis" *Br J Nutr*, 107, 1–6.

Dotterud, C. K., Storro, O., Johnsen, R. and Oien, T. (2010) "Probiotics in pregnant women to prevent allergic disease: a randomized, double-blind trial" *Br J Dermatol*, 163, 616–623.

Falagas, M. E., Betsi, G. I. and Athanasiou, S. (2006) "Probiotics for prevention of recurrent vulvovaginal candidiasis: a review" *J Antimicrob Chemother*, 58, 266–272.

Ferrer, J. (2000) "Vaginal candidosis: epidemiological and etiological factors" *Int J Gynaecol Obstet*, 71 Suppl 1, S21–S27.

Finer, G. and Landau, D. (2004) "Pathogenesis of urinary tract infections with normal female anatomy" *Lancet Infect Dis*, 4, 631–635.

Forsythe, P. (2011) "Probiotics and lung diseases" *Chest*, 139, 901–908.

Giovannini, M., Agostoni, C., Riva, E., Salvini, F., Ruscitto, A., Zuccotti, G. V. and Radaelli, G. (2007) "A randomized prospective double blind controlled trial on effects of long-term consumption of fermented milk containing Lactobacillus casei in pre-school children with allergic asthma and/or rhinitis" *Pediatr Res*, 62, 215–220.

Gluck, U. and Gebbers, J. O. (2003) "Ingested probiotics reduce nasal colonization with pathogenic bacteria (Staphylococcus aureus, Streptococcus pneumoniae, and beta-hemolytic streptococci)" *Am J Clin Nutr*, 77, 517–520.

Grin, P. M., Kowalewska, P. M., Alhazzan, W. and Fox-Robichaud, A. E. (2013) "Lactobacillus for preventing recurrent urinary tract infections in women: meta-analysis" *Can J Urol*, 20, 6607–6614.

Gu, W. J., Wei, C. Y. and Yin, R. X. (2012) "Lack of efficacy of probiotics in preventing ventilator-associated pneumonia probiotics for ventilator-associated pneumonia: a systematic review and meta-analysis of randomized controlled trials" *Chest*, 142, 859–868.

Hao, Q., Lu, Z., Dong, B. R., Huang, C. Q. and Wu, T. (2011) "Probiotics for preventing acute upper respiratory tract infections" *Cochrane Database Syst Rev*, CD006895.

Hao, W. L. and Lee, Y. K. (2004) "Microflora of the gastrointestinal tract: a review" *Methods Mol Biol*, 268, 491–502.

Hatakka, K., Savilahti, E., Pönkä, A., Meurman, J. H., Poussa, T., Näse, L., Saxelin, M. and Korpela, R. (2001b) "Effect of long term consumption of probiotic milk on infections in children attending day care centres: double blind, randomised trial" *BMJ*, 322, 1327.

Helin, T., Haahtela, S. and Haahtela, T. (2002) "No effect of oral treatment with an intestinal bacterial strain, Lactobacillus rhamnosus (ATCC 53103), on birch-pollen allergy: a placebo-controlled double-blind study" *Allergy*, 57, 243–246.

Hilton, E., Rindos, P. and Isenberg, H. D. (1995) "Lactobacillus GG vaginal suppositories and vaginitis" *J Clin Microbiol*, 33, 1433.

Hojsak, I., Abdovic, S., Szajewska, H., Milosevic, M., Krznaric, Z. and Kolacek, S. (2010) "Lactobacillus GG in the prevention of nosocomial gastrointestinal and respiratory tract infections" *Pediatrics*, 125, e1171-1177.
Hol, J., Van Leer, E. H., Elink Schuurman, B. E., De Ruiter, L. F., Samsom, J. N., Hop, W., Neijens, H. J., De Jongste, J. C. and Nieuwenhuis, E. E. (2008) "The acquisition of tolerance toward cow's milk through probiotic supplementation: a randomized, controlled trial" *J Allergy Clin Immunol*, 121, 1448–1454.
Holtzman, M. J., Byers, D. E., Benoit, L. A., Battaile, J. T., You, Y. J., Agapov, E., Park, C., Grayson, M. H., Kim, E. Y. and Patel, A. C. (2009) "Immune pathways for translating viral infection into chronic airway disease" *Adv Immunol, Vol 102*, 102, 245–276.
Huurre, A., Laitinen, K., Rautava, S., Korkeamaki, M. and Isolauri, E. (2008) "Impact of maternal atopy and probiotic supplementation during pregnancy on infant sensitization: a double-blind placebo-controlled study" *Clin Exp Allerg*, 38, 1342–1348.
Jeavons, H. S. (2003) "Prevention and treatment of vulvovaginal candidiasis using exogenous Lactobacillus" *Jognn-J Obstet Gynecol Neonatal Nurs*, 32, 287–296.
Johansson, M. A., Sjogren, Y. M., Persson, J. O., Nilsson, C. and Sverremark-Ekstrom, E. (2011) "Early colonization with a group of Lactobacilli decreases the risk for allergy at five years of age despite allergic heredity" *PLoS One*, 6, e23031.
Kalliomaki, M., Salminen, S., Arvilommi, H., Kero, P., Koskinen, P. and Isolauri, E. (2001) "Probiotics in primary prevention of atopic disease: a randomised placebo-controlled trial" *Lancet*, 357, 1076–1079.
Kalliomaki, M., Salminen, S., Poussa, T. and Isolauri, E. (2007) "Probiotics during the first 7 years of life: a cumulative risk reduction of eczema in a randomized, placebo-controlled trial" *J Allergy Clin Immunol*, 119, 1019–1021.
Kim, J. Y., Kwon, J. H., Ahn, S. H., Lee, S. I., Han, Y. S., Choi, Y. O., Lee, S. Y., Ahn, K. M. and Ji, G. E. (2010) "Effect of probiotic mix (Bifidobacterium bifidum, Bifidobacterium lactis, Lactobacillus acidophilus) in the primary prevention of eczema: a double-blind, randomized, placebo-controlled trial" *Pediatr Allergy Immunol*, 21, e386-393.
Kopp, M. V., Hennemuth, I., Heinzmann, A. and Urbanek, R. (2008) "Randomized, double-blind, placebo-controlled trial of probiotics for primary prevention: no clinical effects of Lactobacillus GG supplementation" *Pediatrics*, 121, e850-856.
Kukkonen, K., Savilahti, E., Haahtela, T., Juntunen-Backman, K., Korpela, R., Poussa, T., Tuure, T. and Kuitunen, M. (2007) "Probiotics and prebiotic galacto-oligosaccharides in the prevention of allergic diseases: a randomized, double-blind, placebo-controlled trial" *J Allergy Clin Immunol*, 119, 192–198.
Kurutepe, S., Surucuoglu, S., Sezgin, C., Gazi, H., Gulay, M. and Ozbakkaloglu, B. (2005) "Increasing antimicrobial resistance in Escherichia coli isolates from community-acquired urinary tract infections during 1998–2003 in Manisa, Turkey" *Jpn J Infect Dis*, 58, 159–161.
Lee, J., Seto, D. and Bielory, L. (2008) "Meta-analysis of clinical trials of probiotics for prevention and treatment of pediatric atopic dermatitis" *J Allergy Clin Immunol*, 121, 116–121 e111.
Majamaa, H. and Isolauri, E. (1997) "Probiotics: a novel approach in the management of food allergy" *J Allerg Clin Immunol*, 99, 179–185.
Makino, S., Ikegami, S., Kume, A., Horiuchi, H., Sasaki, H. and Orii, N. (2010) "Reducing the risk of infection in the elderly by dietary intake of yoghurt fermented with Lactobacillus delbrueckii ssp. bulgaricus OLL1073R-1" *Br J Nutr*, 104, 998–1006.
Manns-James, L. (2011) "Bacterial vaginosis and preterm birth" *J Midwifery Womens Health*, 56, 575–583.

Niers, L., Martin, R., Rijkers, G., Sengers, F., Timmerman, H., Van Uden, N., Smidt, H., Kimpen, J. and Hoekstra, M. (2009) "The effects of selected probiotic strains on the development of eczema (the PandA study)" *Allergy*, 64, 1349–1358.

Osset, J., Garcia, E., Bartolome, R. M. and Andreu, A. (2001) "Role of Lactobacillus as protector against vaginal candidiasis" *Med Clin (Barc)*, 117, 285–288.

Othman, M., Neilson, J. P. and Alfirevic, Z. (2007) "Probiotics for preventing preterm labour" *Cochrane Database Syst Rev*, CD005941.

Ouwehand, A. C., Isolauri, E., He, F., Hashimoto, H., Benno, Y. and Salminen, S. (2001) "Differences in Bifidobacterium flora composition in allergic and healthy infants" *J Allergy Clin Immunol*, 108, 144–145.

Pelto, L., Isolauri, E., Lilius, E. M., Nuutila, J. and Salminen, S. (1998) "Probiotic bacteria down-regulate the milk-induced inflammatory response in milk-hypersensitive subjects but have an immunostimulatory effect in healthy subjects" *Clin Exp Allerg*, 28, 1474–1479.

Pelucchi, C., Chatenoud, L., Turati, F., Galeone, C., Moja, L., Bach, J. F. and La Vecchia, C. (2012) "Probiotics supplementation during pregnancy or infancy for the prevention of atopic dermatitis: a meta-analysis" *Epidemiology*, 23, 402–414.

Penders, J., Thijs, C., Van Den Brandt, P. A., Kummeling, I., Snijders, B., Stelma, F., Adams, H., Van Ree, R. and Stobberingh, E. E. (2007) "Gut microbiota composition and development of atopic manifestations in infancy: the KOALA Birth Cohort Study" *Gut*, 56, 661–667.

Pirotta, M., Gunn, J., Chondros, P., Grover, S., O'Malley, P., Hurley, S. and Garland, S. (2004) "Effect of lactobacillus in preventing post-antibiotic vulvovaginal candidiasis: a randomised controlled trial" *BMJ*, 329, 548.

Rahn, D. D. (2008) "Urinary tract infections: contemporary management" *Urol Nurs*, 28, 333–341; quiz 342.

Rautava, S., Arvilommi, H. and Isolauri, E. (2006) "Specific probiotics in enhancing maturation of IgA responses in formula-fed infants" *Pediatr Res*, 60, 221–224.

Reid, G. (2001) "Probiotic agents to protect the urogenital tract against infection" *Am J Clin Nutr*, 73, 437S-443S.

Reid, G., Beuerman, D., Heinemann, C. and Bruce, A. W. (2001a) "Probiotic Lactobacillus dose required to restore and maintain a normal vaginal flora" *FEMS Immunol Med Microbiol*, 32, 37–41.

Reid, G. and Bruce, A. W. (2001) "Selection of lactobacillus strains for urogenital probiotic applications" *J Infect Dis*, 183 Suppl 1, S77-80.

Reid, G., Bruce, A. W., Fraser, N., Heinemann, C., Owen, J. and Henning, B. (2001b) "Oral probiotics can resolve urogenital infections" *FEMS Immunol Med Microbiol*, 30, 49–52.

Reid, G., Charbonneau, D., Erb, J., Kochanowski, B., Beuerman, D., Poehner, R. and Bruce, A. W. (2003) "Oral use of Lactobacillus rhamnosus GR-1 and L. fermentum RC-14 significantly alters vaginal flora: randomized, placebo-controlled trial in 64 healthy women" *FEMS Immunol Med Microbiol*, 35, 131–134.

Schultz, M. J. and Haas, L. E. (2011) "Antibiotics or probiotics as preventive measures against ventilator-associated pneumonia."

Senok, A. C., Verstraelen, H., Temmerman, M. and Botta, G. A. (2009) "Probiotics for the treatment of bacterial vaginosis" *Cochrane Database Syst Rev*, CD006289.

Shalev, E., Battino, S., Weiner, E., Colodner, R. and Keness, Y. (1996) "Ingestion of yogurt containing Lactobacillus acidophilus compared with pasteurized yogurt as prophylaxis for recurrent candidal vaginitis and bacterial vaginosis" *Arch Fam Med*, 5, 593–596.

Sobel, J. D. (1985) "Epidemiology and pathogenesis of recurrent vulvovaginal candidiasis" *Am J Obstet Gynecol,* 152, 924–935.
Sobel, J. D. and Chaim, W. (1996) "Vaginal microbiology of women with acute recurrent vulvovaginal candidiasis" *J Clin Microbiol,* 34, 2497–2499.
Soh, S. E., Aw, M., Gerez, I., Chong, Y. S., Rauff, M., Ng, Y. P. M., Wong, H. B., Pai, N., Lee, B. W. and Shek, L. P. C. (2009) "Probiotic supplementation in the first 6 months of life in at risk Asian infants – effects on eczema and atopic sensitization at the age of 1 year" *Clin Exp Allerg,* 39, 571–578.
Strus, M., Kucharska, A., Kukla, G., Brzychczy-Wloch, M., Maresz, K. and Heczko, P. B. (2005) "The in vitro activity of vaginal Lactobacillus with probiotic properties against Candida" *Infect Dis Obstet Gynecol,* 13, 69–75.
Tang, M. L., Lahtinen, S. J. and Boyle, R. J. (2010) "Probiotics and prebiotics: clinical effects in allergic disease" *Curr Opin Pediatr,* 22, 626–634.
Taylor, A. L., Dunstan, J. A. and Prescott, S. L. (2007) "Probiotic supplementation for the first 6 months of life fails to reduce the risk of atopic dermatitis and increases the risk of allergen sensitization in high-risk children: a randomized controlled trial" *J Allergy Clin Immunol,* 119, 184–191.
Toh, Z. Q., Anzela, A., Tang, M. L. and Licciardi, P. V. (2012) "Probiotic therapy as a novel approach for allergic disease" *Front Pharmacol,* 3, 171.
Van De Pol, M. A., Lutter, R., Smids, B. S., Weersink, E. J. and Van Der Zee, J. S. (2011) "Synbiotics reduce allergen-induced T-helper 2 response and improve peak expiratory flow in allergic asthmatics" *Allergy,* 66, 39–47.
Van Gossum, A., Dewit, O., Louis, E., De Hertogh, G., Baert, F., Fontaine, F., Devos, M., Enslen, M., Paintin, M. and Franchimont, D. (2007) "Multicenter randomized-controlled clinical trial of probiotics (Lactobacillus johnsonii, LA1) on early endoscopic recurrence of Crohn's disease after Ileo-caecal resection" *Inflamm Bowel Dis,* 13, 135–142.
Van Niel, C. W., Feudtner, C., Garrison, M. M. and Christakis, D. A. (2002) "Lactobacillus therapy for acute infectious diarrhea in children: a meta-analysis" *Pediatrics,* 109, 678–684.
Van Nimwegen, F. A., Penders, J., Stobberingh, E. E., Postma, D. S., Koppelman, G. H., Kerkhof, M., Reijmerink, N. E., Dompeling, E., Van Den Brandt, P. A., Ferreira, I., Mommers, M. and Thijs, C. (2011) "Mode and place of delivery, gastrointestinal microbiota, and their influence on asthma and atopy" *J Allergy Clin Immunol,* 128, 948–955 e941-943.
Viljanen, M., Savilahti, E., Haahtela, T., Juntunen-Backman, K., Korpela, R., Poussa, T., Tuure, T. and Kuitunen, M. (2005) "Probiotics in the treatment of atopic eczema/dermatitis syndrome in infants: a double-blind placebo-controlled trial" *Allergy,* 60, 494–500.
Villena, J., Oliveira, M. L., Ferreira, P. C., Salva, S. and Alvarez, S. (2011) "Lactic acid bacteria in the prevention of pneumococcal respiratory infection: future opportunities and challenges" *Int Immunopharmacol,* 11, 1633–1645.
Wagenlehner, F. M., Vahlensieck, W., Bauer, H. W., Weidner, W., Piechota, H. J. and Naber, K. G. (2013) "Prevention of recurrent urinary tract infections" *Minerva Urol Nefrol,* 65, 9–20.
Watanabe, S., Narisawa, Y., Arase, S., Okamatsu, H., Ikenaga, T., Tajiri, Y. and Kumemura, M. (2003) "Differences in fecal microflora between patients with atopic dermatitis and healthy control subjects" *J Allergy Clin Immunol,* 111, 587–591.
West, C. E., Hammarstrom, M. L. and Hernell, O. (2009) "Probiotics during weaning reduce the incidence of eczema" *Pediatr Allergy Immunol,* 20, 430–437.

Wheeler, J. G., Shema, S. J., Bogle, M. L., Shirrell, M. A., Burks, A. W., Pittler, A. and Helm, R. M. (1997) "Immune and clinical impact of Lactobacillus acidophilus on asthma" *Ann Allergy Asthma Immunol,* 79, 229–233.

Wickens, K., Black, P. N., Stanley, T. V., Mitchell, E., Fitzharris, P., Tannock, G. W., Purdie, G. and Crane, J. (2008) "A differential effect of 2 probiotics in the prevention of eczema and atopy: a double-blind, randomized, placebo-controlled trial" *J Allergy Clin Immunol,* 122, 788–794.

Williams, A. B., Yu, C., Tashima, K., Burgess, J. and Danvers, K. (2001) "Evaluation of two self-care treatments for prevention of vaginal candidiasis in women with HIV" *J Assoc Nurses AIDS Care,* 12, 51–57.

Zuercher, A. W., Fritsche, R., Corthesy, B. and Mercenier, A. (2006) "Food products and allergy development, prevention and treatment" *Curr Opin Biotechnol,* 17, 198–203.

Reviewing clinical studies of probiotics as dietary supplements: probiotics for oral healthcare, rheumatoid arthritis, cancer prevention, metabolic diseases and postoperative infections

M. Lunder
University of Ljubljana, Ljubljana, Slovenia

11.1 Introduction

As noted in Chapter 9, the modern idea of probiotics, prebiotics and synbiotics is to produce food or food supplements which, after ingestion, augment healthy intestinal microbiota, by either adding probiotic microorganisms, indigestible but fermentable prebiotic carbohydrates or both constituents combined in synbiotics. However, many professed probiotic products have not been properly characterized, documented, proven clinically effective and manufactured under good manufacturing practices.

Together with chapters 9 and 10, this chapter reviews clinical studies of the effectiveness of probiotics in treating a number of diseases and medical conditions. This chapter reviews the use of probiotics in:

- oral healthcare (including alleviation of tonsillitis and dental caries)
- rheumatoid arthritis
- cancer prevention (for example, colorectal cancer)
- metabolic diseases and conditions (such as diabetes, obesity and plasma lipid profile)
- postoperative infections (for example, after abdominal surgery).

The chapter provides detailed references to allow further investigation of the therapeutic role of probiotics in treating or alleviating these conditions.

11.2 Probiotics for oral healthcare

Dietary probiotics (lactobacilli) and streptococcal population of the oral cavity (*Streptococcus salivarius*, *Streptococcus sanguinis*, *Streptococcus mitis*, *Streptococcus oralis*) have been studied in the context of prevention and treatment of oropharyngeal infections, such as otitis media (Hatakka *et al.*, 2007b; Roos *et al.*, 2001; Tano *et al.*, 2002) and streptococcal pharyngotonsillitis (Di Pierro *et al.*, 2013; Falck *et al.*, 1999; Roos *et al.*, 1992, 1993, 1996), as well as in the context of caries (reviewed in (Twetman and Keller, 2012)), halitosis (Burton *et al.*, 2005; Kang *et al.*, 2006b) and periodontal infection management (Hatakka *et al.*, 2007a; Kang *et al.*, 2006a, Krasse *et al.*, 2006; Mayanagi *et al.*, 2009).

There are some promising results regarding otitis media in children reviewed (Niittynen *et al.*, 2012). However, the lack of confirmative studies makes it difficult to draw any strong conclusions. More studies are needed to identify the most promising probiotic strains and study populations, and to evaluate the mechanisms behind the possible effects of probiotics on otitis media. Studies with pharyngotonsillitis-prone patients (Roos *et al.*, 1992, 1993, 1996) showed significantly less recurrences of streptococcal tonsillitis in probiotic groups versus placebo. Mostly commensal *S. mitis* and *S sanguinis* were used to restore the normal alpha-streptococcal flora. Probiotics might also offer an opportunity for periodontal infection management (gingivitis, periodontitis) by either direct microbiological interactions or by immunomodulatory interactions. However, it is currently premature to draw any conclusions as to the clinical significance (Teughels *et al.*, 2011).

Whether probiotic bacterial interference applies to dental caries is also an open question. A search for relevant clinical trials on the use of probiotic bacteria as a potential and clinically applicable anti-caries measure was performed by Twetman and Keller (2012). Two animal and 19 human studies were retrieved. Most studies were short-term and restricted to microbiological endpoints, and only three human studies reported a caries endpoint. A high degree of heterogeneity among the included investigations hindered the analysis. Significant reductions of *Streptococcus mutans* in saliva or plaque following daily intake of probiotic lactobacilli or bifidobacteria were reported in 12 out of 19 papers, whereas three reported an increase of lactobacilli. Three caries trials in preschool children and the elderly demonstrated prevented fractions of between 21% and 75% following regular intakes of milk supplemented with *Lactobacillus rhamnosus*. No adverse effects or potential risks were reported.

Currently available literature does not exclude the possibility that probiotic bacteria can interfere with the oral biofilm, but any clinical recommendation would be premature. Considering the complex oral biofilm and the unique ecological environment that exists in the oral cavity, adopting strains isolated or developed for intestinal applications and gastrointestinal health for dental research might not be optimal. Large-scale clinical studies with orally derived specific anti-caries candidates are still lacking (Twetman and Keller, 2012).

11.3 Probiotics for rheumatoid arthritis

It has been shown that patients with inflammatory arthritis have increased permeability of the gut due to inflammation of the gastrointestinal tract (Mielants *et al.*,

1996). This allows food antigens and potentially harmful microorganisms to enter the bloodstream. Patients with inflammatory arthritis have been shown to have elevated antibodies to these antigens, in some cases leading to immune complexes in capillaries supplying the joint capsule (Hvatum *et al.*, 2006). A meta-analysis found a statistically and long-term clinically significant benefit of fasting and a vegetarian diet in rheumatoid arthritis patients (Muller *et al.*, 2001). Since this approach altered the intestinal flora (Peltonen *et al.*, 1997), the benefit of probiotics as an adjunctive therapy for the treatment of rheumatoid arthritis remains an unanswered question.

The use of probiotics to prevent or treat arthritis is quite unexplored, but some studies have indicated the potential benefit. Within the scope of animal models, oral treatment with probiotics has been shown to decrease the clinical severity in arthritic changes (Kano *et al.*, 2002; Rovensky *et al.*, 2009, 2005). A clinical study that was notably underpowered ($n = 21$ patients), and looked at only mild rheumatoid arthritis, did not find a statistically significant difference in the activity of the disease with the use of *L. rhamnosus* GG, although more subjects in the probiotic group reported improvement in subjective well-being (Hatakka *et al.*, 2003). A recent pilot study examined the utility of probiotics *L. rhamnosus* GR-1 and *Lactobacillus reuteri* RC-14 as an adjunctive therapy for the treatment of rheumatoid arthritis (Pineda Mde *et al.*, 2011). While probiotics were well tolerated and suppressed production of several inflammatory cytokines systemically, their activity was not better than placebo and no overall clinical improvement was achieved.

11.4 Probiotics for cancer prevention

Chronic disruption of intestinal microbiota homeostasis, "dysbiosis," could promote many diseases, including cancer. The mechanisms by which bacteria may stimulate carcinogenesis include chronic inflammation, immune evasion, and immune suppression (Azcarate-Peril *et al.*, 2011). Cancer-preventing properties are attributed to probiotic bacteria in fermented milk products and also in genuine yoghurt cultures (Pala *et al.*, 2011). Most studies dealt with the effect of probiotics on colorectal cancer. It is one of the most common cancers worldwide. Several molecular and cellular steps in the carcinogenic pathways have been defined, and evidence indicates a causative role for environmental factors, including obesity and diet, which are closely associated with changes in the gut microbiota (Sanders *et al.*, 2013).

Analysis of the microbiology in patients with colorectal cancer suggests that the bacterial diversity is reduced (Chen *et al.*, 2012), altered (Marchesi *et al.*, 2011; Sobhani *et al.*, 2011), or accompanied by high levels of *Fusobacterium nucleatum* sequences (Castellarin *et al.*, 2012). Several potential mechanisms have been described, including changes in colonic pH, binding or inactivation of carcinogens, enhanced immune responses, reduced colonic inflammation, lowered epithelial proliferation and increased apoptosis (Azcarate-Peril *et al.*, 2011). However, the relevance of these mechanisms of action on cancer risk in humans remains unknown. A single consistent observation is that a synbiotic preparation appears to be more effective in altering biomarkers of colorectal cancer risk than a single probiotic or prebiotic (Rafter et al., 2007; Worthley et al., 2009).

One human study showed a reduced rate of recurrence of adenoma after 4 years of *Lactobacillus casei* administration (Ishikawa et al., 2005). Furthermore, a 12-year follow-up of over 45 000 volunteers with a high intake of yoghurt in an Italian cohort reported a reduction in colorectal cancer, but there was no comparator group in this study (Pala et al., 2011). Although the few studies conducted on cancer end points in humans are encouraging, the end points are diverse, and more answers need to be resolved before clinical recommendations can be made.

Next, patients with colorectal cancer undergoing colectomy may benefit from pre- or peri-operative application of probiotics. Majority of clinical studies indicate that this can improve the integrity of gut mucosal barrier by benefiting the faecal microbiota, and decreasing infectious complications (Liu et al., 2011, 2013, Xia et al., 2010; Zhang et al., 2010a, 2012); however, one study suggests that preoperative administration of prebiotics in elective colorectal surgery appears to have the same protective effect in preventing a postoperative inflammatory response as mechanical bowel cleaning (Horvat et al., 2010).

Probiotics have also been evaluated to help manage the side effects of radiotherapy and chemotherapy, widely used either alone or in combination for the management of intra-abdominal and intrapelvic cancers. Beneficial effects of different probiotics given to patients receiving chemotherapy (Osterlund et al., 2007) or radiation (Delia et al., 2007) have been described. These studies point to the potential beneficial effect of probiotics in damage (radiation-induced diarrhoea) amelioration in the small bowel and large intestine of patients being treated for cancers.

11.5 Probiotics for metabolic diseases

This section focuses on the evidence and prospects for use of probiotics for the interventions in metabolic diseases.

11.5.1 Diabetes

Genetic predisposition, environmental and lifestyle factors, as well as epigenetic changes, contribute to the pathogenesis of type 2 diabetes. Gut microbiota is considered one of the most important environmental factors with impact on host physiology and metabolism. Moreover, gut microbiota has also been reported to play an important role in pathogenesis of obesity and related inflammatory metabolic disorders. Accumulating evidence supports the new hypothesis that metabolic diseases such as obesity and type 2 diabetes develop because of low-grade, systemic and chronic inflammation by disruption of the normal intestinal microbiota induced by dietary intake of high-fat and fructose diet (Cani et al., 2008b; Zhao and Shen, 2010). Data that emerged from various studies by different investigators provided evidence that modulating intestinal microbiota through dietary interventions may contribute to the prevention and control of mentioned inflammatory metabolic disorders (Panwar et al., 2013).

The indications that emerged from *in vitro* cell culture and *in vivo* animal studies (reviewed in (Panwar et al., 2013)) clearly demonstrate that probiotics do have the potential to control diabetes; however, the purported effects have not been adequately validated in the target human population. Double-blind, placebo-controlled, randomized clinical trials that assessed blood glucose, lipid profile and antioxidant status in target human population have produced mixed results.

Two studies performed by Ejtahed et al. (2011, 2012) showed that consumption of probiotic yoghurt significantly improved the antioxidant status and lipid profile in the intervention group. Patients in the probiotic intervention group consumed probiotic yoghurt containing *Lactobacillus acidophilus* La5 and *Bifidobacterium lactis* Bb12300 for 6 weeks, while those in the control group consumed conventional yoghurt. The probiotic groups in these studies showed a significant decrease in fasting blood glucose, HbA1c, and increased erythrocyte superoxide dismutase and glutathione peroxidase activities and total antioxidant status compared with the control group. The probiotic yoghurt consumption also decreased the total cholesterol by 4.54%, and low-density lipoprotein (LDL) cholesterol by 7.45% in the intervention group.

Another recent study evaluated the effect of the consumption of a symbiotic shake, containing *L. acidophilus*, *Bifidobacterium bifidum* and 2 g oligofructose, on glycaemia and cholesterol levels in elderly people. The symbiotic group showed a significant increase in high-density lipoprotein (HDL) cholesterol, non-significant reduction in total cholesterol and triglycerides, and a significant reduction in fasting glycaemia. No significant changes were recorded in the placebo group (Moroti et al., 2012). On the other hand, conflicting results were recorded in one randomized, double-blinded clinical trial assessing the effects of probiotic *L. acidophilus* NCFM in reducing systemic inflammation and improving insulin sensitivity in a group of 45 men with diabetes after a period of 4 weeks. No changes in the expression of baseline inflammatory markers and the systemic inflammatory response were observed, indicating ineffectiveness of the probiotic therapy in diabetic patients (Andreasen et al., 2010).

Pregnancy is sometimes associated with elevated insulin resistance, due to excess body weight and increased secretion of inflammatory cytokines especially during the third trimester. A Finnish study showed that ingestion of specific probiotics altered the composition of the gut microbiota and thereby metabolism from early gestation and decreased rates of gestational diabetes in normal weight women (Luoto et al., 2010). Another study is underway that will assess the effectiveness of probiotic ingestion for the prevention of gestational diabetes in overweight and obese women (Nitert et al., 2013). Asemi et al. determined the effects of daily consumption of probiotic yoghurt on insulin resistance and serum insulin levels of Iranian pregnant women (Asemi et al., 2013). Although consumption of probiotic yoghurt for 9 weeks did not affect serum insulin levels and homeostatic model assessment of insulin resistance (HOMA-IR) score, significant differences were found comparing changes in these variables between probiotic and conventional yoghurts.

11.5.2 Obesity

Intestinal microbiota has been proposed to play a role in obesity development (Ley *et al.*, 2006; Turnbaugh *et al.*, 2006). There are good indications that the intestinal microbiota undergoes changes in response to a high-fat diet resulting, for example, in a decrease of bifidobacteria. Possible explanations for the ability of the gut microbiota to affect obesity development include an improved energy harvest from the diet, stimulation of fat storage by influencing lipoprotein lipase activity mediated by fasting-induced adipose factor (Backhed *et al.*, 2004) and a fat-induced systemic low-grade inflammation (Cani *et al.*, 2008b) accompanied by endotoxaemia and insulin resistance (Cani *et al.*, 2008a). Whether the oral application of exogenous bifidobacteria could help improve symptoms of the metabolic syndrome and promote weight loss in humans needs to be further investigated (Blaut and Bischoff, 2010).

11.5.3 Lipid profile

Human clinical studies have yielded mixed results regarding the effects of consumption of probiotics on the plasma lipid profile. Guo *et al.* meta-analysed data from 13 trials including 485 participants. The results showed that a diet rich in probiotics decreases total cholesterol and LDL cholesterol concentration in plasma for participants with high, borderline high and normal cholesterol levels (Guo *et al.*, 2011). The exact mechanism for cholesterol removal is poorly understood. Several possible mechanisms for cholesterol removal by probiotics have been suggested, including assimilation of cholesterol by growing cells, binding of cholesterol to cellular surface, incorporation of cholesterol into the cellular membrane, deconjugation of bile via bile salt hydrolase, and coprecipitation of cholesterol with deconjugated bile. However, some of these mechanisms are strain dependent, and demonstrated under laboratory conditions which cannot be extrapolated to *in vivo* systems (Kumar *et al.*, 2012).

11.6 Probiotics for postoperative infections

In surgical patients there are several reasons for an altered gut microbiota. This is combined with an altered barrier function that may lead to an enhanced inflammatory response to surgery. Perioperative nutrition-based modulation of gut microbiota is increasingly used as a strategy for reducing the infective complications of elective surgery (Jeppsson *et al.*, 2011). Studies are indicating that patients undergoing abdominal surgery have fewer postoperative infections when prophylactic probiotic strains in combination with different prebiotics are administered perioperatively (Kinross *et al.*, 2013).

Two meta-analyses tried to identify the potential benefits of perioperative administration of probiotics/synbiotics to patients undergoing elective abdominal surgery (such as biliary cancer surgery, liver transplantation, pancreaticoduodenectomy, colectomy). The recent study of Kinross *et al.* included 13 randomized controlled trials totalling 962 patients (304 received synbiotics and 182 received probiotics).

The incidence of postoperative sepsis was reduced in the probiotic group versus the control (pooled odds ratio [OR] = 0.42; 95% confidence interval [CI], 0.23–0.75; $P = 0.003$) and in the synbiotic group versus the control (pooled OR = 0.25; 95% CI, 0.1–0.6; $P = 0.002$). Moreover, synbiotics reduced the length of postoperative antibiotic use (weighted mean differences = –1.71; 95% CI, –3.2 to –0.21; $P = 0.03$). The authors concluded that probiotic and synbiotic nutrition strategies reduce the incidence of postoperative sepsis in the elective general surgery setting and that effect is more pronounced with the use of synbiotics. The other early study of Pitsouni et al. (Pitsouni et al., 2009) also concluded that the use of probiotics/synbiotics may reduce postoperative infections after abdominal surgery. However, due to the significant heterogeneity of the studies included in both meta-analyses, the results should be interpreted with caution.

Benefits of preoperative and perioperative application of probiotics in colorectal cancer patients undergoing colectomy has already been discussed above. The results relating to reduction in postoperative infections with the use of probiotics in patients undergoing liver transplantation are also convincing. In three clinical trials there was a significant reduction in postoperative sepsis and wound infection rate (Eguchi et al., 2011; Rayes et al., 2002, 2005).

The effect of enteral nutrition and synbiotics versus prebiotic (fibre) on bacterial infection rates after pylorus-preserving pancreaticoduodenectomy was evaluated in a prospective randomized double-blind trial in 80 patients (Rayes et al., 2007). The incidence of postoperative bacterial infections was significantly lower with synbiotics (12.5%) than with fibres only (40%). The use of perioperative probiotics also reduced the incidence of infectious complications in patients after pancreaticoduodenectomy in the clinical study by Nomura et al. (2007).

When live bacteria are administered to patients undergoing surgery, safety must be carefully monitored. Patients with depression of immune function may be more susceptible to complications than healthy individuals. Although only a few reports on sepsis induced by administration of probiotics exist, this possibility must be carefully monitored. Furthermore, recent reports indicating increased morbidity and mortality when used in patients with severe pancreatitis also highlight safety concerns (Zhang et al., 2010b). These groups of patients with an ongoing severe inflammation are probably different from patients undergoing elective operations. The results of controlled trials performed so far indicate that therapy with probiotics seems safe and without any reported serious side effects. Further studies are warranted, to elucidate potential mechanisms of action and optimize its use.

11.7 Conclusions

Awareness of the intestinal microbiota's role in nutrition, health, and disease has increased significantly.

As discussed in chapters 4, 5 and this chapter, the current and proposed uses of probiotics cover a wide range of diseases and conditions. Only a few have significant research to back up the claims. Promising applications discussed in this chapter include reduction of postoperative infections in elective abdominal surgery and lowering of cholesterol levels. Some proposed future applications include the treatment of rheumatoid arthritis, cancer prevention, prevention and treatment of diabetes and prevention of dental caries.

References

Andreasen, A. S., Larsen, N., Pedersen-Skovsgaard, T., Berg, R. M., Moller, K., Svendsen, K. D., Jakobsen, M. and Pedersen, B. K. (2010) "Effects of Lactobacillus acidophilus NCFM on insulin sensitivity and the systemic inflammatory response in human subjects" *Br J Nutr*, 104, 1831–1838.

Asemi, Z., Samimi, M., Tabassi, Z., Naghibi Rad, M., Rahimi Foroushani, A., Khorammian, H. and Esmaillzadeh, A. (2013) "Effect of daily consumption of probiotic yoghurt on insulin resistance in pregnant women: a randomized controlled trial" *Eur J Clin Nutr*, 67, 71–74.

Azcarate-Peril, M. A., Sikes, M. and Bruno-Barcena, J. M. (2011) "The intestinal microbiota, gastrointestinal environment and colorectal cancer: a putative role for probiotics in prevention of colorectal cancer?" *Am J Physiol Gastrointest Liver Physiol*, 301, G401-424.

Backhed, F., Ding, H., Wang, T., Hooper, L. V., Koh, G. Y., Nagy, A., Semenkovich, C. F. and Gordon, J. I. (2004) "The gut microbiota as an environmental factor that regulates fat storage" *Proceedings of the National Academy of Sciences of the United States of America*, 101, 15718–15723.

Blaut, M. and Bischoff, S. C. (2010) "Probiotics and obesity" *Ann Nutr Metab*, 57 Suppl, 20–23.

Burton, J. P., Chilcott, C. N. and Tagg, J. R. (2005) "The rationale and potential for the reduction of oral malodour using Streptococcus salivarius probiotics" *Oral Dis*, 11 Suppl 1, 29–31.

Cani, P. D., Bibiloni, R., Knauf, C., Waget, A., Neyrinck, A. M., Delzenne, N. M. and Burcelin, R. (2008a) "Changes in gut microbiota control metabolic endotoxemia-induced inflammation in high-fat diet-induced obesity and diabetes in mice" *Diabetes*, 57, 1470–1481.

Cani, P. D., Delzenne, N. M., Amar, J. and Burcelin, R. (2008b) "Role of gut microflora in the development of obesity and insulin resistance following high-fat diet feeding" *Pathol Biol (Paris)*, 56, 305–309.

Cassani, E., Privitera, G., Pezzoli, G., Pusani, C., Madio, C., Iorio, L. and Barichella, M. (2011) "Use of probiotics for the treatment of constipation in Parkinson's disease patients" *Minerva gastroenterol e dietol*, 57, 117.

Castellarin, M., Warren, R. L., Freeman, J. D., Dreolini, L., Krzywinski, M., Strauss, J., Barnes, R., Watson, P., Allen-Vercoe, E., Moore, R. A. and Holt, R. A. (2012) "Fusobacterium nucleatum infection is prevalent in human colorectal carcinoma" *Genome Res*, 22, 299–306.

Chen, W. G., Liu, F. L., Ling, Z. X., Tong, X. J. and Xiang, C. (2012) "Human intestinal lumen and mucosa-associated microbiota in patients with colorectal cancer" *PLoS One*, 7.

Chen, Y. S., Jan, R. L., Lin, Y. L., Chen, H. H. and Wang, J. Y. (2010) "Randomized placebo-controlled trial of lactobacillus on asthmatic children with allergic rhinitis" *Pediatr Pulmonol*, 45, 1111–1120.

Delia, P., Sansotta, G., Donato, V., Frosina, P., Messina, G., De Renzis, C. and Famularo, G. (2007) "Use of probiotics for prevention of radiation-induced diarrhea" *World J Gastroenterol,* 13, 912–915.

Di Pierro, F., Adami, T., Rapacioli, G., Giardini, N. and Streitberger, C. (2013) "Clinical evaluation of the oral probiotic Streptococcus salivarius K12 in the prevention of recurrent pharyngitis and/or tonsillitis caused by Streptococcus pyogenes in adults" *Expert Opin Biol Ther,* 13, 339–343.

Eguchi, S., Takatsuki, M., Hidaka, M., Soyama, A., Ichikawa, T. and Kanematsu, T. (2011) "Perioperative synbiotic treatment to prevent infectious complications in patients after elective living donor liver transplantation: a prospective randomized study" *Am J Surg,* 201, 498–502.

Ejtahed, H. S., Mohtadi-Nia, J., Homayouni-Rad, A., Niafar, M., Asghari-Jafarabadi, M. and Mofid, V. (2012) "Probiotic yogurt improves antioxidant status in type 2 diabetic patients" *Nutrition,* 28, 539–543.

Ejtahed, H. S., Mohtadi-Nia, J., Homayouni-Rad, A., Niafar, M., Asghari-Jafarabadi, M., Mofid, V. and Akbarian-Moghari, A. (2011) "Effect of probiotic yogurt containing Lactobacillus acidophilus and Bifidobacterium lactis on lipid profile in individuals with type 2 diabetes mellitus" *J Dairy Sci,* 94, 3288–3294.

FAO/WHO (2002), *Guidelines for the Evaluation of Probiotics in Food: Report of a Joint FAO/ WHO Working Group* London Ontario, Canada. Available from: ftp://ftp.fao.org/es/esn/food/wgreport2.pdf (Accessed 28 August 2013).

Falck, G., Grahn-Håkansson, E., Holm, S., Roos, K. and Lagergren, L. (1999) "Tolerance and efficacy of interfering alpha-streptococci in recurrence of streptococcal pharyngotonsillitis: a placebo-controlled study" *Acta laryngol,* 119, 944–948.

Guo, Z., Liu, X. M., Zhang, Q. X., Shen, Z., Tian, F. W., Zhang, H., Sun, Z. H., Zhang, H. P. and Chen, W. (2011) "Influence of consumption of probiotics on the plasma lipid profile: a meta-analysis of randomised controlled trials" *Nutr Metab Cardiovasc Dis,* 21, 844–850.

Hatakka, K., Ahola, A. J., Yli-Knuuttila, H., Richardson, M., Poussa, T., Meurman, J. H. and Korpela, R. (2007a) "Probiotics reduce the prevalence of oral Candida in the elderly – A randomized controlled trial" *J Dental Res,* 86, 125–130.

Hatakka, K., Blomgren, K., Pohjavuori, S., Kaijalainen, T., Poussa, T., Leinonen, M., Korpela, R. and Pitkaranta, A. (2007b) "Treatment of acute otitis media with probiotics in otitis-prone children—a double-blind, placebo-controlled randomised study" *Clin Nutr,* 26, 314–321.

Hatakka, K., Martio, J., Korpela, M., Herranen, M., Poussa, T., Laasanen, T., Saxelin, M., Vapaatalo, H., Moilanen, E. and Korpela, R. (2003) "Effects of probiotic therapy on the activity and activation of mild rheumatoid arthritis – a pilot study" *Scand J Rheumatol,* 32, 211–215.

Hatakka, K., Savilahti, E., Ponka, A., Meurman, J. H., Poussa, T., Nase, L., Saxelin, M. and Korpela, R. (2001a) "Effect of long term consumption of probiotic milk on infections in children attending day care centres: double blind, randomised trial" *BMJ,* 322, 1327.

Hatakka, K., Savilahti, E., Pönkä, A., Meurman, J. H., Poussa, T., Näse, L., Saxelin, M. and Korpela, R. (2001b) "Effect of long term consumption of probiotic milk on infections in children attending day care centres: double blind, randomised trial" *BMJ,* 322, 1327.

Horvat, M., Krebs, B., Potrc, S., Ivanecz, A. and Kompan, L. (2010) "Preoperative synbiotic bowel conditioning for elective colorectal surgery" *Wien Klin Wochenschr,* 122 Suppl 2, 26–30.

Hvatum, M., Kanerud, L., Hallgren, R. and Brandtzaeg, P. (2006) "The gut-joint axis: cross reactive food antibodies in rheumatoid arthritis" *Gut,* 55, 1240–1247.

Ishikawa, H., Akedo, I., Otani, T., Suzuki, T., Nakamura, T., Takeyama, I., Ishiguro, S., Miyaoka, E., Sobue, T. and Kakizoe, T. (2005) "Randomized trial of dietary fiber and Lactobacillus casei administration for prevention of colorectal tumors" *Int J Cancer,* 116, 762–767.

Ishikawa, H., Akedo, I., Umesaki, Y., Tanaka, R., Imaoka, A. and Otani, T. (2003) "Randomized controlled trial of the effect of bifidobacteria-fermented milk on ulcerative colitis" *J Am Coll Nutr,* 22, 56–63.

Jeppsson, B., Mangell, P. and Thorlacius, H. (2011) "Use of probiotics as prophylaxis for postoperative infections" *Nutrients,* 3, 604–612.

Kang, M. S., Chung, J., Kim, S. M., Yang, K. H. and Oh, J. S. (2006a) "Effect of Weissella cibaria isolates on the formation of Streptococcus mutans biofilm" *Caries Res,* 40, 418–425.

Kang, M. S., Kim, B. G., Chung, J., Lee, H. C. and Oh, J. S. (2006b) "Inhibitory effect of Weissella cibaria isolates on the production of volatile sulphur compounds" *J Clin Periodontol,* 33, 226–232.

Kano, H., Kaneko, T. and Kaminogawa, S. (2002) "Oral intake of Lactobacillus delbrueckii subsp. bulgaricus OLL1073R-1 prevents collagen-induced arthritis in mice" *J Food Prot,* 65, 153–160.

Kinross, J. M., Markar, S., Karthikesalingam, A., Chow, A., Penney, N., Silk, D. and Darzi, A. (2013) "A meta-analysis of probiotic and synbiotic use in elective surgery: does nutrition modulation of the gut microbiome improve clinical outcome?" *J Parenter Enteral Nutr,* 37, 243–253.

Krasse, P., Carlsson, B., Dahl, C., Paulsson, A., Nilsson, A. and Sinkiewicz, G. (2006) "Decreased gum bleeding and reduced gingivitis by the probiotic Lactobacillus reuteri" *Swed Dent J,* 30, 55–60.

Kumar, M., Nagpal, R., Kumar, R., Hemalatha, R., Verma, V., Kumar, A., Chakraborty, C., Singh, B., Marotta, F., Jain, S. and Yadav, H. (2012) "Cholesterol-lowering probiotics as potential biotherapeutics for metabolic diseases" *Exp Diabetes Res*, 2012, Article ID 902917, p 14.

Ley, R. E., Turnbaugh, P. J., Klein, S. and Gordon, J. I. (2006) "Microbial ecology: human gut microbes associated with obesity" *Nature,* 444, 1022–1023.

Liu, Z., Qin, H., Yang, Z., Xia, Y., Liu, W., Yang, J., Jiang, Y., Zhang, H., Wang, Y. and Zheng, Q. (2011) "Randomised clinical trial: the effects of perioperative probiotic treatment on barrier function and post-operative infectious complications in colorectal cancer surgery – a double-blind study" *Aliment Pharmacol Ther,* 33, 50–63.

Liu, Z. H., Huang, M. J., Zhang, X. W., Wang, L., Huang, N. Q., Peng, H., Lan, P., Peng, J. S., Yang, Z., Xia, Y., Liu, W. J., Yang, J., Qin, H. L. and Wang, J. P. (2013) "The effects of perioperative probiotic treatment on serum zonulin concentration and subsequent postoperative infectious complications after colorectal cancer surgery: a double-center and double-blind randomized clinical trial" *Am J Clin Nutr,* 97, 117–126.

Luoto, R., Laitinen, K., Nermes, M. and Isolauri, E. (2010) "Impact of maternal probiotic-supplemented dietary counselling on pregnancy outcome and prenatal and postnatal growth: a double-blind, placebo-controlled study" *Br J Nutr,* 103, 1792–1799.

Marchesi, J. and Shanahan, F. (2007) "The normal intestinal microbiota" *Curr Opin Infect Dis,* 20, 508–513.

Marchesi, J. R., Dutilh, B. E., Hall, N., Peters, W. H. M., Roelofs, R., Boleij, A. and Tjalsma, H. (2011) "Towards the human colorectal cancer microbiome" *PLoS One,* 6.

Mayanagi, G., Kimura, M., Nakaya, S., Hirata, H., Sakamoto, M., Benno, Y. and Shimauchi, H. (2009) "Probiotic effects of orally administered Lactobacillus salivarius WB21-containing tablets on periodontopathic bacteria: a double-blinded, placebo-controlled, randomized clinical trial" *J Clin Periodontol,* 36, 506–513.

Mielants, H., Devos, M., Cuvelier, C. and Veys, E. M. (1996) "The role of gut inflammation in the pathogenesis of spondyloarthropathies" *Acta Clinica Belgica,* 51, 340–349.

Moroti, C., Magri, L. F. S., Costa, M. D., Cavallini, D. C. U. and Sivieri, K. (2012) "Effect of the consumption of a new symbiotic shake on glycemia and cholesterol levels in elderly people with type 2 diabetes mellitus" *Lipids in Health and Disease,* 11.

Muller, H., De Toledo, F. W. and Resch, K. L. (2001) "Fasting followed by vegetarian diet in patients with rheumatoid arthritis: a systematic review" *Scand J Rheumatol,* 30, 1–10.

Niittynen, L., Pitkaranta, A. and Korpela, R. (2012) "Probiotics and otitis media in children" *Int J Pediatr Otorhinolaryngol,* 76, 465–470.

Nitert, M. D., Barrett, H. L., Foxcroft, K., Tremellen, A., Wilkinson, S., Lingwood, B., Tobin, J. M., Mcsweeney, C., O'Rourke, P., Mcintyre, H. D. and Callaway, L. K. (2013) "SPRING: an RCT study of probiotics in the prevention of gestational diabetes mellitus in overweight and obese women" *BMC Pregnancy Childbirth,* 13, 50.

Nomura, T., Tsuchiya, Y., Nashimoto, A., Yabusaki, H., Takii, Y., Nakagawa, S., Sato, N., Kanbayashi, C. and Tanaka, O. (2007) "Probiotics reduce infectious complications after pancreaticoduodenectomy" *Hepatogastroenterology,* 54, 661–663.

Pala, V., Sieri, S., Berrino, F., Vineis, P., Sacerdote, C., Palli, D., Masala, G., Panico, S., Mattiello, A., Tumino, R., Giurdanella, M. C., Agnoli, C., Grioni, S. and Krogh, V. (2011) "Yogurt consumption and risk of colorectal cancer in the Italian European Prospective Investigation into Cancer and Nutrition cohort" *Int J Cancer,* 129, 2712–2719.

Panwar, H., Rashmi, H. M., Batish, V. K. and Grover, S. (2013) "Probiotics as potential biotherapeutics in the management of type 2 diabetes – prospects and perspectives" *Diabetes-Metabol Rese Rev,* 29, 103–112.

Peltonen, R., Nenonen, M., Helve, T., Hanninen, O., Toivanen, P. and Eerola, E. (1997) "Faecal microbial flora and disease activity in rheumatoid arthritis during a vegan diet" *Br J Rheumatol,* 36, 64–68.

Pineda Mde, L., Thompson, S. F., Summers, K., De Leon, F., Pope, J. and Reid, G. (2011) "A randomized, double-blinded, placebo-controlled pilot study of probiotics in active rheumatoid arthritis" *Med Sci Monit,* 17, CR347–CR354.

Pitsouni, E., Alexiou, V., Saridakis, V., Peppas, G. and Falagas, M. E. (2009) "Does the use of probiotics/synbiotics prevent postoperative infections in patients undergoing abdominal surgery? A meta-analysis of randomized controlled trials" *Eur J Clin Pharmacol,* 65, 561–570.

Rafter, J., Bennett, M., Caderni, G., Clune, Y., Hughes, R., Karlsson, P. C., Klinder, A., O'Riordan, M., O'Sullivan, G. C., Pool-Zobel, B., Rechkemmer, G., Roller, M., Rowland, I., Salvadori, M., Thijs, H., Van Loo, J., Watzl, B. and Collins, J. K. (2007) "Dietary synbiotics reduce cancer risk factors in polypectomized and colon cancer patients" *Am J Clin Nutr,* 85, 488–496.

Rayes, N., Seehofer, D., Hansen, S., Boucsein, K., Muller, A. R., Serke, S., Bengmark, S. and Neuhaus, P. (2002) "Early enteral supply of lactobacillus and fiber versus selective bowel decontamination: a controlled trial in liver transplant recipients" *Transplantation,* 74, 123–127.

Rayes, N., Seehofer, D., Theruvath, T., Mogl, M., Langrehr, J. M., Nussler, N. C., Bengmark, S. and Neuhaus, P. (2007) "Effect of enteral nutrition and synbiotics on bacterial infection rates after pylorus-preserving pancreatoduodenectomy: a randomized, double-blind trial" *Ann Surg,* 246, 36–41.

Rayes, N., Seehofer, D., Theruvath, T., Schiller, R. A., Langrehr, J. M., Jonas, S., Bengmark, S. and Neuhaus, P. (2005) "Supply of pre- and probiotics reduces bacterial infection rates after liver transplantation – A randomized, double-blind trial" *Am J Transplant,* 5, 125–130.

Roos, K., Hakansson, E. G. and Holm, S. (2001) "Effect of recolonisation with 'interfering' alpha streptococci on recurrences of acute and secretory otitis media in children: randomised placebo controlled trial" *BMJ,* 322, 210–212.

Roos, K., Holm, S. E., Grahn, E. and Lind, L. (1992) "Interfering alpha-streptococci as a protection against recurrent streptococcal pharyngotonsillitis" *Adv Otorhinolaryngol,* 47, 142–145.

Roos, K., Holm, S. E., Grahn, E. and Lind, L. (1993) "Alpha-streptococci as supplementary treatment of recurrent streptococcal tonsillitis: a randomized placebo-controlled study" *Scand J Infect Dis,* 25, 31–35.

Roos, K., Holm, S. E., Grahnhakansson, E. and Lagergren, L. (1996) "Recolonization with selected alpha-streptococci for prophylaxis of recurrent streptococcal pharyngotonsillitis – A randomized placebo-controlled multicentre study" *Scand J Infec Dis,* 28, 459–462.

Rovensky, J., Stancikova, M., Svik, K., Uteseny, J., Bauerova, K. and Jurcovicova, J. (2009) "Treatment of adjuvant-induced arthritis with the combination of methotrexate and probiotic bacteria Escherichia coli O83 (ColinfantA (R))" *Folia Microbiol,* 54, 359–363.

Rovensky, J., Svik, K., Matha, V., Istok, R., Kamarad, V., Ebringer, L., Ferencik, M. and Stancikova, M. (2005) "Combination treatment of rat adjuvant-induced arthritis with methotrexate, probiotic bacteria Enterococcus faecium, and selenium" *Ann N Y Acad Sci,* 1051, 570–581.

Sanders, M. E. (2003) "Probiotics: considerations for human health" *Nutr Rev,* 61, 91–99.

Sanders, M. E., Guarner, F., Guerrant, R., Holt, P. R., Quigley, E. M. M., Sartor, R. B., Sherman, P. M. and Mayer, E. A. (2013) "An update on the use and investigation of probiotics in health and disease" *Gut,* 62, 787–796.

Shen, B., Brzezinski, A., Fazio, V. W., Remzi, F. H., Achkar, J. P., Bennett, A. E., Sherman, K. and Lashner, B. A. (2005) "Maintenance therapy with a probiotic in antibiotic-dependent pouchitis: experience in clinical practice" *Aliment Pharmacol Ther,* 22, 721–728.

Sobhani, I., Tap, J., Roudot-Thoraval, F., Roperch, J. P., Letulle, S., Langella, P., Corthier, G., Jeanne, T. V. N. and Furet, J. P. (2011) "Microbial dysbiosis in colorectal cancer (CRC) patients" *PLoS One,* 6.

Starzynska, T. and Malfertheiner, P. (2006) "Helicobacter and digestive malignancies" *Helicobacter,* 11 Suppl 1, 32–35.

Tano, K., Grahn Hakansson, E., Holm, S. E. and Hellstrom, S. (2002) "A nasal spray with alpha-haemolytic streptococci as long term prophylaxis against recurrent otitis media" *Int J Pediatr Otorhinolaryngol,* 62, 17–23.

Teughels, W., Loozen, G. and Quirynen, M. (2011) "Do probiotics offer opportunities to manipulate the periodontal oral microbiota?" *J Clin Periodontol,* 38, 159–177.

Turnbaugh, P. J., Ley, R. E., Mahowald, M. A., Magrini, V., Mardis, E. R. and Gordon, J. I. (2006) "An obesity-associated gut microbiome with increased capacity for energy harvest" *Nature,* 444, 1027–1031.

Twetman, S. and Keller, M. K. (2012) "Probiotics for caries prevention and control" *Adv Dent Res,* 24, 98–102.

Worthley, D. L., Le Leu, R. K., Whitehall, V. L., Conlon, M., Christophersen, C., Belobrajdic, D., Mallitt, K. A., Hu, Y., Irahara, N., Ogino, S., Leggett, B. A. and Young, G. P. (2009)

"A human, double-blind, placebo-controlled, crossover trial of prebiotic, probiotic, and synbiotic supplementation: effects on luminal, inflammatory, epigenetic, and epithelial biomarkers of colorectal cancer" *Am J Clin Nutr,* 90, 578–586.

Xia, Y., Yang, Z., Chen, H. Q. and Qin, H. L. (2010) "Effect of bowel preparation with probiotics on intestinal barrier after surgery for colorectal cancer" *Zhonghua Wei Chang Wai Ke Za Zhi,* 13, 528–531.

Zhang, J. W., Du, P., Chen, D. W., Cui, L. and Ying, C. M. (2010a) "Effect of viable Bifidobacterium supplement on the immune status and inflammatory response in patients undergoing resection for colorectal cancer" *Zhonghua Wei Chang Wai Ke Za Zhi,* 13, 40–43.

Zhang, J. W., Du, P., Gao, J., Yang, B. R., Fang, W. J. and Ying, C. M. (2012) "Preoperative probiotics decrease postoperative infectious complications of colorectal cancer" *Am J Med Sci,* 343, 199–205.

Zhang, M. M., Cheng, J. Q., Lu, Y. R., Yi, Z. H., Yang, P. and Wu, X. T. (2010b) "Use of pre-, pro- and synbiotics in patients with acute pancreatitis: a meta-analysis" *World J Gastroenterol,* 16, 3970–3978.

Zhao, L. and Shen, J. (2010) "Whole-body systems approaches for gut microbiota-targeted, preventive healthcare" *J Biotechnol,* 149, 183–190.

Zhu, D., Chen, X., Wu, J., Ju, Y., Feng, J., Lu, G., Ouyang, M., Ren, B. and Li, Y. (2012) "Effect of perioperative intestinal probiotics on intestinal flora and immune function in patients with colorectal cancer" *Nan Fang Yi Ke Da Xue Xue Bao,* 32, 1190–1193.

Index

absorption, 60, 76
acid suppressive therapy, 179
acute diarrhoea, 173–5, 186
adenoma, 151, 214
adenosine triphosphate (ATP), 142, 145
alkaloids, 59
allergic disorders, 199–202
Allium sativum, 51, 131–2
aloe, 60–1
alpha (α)-lipoic acid, 145
amino acids, 91–2
    pharmacokinetic drug interactions, 94–6
aminosalicylates, 181
animal assays, 41
anti-tumour necrosis factor antibodies, 181
antibiotic associated diarrhoea (AAD), 176–7
antibodies, 41–2
anticoagulants, 60, 131–2
antimicrobials, 179
antineoplastic agents, 133
antioxidants, 133, 142, 151–2
atopic dermatitis, 201
    probiotics, 199–201

bacterial degradation, 72–3
bacterial vaginosis (BV), 202
Bifidobacterium adolescentis, 200
Bifidobacterium animalis, 184
Bifidobacterium breve, 200
Bifidobacterium lactis Bb12300, 215
Bifidobacteruim longum, 200
bioavailability, 58, 91
biochemical deficiency, 146
black cohosh *see Cimicifuga racemosa*
blood pressure reduction, 157–8
borderline substances
    foods and medicine, 18–20

botanicals, 19–20
drug compounds, 19
vitamins, minerals and other natural compounds, 18–19
botanicals, 9, 19–20
British Dental Association (BDA), 158
British Medical Journal (BMJ), 160

calcitriol, 154, 156
calcium, 129–30, 153–7
    homeostasis, 154
Camellia sinensis, 59–60
cancer mortality, 151–2
cancer prevention, 213–14
Candida albicans, 202
candidal vaginitis (CV), 202–3
capillary electrophoresis (CE), 39–40
capillary zone electrophoresis (CZE), 39
capillary zone electrophoresis-laser induced fluorescence (CE-LIF), 40
carbohydrates, 91
    dietary supplements, 85–90
        active substances and their impact on drug PK, 87–9
        PK and transporters involved in sugar transport and uptake, 86
    pharmaceutical excipients and prodrugs, 90–1
carcinogenesis, 213
choline, 145–6
Cimicifuga racemosa, 59
clinical studies
    vitamins and minerals as dietary supplements, 139–61
        ACE vitamins and selenium reduce cancer and heart disease mortality, 151–2
        essential minerals reduce blood pressure, 157–8

clinical studies (*cont.*)
  fluoride supplements for children in areas without fluoridated water, 158–9
  folic acid supplements prevent neural tube defects (NTD), 149–51
  micronutrients improve immune function in elderly, 159–60
  natural metabolites conditionally essential nutrients, 141–6
  supplements usage to improve micronutrient adequacy, 146–9
  Vitamin C supplements prevent or ameliorate common cold, 152–3
  vitamin D supplements improve bone health and have wider benefits, 153–7
Clostridium difficile, 200
  associated diarrhoea (CDAD), 176–7
Codex Alimentarius, 26
coenzyme Q_{10}, 142
colon
  drug delivery system, 71
  physiology, 69
colorectal cancer, 213–14, 217
common cold, 152–3, 205
competitive protein binding assays (CPBA), 42
constipation, 177–8
continuous antibiotic prophylaxis, 203
conventional drug delivery system, 90
coulochemical, 38
cranberry *see Vaccinium macroparon*
creatine, 145
Crohn's disease (CD), 182–3
Cryptosporidium, 174
Curcuma longa, 60–1

diabetes, 156, 214–15
diarrhoea, 173
  acute *see* acute diarrhoea
  traveller's *see* traveller's diarrhoea
dietary intake, 5
dietary supplements
  health claims, 3–21
    borderline substances between foods and medicine, 18–20
    nutrition claims, 6
    requirements, 4–6
  pharmacodynamic interactions of drugs, 127–33
    antioxidants, 133
    herbal supplements, 130–3
    minerals, 129–30
    vitamins, 128–9
  pharmacokinetic interactions between drugs and carbohydrate, protein, vitamin and mineral supplements, 85–117
    carbohydrates, 85–90
    carbohydrates as pharmaceutical excipients and prodrugs, 90–1
    impact of proteins on drug pharmacokinetics and their usage as prodrugs, 92–3
    minerals and oligoelements, 106–17
    proteins, peptides and amino acids, 91–2
    summary of carbohydrates, 91
    summary of minerals, 117
    summary of proteins, 93
    summary of vitamins, 97
    vitamins, 96–7
  pharmacokinetic interactions of drugs and herbal supplements, 47–62
    allium sativum, 51
    Echinacea purpurea, Vaccinium macroparon and *Silybum marianum*, 58–9
    Ginkgo biloba, 56
    Glycine max, Camellia sinensis and *Zingiber officinale*, 59–60
    herbals, 49–50
    Hydrastis canadensis, Valeriana officinalis and *Cimicifuga racemosa*, 59
    Hypericum perforatum, 51
    Morinda citrifolia, Aloe vera, Vitis vinifera and *Curcuma longa*, 60–1
    Panax ginseng, *Piper methysticum* and *Serenoa repens*, 57–8
    Stevia rebaudiana, Lepidium meyenii and *Garcinia mangostana*, 61–2
    summary, 62
  pharmacokinetic interactions of drugs and probiotic and lipid supplements, 69–77
    drug delivery in colon, 69–71

drug-lipid interactions, 76–7
drugs interaction, 72–3
interactions between drugs, prodrugs
    and plant polyphenols, 71–2
lipidic excipients and drug release,
    74–6
lipids and drug delivery, 74
production and good manufacturing
    practice (GMP), 25–35
    benefits and drawbacks of usage in
        organisations, 32–4
    documentation, 30–2
    key issues related to GMP/GHP
        implementation, 26–30
vitamins and minerals and review of
    clinical studies, 139–61
    ACE vitamins and selenium reduce
        cancer and heart disease mortality,
        151–2
    essential minerals reduce blood
        pressure, 157–8
    folic acid supplements prevent neural
        tube defects (NTD), 149–51
    micronutrients improve immune
        function in elderly, 159–60
    natural metabolites conditionally
        essential nutrients, 141–6
    parents in areas without fluoridated
        water give their children fluoride
        supplements, 158–9
    supplements usage to improve
        micronutrient adequacy, 146–9
    Vitamin C supplements prevent or
        ameliorate common cold, 152–3
    vitamin D supplements improve
        bone health and have wider
        benefits, 153–7
dihyhrofolate reductase, 149
DNA reporters, 42
documentation, 30–2
drug compounds, 19
drug enterohepatic cycling, 73
drug-probiotic interaction, 72–3
drug release, 71, 74–6
drug-vitamin PK interactions, 97
drugs
    pharmacodynamic interactions of
        dietary supplements, 127–33
        antioxidants, 133

herbal supplements, 130–3
minerals, 129–30
vitamins, 128–9
pharmacokinetic interactions of dietary
    carbohydrate, protein, vitamin and
    mineral supplements, 85–117
    carbohydrates as dietary
        supplements, 85–90
    carbohydrates as pharmaceutical
        excipients and prodrugs, 90–1
    impact of proteins on drug
        pharmacokinetics and their usage
        as prodrugs, 92–3
    minerals and oligoelements, 106–17
    proteins, peptides and amino acids,
        91–2
    summary of carbohydrates, 91
    summary of minerals, 117
    summary of proteins, 93
    summary of vitamins, 97
    vitamins, 96–7
pharmacokinetic interactions of
    dietary supplements and herbal
    supplements, 47–62
    allium sativum, 51
    Echinacea purpurea, *Vaccinium
        macroparon* and *Silybum
        marianum*, 58–9
    Ginkgo biloba, 56
    Glycine max, *Camellia sinensis* and
        Zingiber officinale, 59–60
    herbals, 49–50
    Hydrastis canadensis, *Valeriana
        officinalis* and *Cimicifuga
        racemosa*, 59
    Hypericum perforatum, 51
    Morinda citrifolia, *Aloe vera*, *Vitis
        vinifera* and *Curcuma longa*, 60–1
    Panax ginseng, *Piper methysticum*
        and *Serenoa repens*, 57–8
    Stevia rebaudiana, *Lepidium meyenii*
        and *Garcinia mangostana*, 61–2
    summary, 62
pharmacokinetic interactions of dietary
    supplements probiotic and lipid
    supplements, 69–77
    drug delivery in colon, 69–71
    drug-lipid interactions, 76–7
    drugs interaction, 72–3

drugs (*cont.*)
  interactions between drugs, prodrugs and plant polyphenols, 71–2
  lipidic excipients and drug release, 74–6
  lipids and drug delivery, 74
dysbiosis, 177, 213

EC Regulations 852/2004 Art. 8, 26
Echinacea, 132
Echinacea purpurea, 58–9
eczema, 200–1
employees' attitude, 34
enzyme immunoassays (EIA), 42
enzyme-linked immunosorbent assays (ELISA), 42
enzyme treatment, 37–8
ergogenic effects, 91
erythrocyte superoxide dismutase, 215
Escherichia coli, 173–4, 203
essential nutrients, 141–2
European Food Standards Authority (EFSA), 4, 9, 155
extraction methods, 37–8

flame ionisation detection (FID), 39
flow injection analyses, 42
fluorescence, 38, 40
fluoride supplements, 158–9
fluorogenic reporters, 42
fluorometry, 40
folate, 148, 149
  intake, 140, 151
  status, 151
folate deficiency, 150
folic acids, 128, 141, 149
  supplements, 149–51, 150
food additives, 85
food borne polyphenols, 72
food industry, 28
food ingredients, 4
food production
  hygienic requirements, 30
  quality assurance, 28
food supplements, 5, 127
  fortified foods composition analysis and case of vitamins, 37–43
  capillary electrophoresis (CE), 39–40
  extraction and purification methods, 37–8
  future methods, 43
  gas chromatography (GC), 39
  high performance liquid chromatography (HPLC), 38
  immunoassays, 41–2
  microbiological methods, 40–1
  other methods, 42
  spectroscopic methods, 40
foods, 18–20
fortified foods
  food supplements composition analysis and case of vitamins, 37–43
  capillary electrophoresis (CE), 39–40
  extraction and purification methods, 37–8
  future methods, 43
  gas chromatography, 39
  high performance liquid chromatography (HPLC), 38
  immunoassays, 41–2
  microbiological methods, 40–1
  other methods, 42
  spectroscopic methods, 40
Fourier transform infrared-photoacoustic (FTIR-PAS), 40
Fourier transform-Raman spectroscopy, 40
fracture risk reduction, 155
free zone capillary electrophoresis (FZCE), 39

Garcinia mangostana, 61–2
garlic, 131–2
gas chromatography-electron capture detector (GC-ECD), 39
gas chromatography (GC), 39
gas chromatography-mass spectrometry (GC-MS), 39
gas chromatography-selected ion monitoring (GC-SIM), 39
gastrointestinal disorders
  probiotics, 173–9
    acute diarrhoea, 173–5
    antibiotic associated and *Clostridium difficile* associated diarrhoea (CDAD), 176–7
    constipation, 177–8

irritable bowel syndrome, 178–9
traveller's diarrhoea, 175–6
gene expression, 56, 74
Generally Regarded As Safe (GRAS), 71
genetic typing, 16
Giardia, 174
ginger *see Zingiber officinale*
Ginkgo biloba, 56
ginseng *see Panax* ginseng
glutathione peroxidase, 215
Glycine max, 59–60
goldenseal *see Hydrastis canadensis*
good distribution practice (GDP), 28
good hygienic practice (GHP), 26
good laboratory practice (GLP), 34
good manufacturing practice (GMP), 31–2
   benefits and drawbacks of usage in organisations, 32–4
     benefits, 32–3
     drawbacks, 33
     implementation in practice, 33–4
   dietary supplements production, 25–35
     key issues related to GMP/GHP implementation, 26–30
   documentation, 30–2
     example of table of contents of GMP code valid for a plant, 32
   hygienic requirements concerning food production, 30
   legal requirements, 26–7
     connections between GHP and GMP, 26
   quality assurance (QA) in food production and industry, 28
   role of management board in quality assurance (QA), 27–8
   stages of implementation, 27
     stage 1, 27
     stage 2, 27
     stage 3, 27
   tasks and scope, 29–30
   ten rules, 29
good manufacturing products (GMP), 19
good storage practice (GSP), 28
good transport practice (GTP), 28
grape seed *see Vitis vinifera*
gravimetry, 41

green tea *see Camellia sinensis*
gut microbiota, 171–2, 214

HbA1c, 215
health claims, 7–18
   approval process and scientific substantiation, 9, 15–18
   characterisation, 16–17
   claimed effect, 17–18
   specific conditions of usage and target population, 17
   wording, 16
   dietary supplement labelling, 3–21
     borderline substances between foods and medicine, 18–20
     nutrition claims, 6
     requirements, 4–6
   labelling requirements when used, 8
   review of authorised claims, 8–9
     chart, 10–15
   types according to EC regulations, 7
healthy diet, 18–19
heart disease mortality, 151–2
Helicobacter pylori, 179–80
hepatic metabolism, 76–7
herb-drug interaction, 49
herbal supplements, 49–50, 130–3
   cranberry, 132
   echinacea, 132
   garlic, 131–2
     interaction with anticoagulants, 131–2
     other interactions, 131–2
   human trials addressing pharmacokinetic herb-drug interactions for best-selling herbal DS, 52–6
   pharmacokinetic destiny of polyphenols in humans, 50
   pharmacokinetic interactions between drugs and dietary supplements, 47–62
     allium sativum, 51
     Echinacea purpurea, Vaccinium macroparon and *Silybum marianum*, 58–9
     generals of pharmacokinetics and possible targets for PK drugs, 48
     Ginkgo biloba, 56

herbal supplements (*cont.*)
  Glycine max, Camellia sinensis and
    Zingiber officinale, 59–60
  Hydrastis canadensis, Valeriana
    officinalis and *Cimicifuga*
    racemosa, 59
  Hypericum perforatum, 51
  Morinda citrifolia, Aloe vera, Vitis
    vinifera and *Curcuma longa*, 60–1
  Panax ginseng, *Piper methysticum*
    and *Serenoa repens*, 57–8
  Stevia rebaudiana, Lepidium meyenii
    and *Garcinia mangostana*, 61–2
  summary, 62
red yeast rice, 133
high fat diets, 74, 216
high magnesium intake, 158
high performance capillary
  electrophoresis (HPCE), 39
high performance liquid chromatography
  (HPLC), 38
high potassium intake, 157–8
highly concentrated carbohydrate sports
  drinks, 90
homeostatic model assessment of insulin
  resistance (HOMA-IR) score, 215
Hydrastis canadensis, 59
hydroxymethyl glutaryl CoA reductase
  (HMG CoA reductase), 142
hygiene hypothesis, 199
hypercalcaemia, 129–30
Hypericum perforatum, 51

immune function, 159–60
immunoassays, 41–2
immunoquantitative polymerase chain
  reaction (iqPCR), 42
immunosenescence, 159
in-capillary enzyme reaction methods, 39
in vivo behaviour, 97
inflammatory bowel disease (IBD)
  probiotics, 181–4
    Crohn's disease (CD), 182–3
    necrotizing enterocolitis (NEC), 184
    pouchitis, 183–4
    ulcerative colitis, 181–2
insulinotropic effects, 91
International Code of Nomenclature, 16
International Codes of Practice, 26

International normalised ratio (INR),
  131–2
iodine, 130
iodine deficiency, 148
ion-exchange (IEC), 38
irritable bowel syndrome (IBS), 17, 178–9
isoflavonoids, 59–60

kava kava *see Piper methysticum*

L-carnitine, 142
labelling requirements, 4–6
  composition, 5–6
    vitamins and minerals which must
      be declared and their nutrient
      reference values, 5
  general, 4–5
Lactitol, 91
Lactobacillus, 179–80, 204
Lactobacillus acidophilus La5, 215
Lactobacillus acidophilus LAVRI-A1, 201
Lactobacillus paracasei F19, 201
Lactobacillus reuteri RC-14, 213
Lactobacillus rhamnosus, 174
Lactobacillus rhamnosus GG, 213
Lactobacillus rhamnosus GR-1, 213
lactose malabsorption, 180
lactulose, 91
lecithin, 145–6
Lepidium meyenii, 61–2
lipid-drug delivery systems (LDDS), 74–6
lipid-drug interactions, 74
lipid profile, 216
lipid supplements
  pharmacokinetic interactions between
    drugs and dietary probiotic
    supplements, 69–77
  drug delivery in colon, 69–71
  drug-lipid interactions, 76–7
  drugs interaction, 72–3
  interactions between drugs, prodrugs
    and plant polyphenols, 71–2
  lipidic excipients and drug release,
    74–6
  lipids and drug delivery, 74
lipidic excipients
  drug release, 74–6
    PKs of dietary lipids, role in
      pharmaceutical formulations, 75

Index

lipids, 74
liquid chromatography-mass spectrometry (LC-MS), 42
low fat diets, 74

maca *see Lepidium meyenii*
malnutrition, 159
management staff, 31
mangosteen *see Garcinia mangostana*
mass spectrometry (MS), 42
medicine, 18–20
metabolic diseases
  probiotics, 214–16
    diabetes, 214–15
    lipid profile, 216
    obesity, 216
micellar electrokinetic capillary chromatography (MECC), 39
micellar electrokinetic chromatography (MEKC), 39
microbiological methods, 40–1
microbiome, 172
microbiota, 72
microemulsion electrokinetic chromatography (MEEKC), 39
micronutrients, 146–9
  usage of supplements to improve adequacy, 146–9
  vitamin and mineral adequacy of adult British diets aged 19–64, 147
microtitre plates, 41
milk thistle *see Silybum marianum*
minerals, 18–19, 106–17, 129–30
  calcium, 129–30
  iodine, 130
  pharmacokinetic drug-mineral interactions and summary of main properties, 108–14
  physico-chemical properties, 115–16
  summary, 117
  vitamins as dietary supplements and review of clinical studies, 139–61
    ACE vitamins and selenium reduce cancer and heart disease mortality, 151–2
    essential minerals reduce blood pressure, 157–8
    folic acid supplements prevent neural tube defects (NTD), 149–51
    micronutrients improve immune function in elderly, 159–60
    natural metabolites conditionally essential nutrients, 141–6
    parents in areas without fluoridated water give their children fluoride supplements, 158–9
    supplements usage to improve micronutrient adequacy, 146–9
    Vitamin C supplements prevent or ameliorate common cold, 152–3
    vitamin D supplements improve bone health and have wider benefits, 153–7
Monascus purpureus see red yeast rice
mucilage polysaccharides, 50

National Osteoporosis Society (NOS), 154
natural food, 157
natural metabolites
  conditionally essential nutrients, 141–6
  structures of L-carnitine, coenzyme Q10, creatinine, SAMe α-lipoic acid and DHLA, 143–4
necrotizing enterocolitis (NEC), 184
neural tube defects (NTD), 149–51
non-essential nutrients, 141–2
non-nucleoside reverse transcriptase inhibitors (NNRTI), 51
normal digestion, 76
normal phase high performance liquid chromatography (NP-HPLC), 38
nutrition claims, 6
  examples, 6
nutritional effect, 18–19

obesity, 216
  control, 86
oligoelements, 106–17
olive oil phenolic compounds, 9
open-label randomised crossover clinical trial, 132
oral healthcare, 211–12
otitis media, 212
over-the-counter supplements, 86

paired ion (PIC), 38
Panax ginseng, 57

peptic ulcer, 179
peptides, 91–2
  pharmacokinetic drug interactions, 94–6
  pharmaceutical excipients, 90–1
pharmacodynamic interactions
  drugs and dietary supplements, 127–33
    antioxidants, 133
    herbal supplements, 130–3
    minerals, 129–30
    vitamins, 128–9
pharmacokinetic drug-lipid interactions, 76–7
pharmacokinetic interactions
  drugs and dietary carbohydrate, protein, vitamin and mineral supplements, 85–117
    carbohydrates as dietary supplements, 85–90
    carbohydrates as pharmaceutical excipients and prodrugs, 90–1
    impact of proteins on drug pharmacokinetics and their usage as prodrugs, 92–3
    minerals and oligoelements, 106–17
    proteins, peptides and amino acids, 91–2
    summary of carbohydrates, 91
    summary of minerals, 117
    summary of proteins, 93
    summary of vitamins, 97
    vitamins, 96–7
  drugs and dietary supplements and herbal supplements, 47–62
    allium sativum, 51
    Echinacea purpurea, Vaccinium macroparon and *Silybum marianum*, 58–9
    Ginkgo biloba, 56
    Glycine max, Camellia sinensis and *Zingiber officinale*, 59–60
    herbals, 49–50
    Hydrastis canadensis, Valeriana officinalis and *Cimicifuga racemosa*, 59
    Hypericum perforatum, 51
    Morinda citrifolia, Aloe vera, Vitis vinifera and *Curcuma longa*, 60–1
    Panax ginseng, *Piper methysticum* and *Serenoa repens*, 57–8
    Stevia rebaudiana, Lepidium meyenii and *Garcinia mangostana*, 61–2
    summary, 62
  drugs and dietary supplements probiotic and lipid supplements, 69–77
    drug delivery in colon, 69–71
    drug-lipid interactions, 76–7
    drugs interaction, 72–3
    interactions between drugs, prodrugs and plant polyphenols, 71–2
    lipidic excipients and drug release, 74–6
    lipids and drug delivery, 74
pharyngotonsillitis, 212
phosphatidyl choline, 145–6
physiological effect
  vitamins, minerals and other natural compounds with nutritional effect, 18–19
  tolerable UL, 18
Piper methysticum, 57–8
plants, 130
plasma distribution, 77
point-of-care survey, 130–1
polymerase chain reaction (PCR), 42
polyphenols, 60, 71–2
  dietary supplements, 72
  pharmacokinetics in humans, 50
postoperative infections, 216–17
postoperative sepsis, 217
potentiometry, 42–3
pouchitis, 183–4
pregnancy, 215
probiotics
  definition, 172–3
  drug delivery in colon, 69–71
    potential PK targets influenced by commensal microbiota, 70
  for atopic and allergic disorders, urinary tract and respiratory infections, 199–205
  for gastrointestinal disorders, *Helicobacter* eradication, lactose malabsorption and inflammatory bowel disease, 171–86
    future trends, 185–6

gastrointestinal disorders, 173–9
Helicobacter eradication, 179–80
inflammatory bowel disease and associated conditions, 181–4
lactose malabsorption, 180
safety, 184–5
oral healthcare, rheumatoid arthritis, cancer prevention, metabolic diseases and postoperative infections, 211–18
pharmacokinetic interactions between drugs and dietary lipid supplements, 69–77
drug-lipid interactions, 76–7
drugs interaction, 72–3
interactions between drugs, prodrugs and plant polyphenols, 71–2
lipidic excipients and drug release, 74–6
lipids and drug delivery, 74
summary, 73–4
prodrugs, 71–2, 90–1
protease inhibitors (PI), 51
protein hydrolysates, 92
protein microarrays, 42
proteins, 91–2
impact on drug pharmacokinetics and their usage as prodrugs, 92–3
pharmacokinetic drug interactions with peptides and amino acids, 94–6
PK of peptides, amino acids and prodrugs that exploit amino acid transporters, 93
summary, 93
pteroylmonoglutamic acid *see* folic acids
purification methods, 37–8
purple coneflower *see Echinacea purpurea*

quality assurance (QA), 27–8

radiometric-microbiological assay, 41
radioreceptor assays (RRA), 42
real-time quantitative polymerase chain reaction (RT qPCR), 42
red yeast rice, 133
Regulation (EC) No 1924/2006, 7
respiratory tract infections, 204–5
retinoid drugs, 128

reversed phase high performance liquid chromatography (RP-HPLC), 38
rheumatoid arthritis
probiotics, 212–13

s-adenosylmethionine (sAME), 145
Saccharomyces boulardii, 174, 180
safety, probiotics, 184–5
saw palmetto *see Serenoa repens*
scientific substantiation, 9
scopoletin, 60
SCORing Atopic Dermatitis (SCORAD), 200
selenium, 151–2
Serenoa repens, 57–8
Silybum marianum, 58–9
small intestine, 69–71
sodium chloride, 157
solid phase extraction (SPE), 38
solvent extraction techniques, 38
soy *see Glycine max*
spectroscopic methods, 40
St John's Wort *see Hypericum perforatum*
Staphylococcus aureus, 200
steroids, 181
Stevia rebaudiana, 61–2
streptococcal pharyngotonsillitis, 212
supercritical fluid extraction (SFE), 38

titrimetry, 42
traditional herbal medicinal products (THMP), 19
traveller's diarrhoea, 175–6
turbidity measurement, 41
turmeric *see Curcuma longa*

ubiquinone *see* coenzyme Q_{10}
UK dietary standards, 148
ulcerative colitis, 181–2
ultraviolet (UV), 38, 153–4
ultraviolet (UV) radiation, 155–6
upper intake levels (UL), 18
urinary tract infections, 203–4
urogenital infections, 202–4
UV-Vis detector, 38

Vaccinium macroparon, 58–9
valepotriates, 59
valerenic acid, 59

Valeriana officinalis, 59
validation process, 31, 34
ventilator-associated pneumonia, 204
vitamin A, 128, 151–2
vitamin B, 40–1
vitamin B3, 129
vitamin B6, 129
vitamin C, 151–2
vitamin C supplements, 152–3
vitamin D, 42
 status, 156–7
vitamin D deficiency, 154
vitamin D supplements
 improve bone health and have wider benefits, 153–7
vitamin dietary supplements, 96–7
vitamin E, 129, 151–2
vitamin K, 129
vitamins, 18–19, 96–7, 128–9
 folic acid, 128
 fortified foods and supplements composition analysis, 37–43
  capillary electrophoresis (CE), 39–40
  extraction and purification methods, 37–8
  future methods, 43
  gas chromatography, 39
  high performance liquid chromatography (HPLC), 38
  immunoassays, 41–2
  microbiological methods, 40–1
  other methods, 42
  spectroscopic methods, 40

minerals as dietary supplements and review of clinical studies, 139–61
 ACE vitamins and selenium reduce cancer and heart disease mortality, 151–2
 essential minerals reduce blood pressure, 157–8
 folic acid supplements prevent neural tube defects (NTD), 149–51
 micronutrients improve immune function in elderly, 159–60
 natural metabolites conditionally essential nutrients, 141–6
 parents in areas without fluoridated water give their children fluoride supplements, 158–9
 supplements usage to improve micronutrient adequacy, 146–9
 Vitamin C supplements prevent or ameliorate common cold, 152–3
 vitamin D supplements improve bone health and have wider benefits, 153–7
pharmacokinetic details, 101–6
pharmacokinetic vitamin-drug interactions, 98–100
pharmacokinetics illustration, 107
Vitis vinifera, 60–1
voltammetry, 42–3
VSL#3, 183

yoghurt, 180, 215

Zingiber officinale, 59–60

CPSIA information can be obtained
at www.ICGtesting.com
Printed in the USA
LVOW01*0009301015
460322LV00004B/21/P

9 781782 420767